DEEP CHINA

1/13

The publisher gratefully acknowledges the generous support of the Sue Tsao Endowment Fund in Chinese Studies of the University of California Press Foundation.

The publisher also gratefully acknowledges the generous contribution to this book provided by Harvard University.

DEEP CHINA · *The Moral Life of the Person*

WHAT ANTHROPOLOGY AND PSYCHIATRY
TELL US ABOUT CHINA TODAY

Arthur Kleinman   Yunxiang Yan
Jing Jun   Sing Lee   Everett Zhang
Pan Tianshu   Wu Fei   Guo Jinhua

University of California Press

Berkeley   Los Angeles   London

University of California Press, one of the most
distinguished university presses in the United States,
enriches lives around the world by advancing scholar-
ship in the humanities, social sciences, and natural
sciences. Its activities are supported by the UC Press
Foundation and by philanthropic contributions from
individuals and institutions. For more information, visit
www.ucpress.edu.

University of California Press
Berkeley and Los Angeles, California

University of California Press, Ltd.
London, England

Library of Congress Cataloging-in-Publication Data

Deep China : the moral life of the person, what
anthropology and psychiatry tell us about China today
/ Arthur Kleinman . . . [et. al.].
    p. cm.
Includes index.
ISBN 978-0-520-26944-6 (cloth : alk. paper) —
ISBN 978-0-520-26945-3 (pbk. : alk. paper)
    1. Medical anthropology—China.   2. Cultural
psychiatry—China.   3. Ethnopsychology—China.
4. Identity (Psychology)—China.   5. Group
identity—China.   6. China—Social conditions.
7. China—Moral conditions.   8. China—Social life
and customs.   I. Kleinman, Arthur.
GN296.5.C6D44 2011
306.0951—dc22   2011012375

27.95

Manufactured in the United States of America

20 19 18 17 16 15 14 13 12 11
10 9 8 7 6 5 4 3 2 1

In keeping with a commitment to support environmen-
tally responsible and sustainable printing practices, UC
Press has printed this book on 50-pound Enterprise, a
30% post-consumer-waste, recycled, deinked fiber that
is processed chlorine-free. It is acid-free and meets all
ANSI/NISO (Z 39.48) requirements.

To Joan Kleinman
September 4, 1939–March 6, 2011
Sinologist and Ancestor
Even after you have entered the
darkness, we feel your deep spirit and
abiding concern for the moral
underpinnings of things Chinese guiding
this book.

CONTENTS

PREFACE

This book is a true collaboration between its eight authors. We jointly contributed to the introduction. Each of the chapters is authored by one of us; yet all of us commented on each of the chapters at meetings in Shanghai and Cambridge. As a result, we feel we are all authors and editors of *Deep China*. We share a passion for the study of Chinese society and its modernization, particularly for understanding the lived experience of Chinese in our times. We are students of how the immense changes in the social life of Chinese have affected their emotional and moral lives. We share the belief that to really understand China and the Chinese, the conventional concerns with economics, politics, and security must be complemented by the study of society and individuals.

All of the contributors, with one exception, Kleinman, are themselves Chinese. Six of us are anthropologists, one a psychiatrist, and one an anthropologist-psychiatrist. Yan, Jing, Pan, Wu, and Guo took their PhDs at Harvard. Lee and Zhang were postdoctoral fellows at Harvard. Kleinman, who has taught at Harvard for thirty-five years, was on the PhD committees of Yan, Jing, Pan, Wu, and Guo at Harvard and Zhang at UC Berkeley. Kleinman supervised the postdoctoral fellowships of Lee and Zhang at Harvard Medical School. Five of us teach in China: Jing Jun at Tsinghua University (Beijing), Pan Tianshu at Fudan University (Shanghai), Wu Fei and Guo Jinghua at Peking University (Beijing), and Sing Lee at the Chinese University of Hong Kong. Yunxiang Yan is a professor at UCLA, Everett Zhang at Princeton, and Arthur Kleinman at Harvard. Yan, Jing, Wu, and Guo have worked principally in rural China; Pan, Lee, and Kleinman mostly in urban China; and Zhang in both settings. Most of us have participated in a long-running seminar Kleinman has taught, called "Deep China: What Medical Anthropology and Psychiatry Contribute to the Study of China Today."

All of us wish to thank Marilyn Goodrich for her unflagging and greatly human assistance as well as Richard Landrigan, Rachel Hall-Clifford, Bridget Hanna, and especially Marty Alexander for their help as research assistants. Special thanks goes to Maria Stalford for coordinating the responses to the author queries and finalizing the manuscript. We are also deeply grateful to the Michael Crichton Fund, Department of Global Health and Social Medicine, Harvard Medical School, and the Asia Center, Harvard University, for funding workshops in Shanghai and Cambridge and contributing a subvention for publication. The Harvard Yenching Institute also funded several of us to participate in this project, for which we also wish to express our appreciation.

Arthur Kleinman, Yunxiang Yan, Jing Jun, Sing Lee, Everett Zhang, Pan Tianshu, Wu Fei, and Guo Jinhua

Remaking the Moral Person
in a New China

In the early years of the new millennium, the image of China is multiplex, consisting variously of a powerful nation with a robust economy; a communist society that has become more capitalist than the West; a strategic competitor to the United States; an unfathomably huge population approaching 1.4 billion people; and a culture that remains distinctive in spite of globalization. Most people in the West are now familiar with the surface facts: China is the second-largest economy in the world and set to become the largest in the lifetime of young adults. China is the world's manufacturing center. Goods of all kinds, available on every continent, are stamped with the "Made in China" label. China not only has the largest reserve of foreign currency (mostly in U.S. dollars—well over a trillion of them!), but its financial system is also different and has so far weathered the global crisis much better than the United States, Europe, and Japan. Indeed, China's economy continues to grow strongly. To deal with weakened exports, the Chinese government has further stimulated an already large and potentially immense domestic consumer market that buys everything from McDonald's hamburgers to the Boeing 777 jet airline, so that it can become increasingly self-reliant. Some economists view China (not the West) as the engine that can—the country that can pull the global economy forward. And the Beijing Olympics and Shanghai World Expo have demonstrated to all the cutting-edge technology, sophisticated design, extraordinary level of infrastructure, and extensive "soft power" of its popular media that the new China can mobilize at a dizzying speed.

The West has invited China to take responsibility for maintaining the global political economic order and Northeast Asian security. Its environmental responsibilities are held to be enormous because it has surpassed the United States as a polluter and its extraction of resources is global. And yet, the Chinese party-state also continues to be accused of violating human rights, imposing authoritarian rule on its people, and posting a challenge to the established U.S.-centered dominance in today's world. The international media have played up the government's suppression of dissenting minorities in Tibet and Xinjiang, while the domestic media blame ethnic discontent on exiles and outsiders who seek to split the nation, thereby creating an unbridgeable chasm between internal nationalism and Han ethnic chauvinism on one side, and international human rights criticism on the other.

These facts, regardless of how they are interpreted, beyond doubt tell us something important about China today. However, for a better and more balanced understanding of China, we also need to know how Chinese themselves see where China is headed, understand who they are, and prioritize what is at stake in their lives. For example, in early 2009, a popular saying traveled widely on the Internet: "In 1949, only socialism can save China; in 1979, only capitalism can save China; in 1989, only China can save socialism; in 2009, only China can save capitalism."

What China can actually do for either socialism or capitalism is beside the point; the real point being made in this saying is that what happens in China and in the world must be understood in the terms that, for cultural, historical, and political economic reasons, are employed by the Chinese themselves and that really matter to them.

When we go beyond the surface facts, we are struck that Chinese individuals, their networks of close ties, and their emotional and moral conditions constitute a crucial complement to our gathering understanding of the remaking of Chinese society and Chinese lives. How did Chinese individuals respond to the institutional shifts of the past decades that have weakened collectivist structures like the work unit while placing greater emphasis on individual capabilities and obligations? How did the responses of Chinese individuals in turn reshape the contours (and legitimacy) of economic reform and the party-state? How do Chinese individuals evaluate and justify their social actions? And, how do individual justifications and evaluations influence the moral landscape in the country, and thereby reshape the moral person in Chinese culture?

These questions are deeply embedded in everyday life and they are crucial; yet, because they are so often unvoiced, they create a large silence amid the dominant voices that project our leading images of China today. Those images distort how we see China. Understanding how Chinese persons from all walks of life answer and reanswer these and related questions transforms the kind of knowledge we possess about China (and the Chinese). If government policies, social institutions, and market activities constitute the *surface* of a changing China, the perceptual, emotional, and moral experiences of Chinese, hundreds of millions of them, make up what we refer to as *deep* China. In this book, our group of social anthropologists and psychiatrists has made a collective effort to take a closer look at one facet of this deep China: the remaking of the person in China's changing emotional and moral context since the 1980s.

THE REMAKING OF THE PERSON AND THE DIVIDED SELF

Notwithstanding their respective social status, Chinese individuals, in a society of unprecedented change at breakneck speed and the highest mobility, simply have been unable to avoid the question: who am I? In the past, the self-identity of the Chinese individual was defined by preordained social relations that revolved around the centrality of the family and descent line in the form of a close-knit kin group. Hence, one was an oldest son, a younger daughter, a concubine's son, the first wife of a first son who is the family head, a peasant, a landlord, a scholar-bureaucrat (Fei [1947] 1992; c.f. Mauss [1938] 1985). The 1949 revolution emancipated the individual to a great extent from the constraints of the family and kinship networks, and even from the traditional hierarchy of social status, but it placed him or her into the all-encompassing system of socialist redistribution and political control. As a result, the individual's identity was, in addition to the family and kinship network, also defined by the collective (either rural commune or urban work unit) and ultimately the socialist state (Yan 2010). It included a new and equally telling hierarchy with cadre, poor peasant, urban worker, and soldier at the top and the former wealthy people at the bottom (Kraus 1981). Only in the post-Mao reform era has the individual found the social conditions that would enable the quest and construction of self-identity outside of the caste-like structure of socialist hierarchy (Hansen and Svarverud 2010; Yan 2009b, 2010; Zhang and Ong 2008).

The development of the private sector in the Chinese economy, which went from nonexistent to accounting for more than two-thirds of GDP output, is clearly the most important new social condition, because it offers individuals the alternative to work outside the state-controlled economic sector in a largely unregulated domain in which relative wealth defines lifestyles and life choices. Moreover, market competition and social mobility encourage and even force the individual to be proactive, rationally calculating about self-interest, and competitive, which has lead to the rise of what Nikolas Rose (2007) calls the "enterprising self." In the late 1980s and early 1990s the party-state had to guide college graduates through educational programs and new regulations to search for a job in the labor market, as they were all used to waiting for job assignments from the state (Hanser 2001; Hoffman 2001). Since the mid-1990s, however, the image of an enterprising self is commonly shared by Chinese youth who not only actively participate in various forms of self-development but also perceive the social world to be inhabited by autonomous and responsible individual actors. A new understanding of meritocracy has led many individuals in socially disadvantaged positions to accept personal responsibility for their failure in career development (Hanser 2001; Hansen and Pang 2008; Pun 2005). The enterprising self, however, is under the restraining power of the Chinese state, which in the new century speaks the language of neoliberalism more often than that of Marxism and Maoism. As Ong and Zhang note: "Alongside the encouragement to be self-reliant and self-enterprising, political control is exercised through the profiling of different groups perceived to be more or less aligned with new forms of competitiveness and profitability" (2008: 14).

In everyday life, the enterprising self is mostly expressed and maintained in terms of consumption and other forms of instant individual gratification. This new trend has been characterized by Lisa Rofel (2007) as the rise of the desiring self. Emotions and desires are certainly not new to Chinese individuals, but in both the traditional and socialist cultures, most of these individual desires were either controlled or stigmatized as improper. More importantly, they could never be openly celebrated in public life. The most interesting drama that has unfolded in the last two decades or so is how desires of various sorts—sexual, material, and affective—have been brought out, elaborated, negotiated, and celebrated in the mass media, Internet chat rooms, courtroom debates, and social interactions in public places. Through the working of these public allegories, a new inner self is constructed, replacing the previous socialist sentiment of class consciousness with a postsocialist sensibility of personal desires (Rofel 2007; see also Liu 2002; and Zheng 2009).

The dream to make it big, to possess and consume more, and to fill out one's personhood as large as one wants through self-effort is no longer limited to the elite and better educated urbanites. Recent studies of migrant workers, especially rural youth working in cities, show that the major motivation for many young migrant workers to leave the countryside is not economic hardship at home; instead, they want to see the outside world and to have the freedom and choices for making a life of their own (see Chang 2008; Hansen and Pang 2008; Pun 2005). As unrealistic as they are, many young migrant workers want to become white-collar professionals, or even rich and famous. As Leslie Chang shows through numerous personal stories, most young girls working on the factory floor have big dreams of becoming somebody, and quite a number of them eventually make it. The key, as a seventeen-year old girl explained, is that you have to discover and develop yourself, and not wait for anyone's help (Chang 2008: 174).

THE DIVIDED SELF

So far we have written about the individual in Chinese society as if his or her selfhood were single and uniform. This is in keeping with the convention of anthropological and sinological writings, but it is quite out of step with depth psychology, psychodynamic psychiatry, and a vast terrain of modernist literature and the arts that present the self as torn between self-interest and collective good, struggling over desire and responsibility, negotiating contradictory emotions, shifting attention between things in and out of awareness, and juxtaposing imagination and practical action. It would indeed be ironic if a book entitled *Deep China* were to articulate a superficial version of the interiority of the person. We propose instead to adopt "the divided self" as a focus for the study of the Chinese today and suggest that the self can be divided by a number of "dividers," such as past versus present, public versus private, moral versus immoral, and so on.[1]

In *What Really Matters*—a book that describes people's lives in their moral context when what is most at stake for the person is not what is most at stake for the group—Arthur Kleinman (2006) presents the case of Yan Zhongshu (a pseudonym for a Chinese physician and clinical academic who experienced the trauma of violence during the Cultural Revolution). Dr. Yan was sent to a remote region in western China for about a decade. His wife committed suicide. His youngest child, a daughter, was separated from him during much of this period, and his two sons, who accompanied him, were not only deprived of an education but also experienced harsh living conditions. This included limited nutrition, which stunted their growth, and contaminated water, which blemished their skin and prematurely whitened their father's hair. Dr. Yan was the victim of brutal public criticism and beatings and for a number of years could neither practice his profession nor return home to Beijing. The experience made him angry and despondent in the 1970s. Even in the first few years of the twenty-first century, when Kleinman completed a decade of interviews with him, he was deeply affected. Even though his career and family prospered, bitter feelings and greatly disturbing memories lay just below the surface of his day-to-day life. Here are excerpts from his conversations with Kleinman that illustrate the long-term emotional and moral consequences of political violence, and through them how the self becomes divided:

> To survive in China you must reveal nothing to others. Or it could be used against you. . . . That's why I've come to think the deepest part of the self is best left unclear. Like mist and clouds in a Chinese landscape painting, hide the private part behind your social persona. Let your public self be like rice in a dinner: bland and inconspicuous, taking on the flavors of its surroundings while giving off no flavor of its own. Too strong a personal flavor and you may entice others to jealousy or hatred. . . . (80)

> Chinese like me—especially those who lived through the political campaigns— learned how to get by. You do what you must do . . . even if you can't stand what you did. But we also learned to be skeptical, skeptical of any ideology, especially Communism, but including Confucianism. It is really much more than skepticism. We feel alienated from any standard of values. Only those that count at the moment to help you get through mean something. (89)

> [Speaking about the Cultural Revolution] So bad that when I think about the dirt, the awful, meager food, the dirty, sour water, I feel that old despair again like a numb, empty feeling, a terrible feeling I don't ever want to relive again. Ah, what a time! (94)

> Now that it has all changed, it makes the past seem false, a big lie. (110)

One doesn't usually hear open expression of these sentiments today, even among Chinese intellectuals like Yan Zhongshu, who are old enough to have experienced the worst of the Cultural Revolution. So where are these sentiments? Have they been displaced by prosperity and happier experiences? Are they entirely forgotten? If you enquire in private, of course, people will share their memories, but troubling memories don't appear to be active in their current lives. Is this really the case?

In 1980 and 1981, memoirs of the traumatic effects of the Cultural Revolution were published in China; they became a genre known as scar literature. This burgeoning literary movement was quickly suppressed by the government, however. It is not politically correct in today's China to spend time commiserating over the traumas of the Cultural Revolution, the famine brought on by the Great Leap Forward, or any of the other violent periods China has witnessed since 1949. People are not prohibited from remembering, but it is as if there were an internal censor restricting what is said. Such an internal censor may be experienced as voluntary and even justifiable. Although the publication of *Prisoner of the State*, the secretly recorded memoir of Zhao Ziyang, former party secretary of the Chinese Communist Party (CCP) who was deposed for being sympathetic to the students at the time of the Tiananmen incident, has received a great deal of attention in the West, its impact among mainland Chinese people has been minimal so far. A Chinese medical researcher in his mid-thirties working in Hong Kong, where the book is freely available, had this to say when asked if he had interest to read the memoir: "I have little interest to read it. Maybe some intellectuals do. It is something only important for some Chinese who somehow believe in idealism. For ordinary people, secular affairs are still the most important."

Yet, interviews with Chinese who have left China for the West, like Dr. Yan, as well as local studies in China that include in-depth interviews, readily show that beneath the surface calm, Chinese do remember the pain and suffering of what they experienced during the years of radical Maoism and in earlier historical periods of brutality and danger. How these emotions of hurt and resentment affect their current lives is not so clear. Given the large number of Chinese who were born after the worst of the Cultural Revolution, these experiences of victimization are shared by an ever diminishing minority of Chinese people. Yet even so, there must be, especially among the elderly, a large reservoir of bitterness, sadness, and anger.

There must be many Chinese whose divided selves harbor these negative but difficult to express and socially inappropriate emotions. Many people find themselves in an uncomfortable moral condition: they are unable to deal with the past or come to terms with themselves. And yet, they may (and probably do) find this new era of prosperity a time of increasing satisfaction with their lives and those of their family members. This is a time, they are told, not to look back in sorrow and anger, but one to appreciate as so very different from the past that it seems, well, past. It is the future of their children and grandchildren that looks bright. And the present is such an unprecedented era of opportunity, wealth, and enjoyment that to be resentful and express negative sentiments seems culturally inappropriate and personally unavailing, along with being politically unwise. (While people outside of China had much to say about the June 4 Tiananmen incident, for example, its twenty-first anniversary has, by and large, gone by rather uneventfully within the country.) Hence, the harmonious society that China's leaders are emphasizing needs to be seen against inner experiences that both support this ideal and simultaneously belie it.

Unlike James C. Scott's (1990) celebrated argument that in authoritarian societies, secret or hidden criticism feeds resistance to political domination, there is little evidence in urban China that this is the case today. Thaxton's (2008) account of the resistance of peasants to local political abuses during the Great Leap Forward and the Cultural Revolution just doesn't seem to describe the experience of China's new middle class in this very different era. And yet, if active political resistance is absent, the divided self still speaks to a public/private division that is central to the life of China's people and that has real consequences for their psychology.

The inability of expressing the true self, according to Xin Liu, is characteristic of the individual in contemporary China. Focusing on the breakdown of social relations in the 1990s, Liu (2000) depicts the collapse of moral economy and the triumph of immoral politics in a rural community and argues that the lack of any ethical order creates a new moral space at large. In this moral space, individuals no longer subscribe to any fixed interpretation of meanings in social life; instead, they skillfully manipulate cultural forms of expression to the best of their personal interests in accordance with a given situation, making the conditions of existence ambiguous, uncertain, and changing all the time (2000: 181–185). In another book Liu (2002) goes on to explore the changing expression of the self among a group of entrepreneurs, local officials, and entertainment service providers. Again, Liu discovers that neither the past-oriented traditional form of the self nor the revolutionary form of the self, oriented toward a utopian future, exists in contemporary Chinese life. Replacing them is a Chinese version of the modern narrative of the self in which the self is no longer connected to the larger society because of a total breakdown of social relations. The typical example of this new Chinese self, according to Liu, can be found among the rich and successful entrepreneurs who feel and express nothing but a strong sense of anomie: timeless, placeless, and meaningless. Although they are busy in endless business deals they often cannot remember what they did or where they were the previous day (Liu 2002). It seems the self among these new elite is divided between the successful surface self and the empty core.

Perceived from a different perspective, the divided self in China also has a much deeper cultural root and operates at a much more serious level as well. There is a long tradition that calls for the individual's sacrifice of personal interest or pleasure for the sake of a larger collectivity, often being portrayed as a more important part of the self. For example, the Chinese individual is motivated to work extra hard only when the self is closely connected to and is part of the family group, argues anthropologist Stevan Harrell (1985). At the turn of the twentieth century, Chinese intellectuals and political reformers saw the necessity of liberating the individual from the small and inward family circle in order to serve the nation-state. Again, they invoked the notion of a divided self. The most well-known example is the call for a new citizen made in the 1910s by Liang Qichao, the enlightenment leader of modern China. Liang argued that the individual has a dual-self, the small self centered on personal interest and the great self based on the interest of the nation; the small self should always be secondary and submissive to the great self (see Chang 1971; Levenson 1959). This version of the divided self, and the inner hierarchy between small and great self, was widely accepted by the Chinese elite from different political camps including the Communists, and was further developed in the name of Maoism after 1949 (see, e.g., Madsen 1984). It continues to be held by the party-state in the post-Mao era.

Interestingly, more often than not the Chinese individual does not see any inner contradictions in the notion of divided self because of this hierarchical order between the small and great self. For example, the current generation of Chinese youth is known for their pursuit of freedom, choice, and self-interest; yet they also accept the official discourse that part of their individual identity is defined by their patriotism, namely, their loyalty to the party and the state. As a result, the self-enterprising individual can also be nationalistic, identifying with the party-state in the name of patriotism and nationalism (Gries 2004; Hoffman 2010). Another interesting and perhaps more telling example is the ideal individual promoted in the popular novel *Wolf Totem* (2004), whose philosophy was quickly dubbed the "way of the wolf" *(langdao)* and widely celebrated in China. The ideal individual promoted in this novel, symbolized by the strong survivor wolf, is a self-reliant, proactive person who, as a member of the group, is self-disciplined and beholden to authority. The behavior patterns within the wolf pack represent an idealized relationship between individual and group or the small and great self that both Mao and the post-Mao leaders like to maintain: "Each member is independent, wild and free at the same time as loyal to its pack and willing to be sacrificed if needed for the survival of the group. It is a strictly hierarchical formation with a strong and wise leader, whose authority is unquestioned" (Wedell-Wedellsborg 2010: 179).

Finally, the divided self can be described at the level of individual morality. In this book, for example, Sing Lee reveals the moral quandary that Chinese psychiatrists went through while working with pharmaceutical firms throughout the 1990s. While many resisted aggressive marketing and maintained professional integrity and ethical standards of practice, they still had to prescribe expensive new drugs to patients and rely on increasingly lavish industry support for activities that accomplished as much marketing as educational purposes. Those doctors in mental hospitals affiliated with the police who allow their professional competence to be suborned by political and institutional pressures offer yet another, if less common, example. In the face of competing moral demands, the average Chinese psychiatrist often yields to local rather than global ethical norms of practice. This is because job security, a better income and standard of living for family members, and opportunity for personal and institutional advancement matter more. How to balance individual interest and professional ethics, therefore, presents a new challenge to the divided self of the Chinese individual, each of whom must find a way to come to terms with herself or himself in actual social performance, as we seek to demonstrate in this book.

THE DIVIDED SELF IN ACTION

Even though the chapters in this volume deal with different topics, they address the issue of the remaking of the person in one way or another. It is our hope that by working together but focusing on different aspects of this transformative process of making and remaking, we may begin to have a better understanding of the Chinese self and what it implies for getting at the new China.

Our collective effort starts with Yan's chapter that highlights three types of profound change in the Chinese moral landscape. First, there has been a shift away from collective moral experience of responsibility and self-sacrifice to a more individualistic morality that emphasizes rights and self-cultivation. Consequently, the meaning of life has been redefined from the individual point of view. Second, this shift in moral life has led to a widespread public perception of moral crisis because of conflicts between individualistic values and the collective values of both the officially endorsed socialist morality and the Confucian tradition. Third, moral practices in everyday life appear to move in two opposing directions, that is, an increase of morally disturbing practices, on the one hand, and the emergence of a new and more promising moral horizon, on the other. The real challenge to the Chinese individual lies precisely here: how to define and remake the self amid these competing and often conflicting ethical values and actual moral practices.

The remaking of the person in the post-Mao reform era started at the most fundamental level—that of sexual desire, as shown in Zhang's chapter. It is no longer news to hear reports of the booming sex industry, the rather rapid development of a homosexuality movement, the public expression of sexual desires among Chinese individuals from all walks of life, and the impact of this sex revolution on marriage and family. Among the most important driving forces for such a sea change is the one-child policy, according to Chinese sociologist Pan Suiming (1995; 2006). Elaborating on Pan's view, Zhang argues that the one-child policy delinked sexual desire from reproduction (e.g., by reinforcing sterilization and promoting the use of condoms) at the juncture of the individual body and the population (social body). This policy had the intended effect of lowering the birth rate, and also the unintentional—yet forceful—effect of encouraging the expression and pursuit of sexual desire. It is noteworthy that Chinese gays and lesbians have begun to publicly engage in identity politics, demanding not sympathy but full social recognition of their rights. At the center of raised consciousness, real claims, and altered practices there is a new moral person who is both more autonomous and unstintingly affirmative of her or his personal happiness. Mao would be horrified!

One of the existential demands that the moral person in any society must negotiate is the pull and push between the pursuit of self-interest and altruistic concern for the common good of others, including strangers. The stories about the collection and transfusion of blood in Jing's chapter disclose a quite complicated picture where both selfishness and altruism are real and in constant interaction. The key, for Jing, is whether the Chinese government can fully recognize the altruistic side of human nature and promote it through proper regulations and programs. The most surprising example is the city of Shenzhen, where the government promoted voluntary blood donation as early as 1994. By 2004 the city basically met its blood needs from free donations by individual citizens. Given that Shenzhen was the first Special Economic Zone and is known for a style of run-away capitalism, the pursuit of self-interest has long been legitimized in public life. Yet, the citizens in this new city, almost all migrants and hence strangers, could be the first to meet the challenge of establishing a new moral practice of social compassion and volunteerism. This vivid example speaks to a decidedly more pro-social moral core of the person and a more promising moral fabric for society under the highly competitive and individualistic mode of the market economy.

Chinese society since the 1980s is characterized by high mobility and the reformation of social groups; consequently, the remaking of the moral person has also undergone a dynamic process of restratifying and repositioning the self. As the word *subject* suggests, the person is "subject" to changing political, economic, and cultural status. From the perspective of locality-based identity, Pan's chapter offers an ethnographic account of self-making in Shanghai neighborhoods. Throughout the city's colonial history, a hierarchy of moral status was established on the basis of the distinction/opposition between the French Concession and International Settlement as upper quarters and the urban slums as lower quarters. The official push for market economy and internationalization of Shanghai in the post-Mao reform era triggered a wave of what Pan calls "Shanghai nostalgia," in which a renewed emphasis on the divide between upper and lower quarters turns out to be central and is actively created both by individuals and local governments alike. As a result, a geographic element is added to the remaking of the moral person in Shanghai, which, ironically, is rooted in the colonial past but oriented toward the future of Shanghai becoming a global city.

Remaking the person is no trivial matter. The self is embodied. Changing it leads to complications and can be painful. In his chapter on neurasthenia and depression in China, Lee, a psychiatrist, brings us into the often troubled inner world of the Chinese person. During the Maoist era, various symptoms of mental and emotional problems were all labeled under the generic category of neurasthenia. It was only after Kleinman discovered the political and social origins of the widespread disease of neurasthenia in China that psychiatrists began to question the accuracy of the simple diagnosis. The deeper reason for this trend of medicalization of mental and emotional problems in public health, however, was the denial of the individual under Maoist socialism. In the past decade, Lee convincingly demonstrates, Chinese psychiatrists stopped using the term *neurasthenia;* its replacement, *depression,* has rapidly become the new term for both medical professionals and, increasingly, patients themselves. As Chinese individuals have become more and more open to expressing themselves, especially in emotional terms, more and more cases have been diagnosed as depression and treated with antidepressant drugs and related therapies. A new market for both antidepressants and psychiatrists emerged, which in turn had the effect of heightening the recognition of depression as a common and acceptable mental disease in modern society. While Lee considers this to be a positive development for recognizing the importance of mental health, he also expresses concern about the commercialization of depression due to the profit-seeking motivation of drug companies and practicing professionals.

Under special circumstances, the remaking of the person might take the extreme form of suicide. Recent studies of suicide in China reveal three differences from patterns of suicide in the United States: a higher rate of suicide (more than twice that in the United States), a concentration of suicide cases among women in rural areas, and a relatively lower rate of depression among those who commit suicide. To better understand these features, Wu offers a cultural interpretation in his chapter. The core of the moral person in Chinese culture, Wu avers, can only be understood via the role of face, a Chinese notion that refers to the embodied moral face of virtues and values that one must retain and the social face of prestige and respect that one must seek out. A person feels humiliated by losing moral face and ashamed for losing social face. Quite often, Chinese individuals go to extremes to rescue or regain lost face—be it moral or social, including going so far as to commit suicide. This is particularly true for suicide cases among rural families where the definition of one's happiness is based on the achievement of harmonious family life. The insignificance of triggering events in rural suicide, such as a conjugal quarrel or wrongful accusation, often puzzles outside legal professionals and scholars alike. The true reason, says Wu, lies in the individual's effort to rescue or regain the lost face and position of relative power in family politics, which appear to be more important than life itself because they are, respectively, the core of the moral person and the fulcrum for balancing the competing micropolitical interests in the family. In this ironic sense, suicide in China carries proactive and positive meanings for the construction of the moral person, even though the act itself destroys personhood, breaks the family, and usually fails to result in a positive outcome. This may be the most tragic consequence of the self and the family's moral division.

The remaking of the moral person can also be seen from the perspective of the nonperson, that is, the social labeling of certain individuals as inadequate, improper, or unacceptable persons. Here the chapter by Guo and Kleinman sheds additional light on our understanding of the Chinese person through a detailed study of the social stigma associated with AIDS and mental illness. The true ghosts in contemporary China are those family members labeled as nonpersons. Once condemned as such, they lose their social network, their social efficacy, and ultimately their socially engendered individuality. Denial and avoidance of becoming a nonperson, like protection of face, at times drive individuals to dangerous acts that on the surface can appear senseless or self-destructive; yet, their deeper significance is that moral status can trump survival in Chinese culture. Courtesy stigma—a stigma acquired as a consequence of being connected with a person who bears a stigma—is particularly common in China and other Asian communities that have been based on collectivistic systems of social life. The rise of individualistic values is in this regard a double-edged sword. It may diminish concealment and ultimately social and structural discrimination via personal advocacy efforts for antistigma interventions. It may also, however, induce family members, colleagues, and friends affected by courtesy stigma to distance, reject, or even abandon caregiving of those with personal stigma arising from HIV or mental illness.

In Kleinman's chapter, which concludes this book, he proposes several quests for meaning that represent how ordinary Chinese are expressing what matters most to them. It is notable that most Chinese interviewed by Kleinman express a quest for personal and family happiness and fortune. A much smaller but insistent group present a quest for social justice that often grows out of grieving over the personal experience of political violence. The quest for meaning further illustrates the divided self, while emphasizing its collective significance as moral affirmation and critique of the way things are in China today. What Kleinman concludes is that these personal and collective quests for making sense of the tumult of Chinese experience turn on the moral stakes of ordinary life. The transformation in the person occurs at the same moment that social life is becoming something new and different; so that individual change in subjectivity and moral change in the community resonate powerfully with each other. A new person is being created in a new world, and both are divided by the political, economic, and cultural processes that constitute twenty-first century China.

CONTEXTUALIZING THE NEW PERSON IN SOCIAL CHANGES SINCE THE 1980S

Obviously, the new moral person is both a product and producer of radical social changes since the 1980s; all dramas of remaking the self that we depict in this book must be understood as part and parcel of China's post-Maoism transition to a highly mobile, increasingly plural and individualized society, as well as its continuing quest for modernity. Among others, the following four social trends are particularly noteworthy.

INSTITUTIONAL CHANGES THAT UNBIND THE INDIVIDUAL

The Chinese term commonly used to describe the 1980s institutional changes is *song-bang*, a verb that literally means "to untie." The rural reform programs including the most radical—decollectivization—were nothing more than the untying of the peasants *(gei nongmin songbang)* from the constraints of the collectives and allowing them to work as individual laborers (Zhou 1996). To stimulate economic growth and raise efficiency, the Chinese party-state restored the private sector in the economy, which in turn required rapid labor-market growth. There had been virtually no labor market under radical Maoist socialism before the late 1970s, since no one worked outside the socialist planned economy; in contrast, 126 million individuals were working in the urban private sector by 2005, plus millions of peasants were engaged in private farming (Tsai 2007).

The most telling example in this connection is the rural-urban labor migration. Those involved in this migration are referred to as "migrant workers" in China because they can only work temporarily in the cities and they do not have a legal right to become permanent city residents. There were an estimated two million migrant laborers in 1980 and by 2006 the number had grown to 132 million. The majority of the migrant workers have to deal with their urban work and lives as individuals, away from both home and family. The other side of the equation is that a large number of elderly people and small children—eighty-eight million by 2004—were left alone at home in the countryside.

Yet, as the market-oriented reforms proceeded further, the party-state began to see the necessity of downsizing the money-losing state-owned enterprises (SOEs) in order to increase efficiency and competitiveness. This was done through bankruptcies, sales and auctions, mergers, and acquisitions. Between 1993 and 2002, more than sixty-three million jobs in SOEs were cut, and by the end of 2005 another ten million were eliminated. Chinese official data reveal that between 1998 and 2003 more than thirty million workers were laid off from SOEs, representing a 40 percent cut in the SOE workforce (Hurst 2009).

The point is that whenever individualization and privatization became necessary, the party-state did not hesitate to use its power to institute institutional changes (Ong and Zhang 2008; Yan 2010). It did so passively in reaction to the rural decollectivization reforms, but it acted proactively and with determination with respect to the restructuring of SOEs. In a similar vein, the three major reform projects after the late 1990s—namely, the privatization of housing, the marketization of education, and the marketization of medical care—are all institutional changes launched by the state to force individuals to shoulder more responsibilities, to more actively engage in market-based competition, and to assume more risks and to become more reflexive. These institutional and policy changes eliminated most of the responsibilities of the state.

Individualization emerged as the developmental strategy adopted by the party-state and inevitably became a highly contested process, since it created losers and winners. Most Chinese individuals had to internalize the negative impacts of individualization by assuming more responsibilities, experiencing greater uncertainty and risk, and working harder. This in turn altered subjectivity. The outcome is the rise of the new kind of enterprising and desiring self, which we have described earlier.

NEW LIFE ASPIRATIONS AND SOCIAL MOBILITY

Along with the institutional reforms that untied the individual from the collective system of work, the increased information flow in the early 1980s opened up new horizons for life aspirations. It started with the visits of overseas Chinese who brought back fashionable commodities, new lifestyles, and life experiences that were so different from their relatives inside China that they shook them out of their taken-for-granted local worlds and fired their imagination for change. Thanks to the technological revolution in communications, Chinese individuals were able to quickly connect with the contemporary world outside China, first by tape recorders, televisions, and VCR machines, and then by CDs, cell phones, email, and the Internet. In the early 1980s, the songs of Taiwanese pop singer Teresa Teng conquered the mainland via brick-like tape-recorders, many of which were brought back by visiting overseas Chinese. While the government was trying to ban Teresa Teng and other pop singers from Hong Kong and Taiwan, millions of individuals were inspired by the emotion-ridden, person-centered, apolitical messages to rethink the meaning of life (Gold 1993).

One of the key challenges that Chinese individuals faced during the early 1980s was more ethical than practical: for what purpose does one live one's life? This question of existential meaning had remarkable political and moral resonance. It led to a nationwide debate over the significance of life. The Cultural Revolution (1966–76) had not only undermined the rhetoric and ideology of Maoism, it had also shaken the Confucian roots of Chinese society, corroding traditional and modern values. This questioning context stimulated another debate in 1988 on the legitimacy of profit-seeking for the individual. Millions of individuals participated during the two national debates and in many others of smaller scale (see Xu 2002: 51–74, 140–147; see also chapter 1 in this volume). The new life aspirations all revolved around the pursuit of individual freedom, prosperity, and happiness, in sharp contrast to the previous emphasis on self-sacrifice (and also self-discipline and self-restraint) for collectives and the state. The new ideal of having a life of one's own replaced the previous call for a life devoted to the socialist cause. The very rhetoric of everyday life expanded to legitimate and express the self. The customary use of an indirect and embodied language of emotions morphed into a psychologically richer, open expression of personhood. To talk directly about one's self-interest and well-being was no longer regarded as vulgar and impolitic (see Zhang and Ong 2008; and Rofel 2007).

At the level of social practice, individuals grasped the opportunities brought about by institutional reforms toward a market economy and pursued a life of their own with their feet—some literally and others symbolically. Millions of villagers left the countryside to seek work in cities, urban residents left their old jobs to seek new opportunities in the emerging private sector, and youth competed with one another to move up through the channel of higher education. Increased social mobility in turn altered the previous makeup of the society and led to a much more open and dynamic system of social stratification.

A simple indicator of increased social mobility is the growth of the Chinese middle class—a group that did not exist during the Maoist era but which has developed during the last three decades. Business people, for example, started from a rather low rank in the early 1980s, when the planned economy dominated and the private sector was regarded as a nondesirable yet necessary complement. They were referred to as *getihu* (literally translated as "individual household," yet connoting entrepreneurship), because the existing system of social stratification could not recognize them. In the 1990s, the party-state began to promote private business, and many civil servants and other elite began to leave the public sector for private businesses, a national fever known as *xiahai* ("jumping into the sea" of the private economy). Gradually, business people were recognized as private entrepreneurs per se and emerged as a new and powerful social group. In the new century, the CCP revised its constitution allowing for the recruitment of private entrepreneurs as party members, on the argument that they represent the most advanced force of production.

In a similar vein, white-collar professionals, especially those working for transnational companies, evolved from a marginal social group in the 1980s to a widely admired new class after the 1990s—the middle class with high income and modern lifestyles. Recent surveys show that the size of the Chinese middle class has grown to just under two hundred million in 2008 (estimated to reach 520 million in 2025), including diverse occupational and social groups. It should be noted that many of these social groups did not exist in the Maoist era, such as lawyers, business consultants, and CEOs; others did not have the kind of wealth and prestige that the market economy offered in the reform era, such as athletes and pop stars; and new occupations like researchers and real estate agents developed higher standards and codes of practice. They professionalized the middle class and thereby simultaneously created new occupations, life aspirations, and status categories. Increasingly freed of the constraints of life lived under the work unit's urban collective, people's careers encouraged individual choice and expression, which in turn invested more symbolic capital in work in the private sector *and* in individual lifestyle. Among others things, home ownership has altered the life experiences, sense of self, form of identity, and the understanding of individual rights among the quickly expanding middle class in urban China, often leading to the collective action of asserting rights among home owners (Read 2008; Zhang 2004, 2010). Automobile ownership on a huge scale has fostered a level of freedom of travel and altered expectations about services to a degree unprecedented in earlier eras. Text messaging has enabled collective action like strikes in factories and protests that transcend established forms of state control. And the state itself is subjected to all kinds of middle-class demands for improved governance that have tangibly changed how the state operates. All of this is a taste of much more to come as China becomes a middle-class society.

Meanwhile, tens of thousands of Chinese have traveled abroad as students, business people, and, most recently, tourists. In the new millennium a reverse migration of Chinese scientists, engineers, and physicians, who had received advanced education and good jobs in the West, returned to China—a new globalized generation who had experiences with civic society and self-development that were unknown in socialist China. And this huge cohort is enriching and remaking civic life.

The market economy, especially the new culture of consumerism, made all kinds of goods available to whoever had the purchasing power, eliminating the previous privilege of the political elite who could enjoy special supplies from the centralized system of redistribution. For example, home telephones were formerly a privilege of the political elite until the early 1980s. Once they were commodified in the second half of the 1980s, however, home telephones quickly became a necessity for every household. A similar change from the official monopoly of symbols of privilege to consumer goods occurred with the automobile. In other words, the market created a certain kind of equality among consumers as long as they had the purchasing power; in addition, the market also created new aspirations for many to acquire more purchasing power so that they could change their social status and redefine who they are through the new lifestyles. Style, in contrast to the plain and often shabby clothes and crude furniture and household accoutrements of the collectivist era, came to express and represent the new subjective freedoms of the market era. And, through a process of cultural interaction, higher styles of cuisine, dress, dwelling, and media created a deepening individual sensibility to the beautiful, the tasteful, and what the French sociologist Pierre Bourdieu (1984) called "distinction," as a thermometer of middle-class élan and panache.

NEW PATTERNS OF SOCIAL INEQUALITIES

The information about new lifestyles and new life aspirations is more or less universal, at least regarding surface values, and it reaches almost every individual thanks to new communication technologies and the marketing-savvy mass media. Yet, the actual changes in realizing one's new aspirations and becoming what one wants to be remain unevenly distributed. New patterns of social inequality have been created throughout the post-Mao reform era. While socialist egalitarianism is regarded as one of the principles in a planned economy, social differentiation, distinction, and hierarchy have been restored and glorified through both the mass media and market promotion of consumerism. Luxury commodities, high-end shops, upscale apartment buildings, and exclusive clubs are widely used to create the new boundaries across social classes, and special societal recognition is given to those who move up the social ladder. The most telling example is the Chinese Communist Party's decision to court successful private entrepreneurs while alienating workers and peasants.

The household registration system, for example, still deprives rural residents, a large part of the Chinese population, of the legal right to permanently live in cities; instead, their work and life in cities, as migrants studying in schools or doing construction or factory work, depend on the renewal of their temporary permits for work and residence. From the cultural perspective, it is as if rural people belonged to a separate (and marginal) caste.

Millions of blue-collar workers were laid off from previously state-owned enterprises without much social welfare support. An increasing number of rural and urban residents became the victims of rapid urbanization and unregulated real-estate development as they were forced to relocate with little compensation or to lose their farmland or urban residence to developers. Gender inequality has been significantly increased as the party-state practically withdrew all its previous programs and policies that fought against discrimination in both the workplace and at home. A new type of equality emerged across the generational line. Many senior citizens contributed to the building of socialism under a system of low wages and high accumulations by the party-state, and their hope for old-age security has been washed away because marketization led to serious shrinkage in medical-care insurance, pensions, housing, and other benefits of socialist welfare programs. Many middle-aged and poorly educated people also were unable to keep pace with the tidal wave of marketization. They were laid off or forced to work as manual laborers at extremely low pay. Along with the intensification of competition for employment and the higher threshold for job placement (now that millions of Chinese graduate each year from universities) in an increasingly complicated and globalized market economy, the gap between the downward-moving older people and upwardly mobile youth in China has been expanding rapidly. This generational gap causes dramatic disjunctions in both public and private spheres of life.

In addition, the development of a youth culture that leans mostly on the ever-changing popular culture and Internet further increases the intergenerational gap, making the meaning and definition of what constitutes a proper person (and an adequate or good life) a much more differentiated and dynamic process than ever before. And marginal groups like the physically handicapped and mentally disabled have experienced a tougher time finding and keeping jobs, now that the welfare net has been shredded.

The emergence of new types of sociality constitutes another novel aspect in the re-making of the person in contemporary China. Along with the increase in mobility—social and geographic—more individuals find themselves interacting in public life with other individuals who are either unrelated or total strangers. Thereby their collective identity and group membership become secondary to individual identity and personal capability.

On the positive side, new types of sociality with unrelated individuals have emerged, ranging from online chatting and socializing with people with similar hobbies to public participation in NGOs and through volunteerism. Although in many cases the new sociality will eventually turn a stranger into an acquaintance or will form a new group membership, such as online dating or NGO work (Roland-sen 2008), in other cases it remains a temporary connection among unrelated individuals. A recent example in this regard was the rise of individual volunteerism in the aftermath of the Sichuan earthquake in May 2008. Shortly after the disaster, more than 250,000 people rushed to the quake areas at their own expense to help the victims. When asked why, many responded that they had been moved by the suffering of the victims and thus they wanted to offer help, with a number of them specifically pointing out that helping others makes their personal lives more meaningful. Such private volunteerism was previously discouraged by the state and was also extremely limited (see chapter 1 in this volume).

The increasing interactions among unrelated individuals has also "individualized" the prevailing moral values and trust in Chinese society. When individuals' identities center on membership in different social groups, they rely on a type of personal trust that only respects people who are in one's own social web, ranging from family and kinship to a wider, yet still well-defined, network of friends. Personal trust derives from long-term interactions with the same group of people and thus is based on low mobility and a narrower scope of social exchanges. In such a local world of acquaintances, moral standards are particularistic because they are determined by the social distance between two parties; strangers are treated with a degree of cautiousness that may border on the paranoid perception that they might be potential enemies and thus are not trustworthy. In contrast, in a highly mobile and open society, most social interactions occur among individuals who are not related to one another by any particularistic ties; in many cases, people do not expect to interact with the other party again in the future. In such a world of strangers, social trust is more important than personal trust and morality is based on more universal values. This kind of local world directly challenges the traditional definition of the person that is based on the divide between in-group and out-group as well as the social distance between the self and all related persons. This atomized status is increasingly the local world experienced by urban Chinese (e.g., Yan 2009a).

The emerging new social relations and the individual pursuit of new types of intimacy, love, and sociality have had an unexpected impact on the Chinese family as well. That is, more and more women have played an active role in dissolving marriages that have stopped working. According to the official statistics of the Ministry of Civil Affairs, the divorce rate in China grew from 4 percent in 1979 to 13.7 percent in 1999 to 21.6 percent in 2008. Moreover, 70 to 80 percent of the filed legal cases of divorce since 2000 were initiated by women. These astonishing developments completely subvert the received wisdom that in Chinese culture marriage is secure and a wife is more dependent on the union than her husband. More importantly, the agency and determination of Chinese women seeking divorce also shook the male-centric foundation of Chinese familial morality that primarily defines a wife as a virtuous and selfless caregiver. So much so that in a recent special report on women's active role in divorce published in *The Southern Weekly of the People,* the headline reads "Why Our Wives No Longer Love Us" (Peng and Ma 2009).

In the PRC's sixty-year history, this is the second wave of divorce that women have advanced. The first wave grew shortly after the promulgation of the 1950 Marriage Law that made free choice and romantic love the base of a marital union. Many women who entered marriage by parental arrangement sought divorce in the name of fighting against feudalism and in the name of socialist construction of a new China (see, e.g., Diamant 2000). The openly acclaimed motivation for the second wave of divorce, however, is entirely individualistic and personal, ranging from irreconcilable differences regarding sexual activities and material life to conflicts over personal character and individual quests for meaning. The newly opened opportunities for women to work and develop themselves outside and, in many cases, far away from the family have been identified as a major contributing factor.

It is also noteworthy that rural China is not lagging behind in this aspect; women initiate the majority of divorce cases in villages and small towns throughout China. A 2005 journalist's investigation of five counties in Hubei Province, for example, revealed that divorce accounted for more than 50 percent of all civil lawsuits, and 90 percent of the divorce cases were initiated by women. Liu Yanwu, a Chinese rural sociologist, carried out a follow-up case study in one of the villages that confirmed the trend with more ethnographic details. Among sixteen divorces, thirteen were initiated by women. Only one of the thirteen wives left because of the unbearable conflicts with a mother-in-law, which has long been the key cause of family conflicts in Chinese culture. The vast majority of these women—twelve out of thirteen—sought divorce because of extramarital affairs or a lack of satisfaction with their husband. Moreover, extramarital affairs are no longer the monopoly of rural males. Seven out of the twelve wives applied for divorce because they first had an extramarital affair and then broke off their marriage. In rural China, for a variety of reasons, most divorced women left their child or children behind. In this case study, for example, fourteen out of the fifteen wives (one woman divorced twice from the same husband) decided not to take their children. Liu also found that fourteen out of the fifteen divorced women remarried quickly, while only five divorced men were able to find a wife again. The general consensus among villagers is that divorced men are difficult to marry off and that this fact further increases the advantage of women who can seek divorce more easily. These new developments led Liu to a highly critical conclusion: more and more rural women have abandoned their family and children for the sake of pursuing personal happiness.

The divorce rate has been constantly on the rise during the post-Mao reform era. Generally speaking, the divorce rate is higher in cities than in the countryside, and higher in the more developed areas along the southeast coast than in the poor and underdeveloped hinterland. Among the divorcees women tend to have a much higher level of education than their male counterparts. For example, as early as 2002 the divorce rate in Beijing rose to 50.9 percent. In other large cities like Shanghai, Guangzhou, and Tianjin, highly educated women who work in government agencies, businesses, or professional fields constitute the majority of female divorcees, many of whom have been accused of dumping their husbands. Yet, as a number of scholars and marital consultants point out, regardless of who initiates the divorce, most women still feel that they are the victim because of their original ideal of a marriage that lasts forever. Moreover, the main reasons for women to seek divorce are either a husband's infidelity or domestic violence, which means they were victimized to begin with. However, another intriguing point is that because of the influence of the male-centric culture, many Chinese men cannot accept the fact that nowadays women are more likely to initiate divorce, and they too feel they are the victims of disorientingly rapid change.

At a deeper level, the new trend of women-initiated divorce has shaken the Chinese notion of what constitutes a moral self and in turn reshapes the construction of the ideal family and gender relations. The transformed gender dynamics could have a more dramatic impact on the moral person, as shown in Wu Fei's insightful analysis of the cultural logic among rural women who took the most radical act to protect the moral self. Recrimination, resentment, grievance, protest, and resistance—all loom large in rural women's suicidal acts. In this sense, suicide needs to be recognized as a coping strategy for young women (and the elderly) in rural China.

All these changes center on the individualization of morality in the domestic sphere in the form of the legitimation of personal happiness and self-realization both for men and for women. Given that the Chinese family institution was founded on patriarchal and collective principles that favor males over females, the ethical shift inevitably creates confusion, tensions, and conflicts between husbands and wives, men and women in general, and younger and older generations. As Ulrich Beck points out for this process globally: "The tension in family life today is the fact that equalization of men and women cannot be created in an institutional family structure which presupposed their inequality" (2001: 204). It remains to be seen what kind of long-term social consequences women seeking divorce may bring about, but one thing is for sure: both men and women must reconsider what it means to be a person, in marriage in particular and for gender relations in general.

WHAT IS AT STAKE FOR THE CHINESE TODAY?

China's extraordinarily fast and compressed modernization may have created a special cultural version of the divided self. This is not the nineteenth-century Confucian-by-day-Taoist-at-night chinoiserie. Instead, it centers on, but reinterprets, an image that achieved fame and controversy in Mao's final period: a painting of an owl with one eye open and the other closed. The painting has been interpreted as a critical wink at the terrible times of the Cultural Revolution, but also as an image of division within the self that speaks to our time. Whatever the intention of the artist Huang Yongyu, who was publicly vilified and privately celebrated at the time for what was believed his temerity in critiquing Mao's leadership, we consider this image emblematic of a deep structural tension in China's moral worlds and in the Chinese individual (Laing 1988; Wang 2000). One eye is open to the technical, financial, and political realities of the time. It is absorbed not only in cell phone calls, emails, and surfing the internet, but also with protocols, audits, and public messages and performances. It is alive with practical self-interest, but also exquisitely attentive to the local politics of life at home and at work. This open eye takes in the "blooming buzzing" world, which in the case of today's China is so complex and confusing that its attractions are, more often than not, surrounded with worries and uncertainty. It sees things as they are, or as they pretend to be.

The other eye is closed, in our interpretation of the image's relevance for today, so as to distance the person from the immediacy, expediency, and sheer practicality of getting on with life and negotiating the constant flow of threats and opportunities. Protecting the privacy of the person, the closed eye helps her or him consider, apart from the powerful pull of context, what really matters. It can encourage care of the self and concern for others. And it can create self-reflective criticism in the service of ethics, aesthetics, and meaning-making. Caregiving, stewardship of the environment, and the responsibilities of the citizen for the common good are thereby animated. This closed eye sees things as they might or should be. But this quiet absorption of the self also encourages memories of things past that have left a residue of unexpressed disappointment, bitterness, resentment, and injustice. Hence the closed eye also sees things with irony, skepticism, and regret. The tension between the eyes is unrelieved and irresolvable. It cannot be predicted how any given person or group will respond. Yet, there seems to us to be as much reason to feel hopeful at the prospects as to see them as troubling. Maybe the picture, despite the painter's denials, is simply a wink, a wink at what we take to be Chinese reality, and the suggestion that there are other, deeper things going on that need to be understood. This is a new moment for China and the Chinese. Our understanding suggests the following things are most at stake.

As we write, China is clearly facing a number of challenges: the widening gap between the rich and the poor, labor unrest, rampant corruption, environmental destruction, a crisis in regulation of food and other products, the clash of values in society that we have described, conflict with ethnic minorities, restriction on communication of dissenting and activist voices, and continued surveillance and repression, now most visibly via the Internet and arrests of dissenters. What is more, the leadership is under pressure to maintain strong economic growth, create jobs, reduce unemployment, and provide greater welfare support for urbanites and introduce such support in rural areas. The demographic transition, moreover, has created more Chinese over sixty than under five for the first time in history, with those over eighty-five growing at the most rapid rate. The upshot is a looming crisis of elder care with greater pressure on singleton adult children in increasingly urban settings among an exploding middle class.

Each of these issues affects, and is affected by, the new subjectivity of Chinese and the changing moral context. Hypermaterialism encourages greed, deepens inequality, contributes to corruption and environmental destruction, and leads people away from acts of protest and resistance. Cynicism defeats reforms. Hyperindividualism ends up blaming the poor, limits concern for public welfare, and leads away from concern with social and health disparities. In contrast, critical self-reflection intensifies concern over these problems and their solutions, while the new emphasis on environmental awareness, caregiving for others, and responsibility for the public good advances both a reformist agenda and resistance to local injustice.

Protest is an old tradition in China. It has long been an ethical obligation of intellectuals, albeit one that has been often overlooked. Popular protest has increased substantially over the past few decades, and, as Elizabeth Perry (2009) notes: "Passed down through folk stories, legends, and local operas, familiar repertoires of resistance were for centuries a major means of alerting an authoritarian political system to the grievances of ordinary people . . . in which savvy protesters frame their grievances in officially approved terms in order to negotiate a better bargain with the authoritarian state." Today's protests are almost always against officials in local governments but at the same time plead for the central government's leaders to address these injustices. (Saich 2011) What is not politically possible is protest against the central government itself.

Whether one believes or not that a new consciousness of human rights is part of China's psychological and moral transformation, there is sufficient evidence in the chapters that follow to support the idea that personhood in today's China includes a deeper sensibility about protecting the natural environment, improving social welfare, volunteering for humanitarian intervention after natural catastrophes, and calling for the state to be on the side of social justice. What seems to be at stake here is an increasing awareness, especially among the young, of global values and that China must engage these values. This recognition informs what is regarded as locally legitimate. That in turn can encourage practices that promote real local reform. Both in moral and psychological spaces, individuals push for changes that in the larger political space may not be realizable. These aspirations—ethical, aesthetic, religious, emotional—center on the everyday social world. It is in that mundane context that the China of the future is being built, every bit as much by moral and psychological change as by state policies and programs.

What is also at stake is individual recognition that Chinese lifestyles and values are more diverse and pluralistic than the state often articulates. Increasing tolerance, decreasing stereotyping, and a willingness to go to bat for others in trouble are widely reported, albeit balanced by habits of the heart that are more selfish and commercial. Yet, in the broad picture, globalization, massive migration, the media, a middle class demanding higher levels of governance, and the other forces of modernity are bending the arc of Chinese history and culture toward recognition that China encompasses multiple identities and belongs to a larger and changing world.

What matters is that the future is seen by many in much more optimistic ways.

And that future is not a European or North American—or, for that matter, Japanese or Korean—ideal, but a Chinese future. Concrete examples are the best way to show what is at stake for Chinese across the very different domains of a vast society.

Young Chinese psychiatrists and social scientists, for instance, see their futures *in* China, even though their professions have been in the past strongly oriented to Western futures. They are building careers and families, but they are often intensely aware that they are building professions and, through these, helping in small but serious ways to create a new China. They are calling for higher standards, opportunities to pursue work that matters, greater concern for professional ethics, and serious attention to forms of social suffering—from poverty to psychosis, unemployment to substance abuse, autism to AIDS—with the aspiration that their work ought to influence policy and programs. And many of them want to promote patient rights and human rights more generally.

But they are concerned (like their peers) with better job conditions, good schools for their children, how to help their elderly parents, ways to maximize family resources, opportunity for travel, and staying in close contact with global developments in their disciplines. Yet while their ethical aspirations may well lead them to support efforts at poverty reduction, improved ethnic relations, enhanced opportunities for women and migrants, and health-care-financing reform, their local worlds at work and at home also preoccupy their attention with highly pragmatic and personal issues of getting on with their lives. This constitutes their local moral experience, and it regularly leads them away from public concerns. It is at the core of the divided self.

Ethical aspirations and actual local moral experience for these professionals on the individual level, as for hundreds of millions of other Chinese, may not be in harmony. The conflicts between the two may seriously limit what they can hope to achieve. Few individuals are able to change their institutions, let alone their societies. Framing individuals as heroes who reform their local worlds is usually inappropriate. For Chinese, like the rest of us, just muddling through is an achievement. Yet, an antiheroic model may be more relevant. Individuals can (and do) perturb and disturb their local worlds, challenging and resisting an ethos that they find wanting and yet not putting themselves at substantial levels of personal danger (see Kleinman 2006). This antiheroic attitude grows out of critical self-reflection, ethical aspiration, and the practical realities surrounding each of us. It builds on recognition of what is politically and socially feasible, as well as the mastery of strategies of handling state agencies and the informal networks of power and influence. We believe it is fostered both by globalization and by China's particular pathway to modernity.

Protest and resistance based in this subjectivity are different than protest and resistance fostered by hatred for authority, resentment over past and present grievances, and the deep sense of a frustrated quest for social justice. It is, to begin with, less a form of political criticism than an experience of moral resistance. Its consequences, for that very reason, are more likely to be changes in moral experience at home, at work, and in the community. Those local changes in moral life have the potential to have larger scale effects, however. Whether they have potential to change the political process and the state is less certain. Yet, in changing society, they are changing how people live, and that change should not be underestimated. A few concrete examples of such change in the areas of rural protest, environmental activism, the role of women, and other of the domains we have identified should put some flesh on this skeletal outline.

Take, for example, reports of a protest in Luliang County, Yunnan Province. In its aftermath, local media used the stock terms of opprobrium for opposition to the Party like "the masses who didn't know the truth," "evil elements with ulterior motives," and "troublemakers" to describe the more than one hundred protesters. In response, the Yunnan Provincial Party Propaganda Department criticized the media, not the protesters, for using unacceptable language. The provincial party's notice stated that (1) mass protests invoke problems in the relationship of the government/party and the people, (2) often the government's policies are at fault, and (3) the people's response is often reasonable and, furthermore, they will listen to reason. Balancing this heartening account are stories of other rural protests that end violently with state oppression of the protesters. Our purpose is not to be naïve but to present what is more promising alongside the much better known troubling examples.

One of us, Jing Jun, works in a small town in Western China where the local population has become increasingly adept at using moral protest to turn a formerly polluted waterway into an ecotourism site for studying and implementing more effective environmental engineering and resource management. This example has been multiplied many times over in the cases of environmental disputes involving forceful protests, collective lawsuits, petition movements, sabotage, and even riots in rural China that have moved ordinary citizens from individual anger and moral resistance to bold acts aimed at changing government policies, reforming polluting enterprises, and influencing court decisions. These cases of local environmental action have increased in frequency over the past ten years. In a number of them, Jing Jun detects a collective revolution in local cognition, sensibility, and behavior that often turns on concrete recognition of the specific dangers in the health consequences of pollution. Jing Jun draws on the idea advanced by Fei Xiaotong—China's greatest social scientist—that villagers' self-respect *(zi zun)*, self-confidence *(zi xin)*, and self-determination *(zi zhu)* are at the basis of the cultural awareness required to instigate such local action as protecting families and communities from unsafe drinking water created by pollution from a powerful fertilizer company. Jing Jun (personal communication) concludes:

> The rise of environmental protests in China is emblematic of the growing consciousness of community and individual rights among ordinary citizens as well as the cumulative effect of newly promulgated laws. In rural areas particularly, the inauguration of drastic economic and administrative changes in the 1980s and 1990s has led to a readjustment of state-society relations. Economic liberalization included agricultural decollectivization, marketization, and the legitimization of geographical mobility and the private sector. Administrative reforms were typified by the promulgation of the Organic Law of Villagers' Committees and the Administrative Litigation Law, in 1987 and 1990, respectively. Greater migration of rural youngsters into cities to find migrant jobs in the 1990s and 2000s exposed young villagers to new ideas of social justice. And they have brought back these ideas to their homes of origin. These changes altered the power relations in village China, sometimes weakening the political base of rural cadres and leading to incidents in which ordinary villagers took upon themselves the task of organizing the local people to defend their community and individual rights.

More generally, over issues of real and pressing concern to local communities, people increasingly take their cases to the courts in the form of lawsuits against local governments, in the so-called *wei quan* ("rights defense") movement, with coalition and support from lawyers, journalists, and so on (see Lee 2007; O'Brien and Li 2006). Is this an emerging civil rights movement in China? One also sees an incipient workers' rights movement of growing size in China despite the strict legal prohibition on forming independent unions. The introduction in 2008 of three new labor laws (the Labor Contract Law, the Law on Employment Promotion, and the Law on Labor Dispute Mediation and Arbitration) that do enhance employment standards and labor rights can be viewed as the state's attempt to preempt and control this new movement, but it also legitimizes a new political-moral reality. The summer of 2010 saw renewed efforts at creating autonomous unions.

A similar sense of opportunity and practical ways to achieve resistance or create desired change was found by Pan Tianshu among deaf people in Shanghai who would not allow the imposition of Chinese Sign Language—a feature of the state's efforts to show to the world its new concern and effectiveness on behalf of "people with special needs"—because a local colloquial form of communication with gestures, facial expressions, and paralanguage served them in more practically useful and group sustaining ways. Pan sees this struggle as yet another illustration of the tension between the party-state's strong desire to beautify and regulate in order to impress global audiences at events like the Beijing Olympics and the Shanghai World Expo *and* the struggle of the aged, the sick, and the disabled for practical on-the-ground improvements in the conditions they must face—conditions that are all-too-often overlooked by the authorities in the process of building a "harmonious society."

The so-called psycho-boom in Shanghai, Beijing, and other major cities in China offers another concrete instance. No one predicted that large numbers of Chinese would become interested in obtaining certificates in counseling and psychotherapy. Yet this is what is happening. There seem to be two motivations. One is a real desire to help others with emotional and relational problems. It has been encouraged by popular TV programs and books that portray the powerful effects of psychological interventions on increasing happiness and reducing distress. The other motivation seems to have to do with a new interest in exploring one's own selfhood and cultivating inner experience. The latter interpretation grows out of the fact that many of the individuals who are receiving diplomas do not go on to practice. The fact that such diplomas can be granted after as little as a weekend training course also makes this movement more worrying.

.The cultivation of subjectivity is also demonstrated by the increasing popularity of personal memoirs, Internet-based chat rooms, television soap operas, a turn in popular religion to more spiritual quests, postretirement education, and development of volunteerism. In these activities, we see a Chinese equivalent to the *Bildungsroman* in the early twentieth-century German novel. The emphasis is on development of the self, moral education of the individual, and the cultivation of a richly affective personality. Even the traditional Chinese emphasis on "nourishing life" through strengthening the body's vital energy via martial arts, exercise, and, especially among the elderly, dance is morphing into a more psychological quest for inner strength. The psychology sections in general bookstores have been, for the past decade, impressive for the number of publications, including translations of European and American authors. And in those sections, besides self-help titles, books on psychoanalysis, psychodynamic psychotherapy, and depth psychology more generally are numerous. All these signs of newly intensified interest in emotions, personality, and self-development speak to a sea change in the cultural orientation of

Chinese from a prioritization of bodily processes to a deepening appreciation of the importance of the subjective, the intimate, and the private. This intensification of popular interest spills over into domains as distinctive as the erotic, the aesthetic, the educational, the sentimental, the athletic, and all those aspects of pop culture that under Maoism were despised.

The upshot would seem to be the emergence of a new and original Chinese bourgeois culture that centers itself on the outer and interior furnishings of a new Chinese self. It is our belief that this is one of the great historical pivots in Chinese society. Will increasing freedom to express the self translate into increasing freedom of speech? Will cultivation of personal satisfaction and happiness spill over into greater social justice? Will the individual aspiration for ethics become a movement for societal ethics? Will middle-class individualism not just make new demands on governance but also go on to reshape the forms of governance? Or will the Chinese self turn out to stand for a very different societal future? And will we be surprised as much by a uniquely Chinese cultural transition to new moral and political realities as we have been by how well the CCP has managed to stay atop this chaotic transition to modernity?

No one can predict the future, but that does not mean we should not explore the future implications and better prepare ourselves for the future. Here, a cross-cultural comparison may help underline why the remaking of the person and the moral context that supports individualization in today's China may hold larger political significance.

Writing about Ethiopia and its problems, Helen Epstein (2010), a distinguished writer on health and social affairs in Africa, concludes: "Both the Ethiopian government and its donors see the people of this country not as individuals with distinct needs, talents and rights but as an undifferentiated mass, to be mobilized, decentralized, vaccinated, given primary education and pit latrines, and freed from the legacy of feudalism, imperialism, and backwardness. It is this rigid focus on the 'backward masses,' rather than the unique human person, that typically justifies appalling cruelty in the name of social progress." Surely the collectivist era under radical Maoism operated with a similar vision.

Hence, the changing subjectivity of Chinese, with a deepening of the sense of self and an emphasis on the individual and his or her quality, especially in the context of a rising middle class, can be understood not just as a remaking of the moral world, but perhaps also as a new political reality—a reality that encourages the development of individuals and that itself involves the reshaping of governance by this new emphasis on individuals. What the longer-term significance of this societal transformation will be, which includes but is not limited to the building of a huge middle class, with its new demands on governance, remains uncertain, and yet the possibility is now real that the political process as much as moral life will become something new and different, and perhaps already has become that, something more availing for human prospects.

Deep China, then, presents evidence to support a pivotal transformation in the moral context and in the personhood of the Chinese today. That transformation has been obscured by the enormous economic, political, and security interests that still dominate our understanding of modern China. Yet, the authors believe that this moral and psychological transition not only provides a deeper understanding of the experiences and lives of the Chinese people, but also suggests that Chinese culture and society are modernizing in such a way as to alter our appreciation of where China is headed. The chapters that follow illustrate in concrete detail this potentially hugely consequential change across diverse domains of life and society. We believe that this new framing for the study of China is what is most important in the knowledge that anthropology and psychiatry have generated about the Chinese. And we also believe that this deep understanding holds significance for our gathering sense of what is happening more broadly at the global level in today's world.

NOTE

1. Of the many theoretical and literary formulations of divided selves, those that come out of the writing of James ([1902] 1985) have particularly inspired our view, as well as those of Brombert (1999), Camus ([1994] 1996), Ellenberger (1981), Freud (1989), Judt (1998), Levi ([1986] 1988), and Rivers (1922), among others.

REFERENCES

Beck, Ulrich, and Elisabeth Beck-Gernsheim. 2001. *Individualization: Institutionalized Individualism and its Social and Political Consequences.* London: Sage Publications.

Bourdieu, Pierre. 1984. *Distinction: A Social Critique of the Judgment of Taste.* Translated by Richard Nice. Cambridge, MA: Harvard University Press.

Brombert, Victor H. 1999. *In Praise of Antiheroes: Figures and Themes in Modern European Literature, 1830–1980.* Chicago: University of Chicago Press.

Camus, Albert. [1994] 1996. *The First Man.* Translated by David Hapgood. New York: Random House.

Chang, Hao. 1971. *Liang Ch'i-ch'ao and Intellectual Transition in China, 1890–1927.* Cambridge, MA: Harvard University Press.

Chang, Leslie T. 2008. *Factory Girls: From Village to City in a Changing China*. New York: Spiegel & Grau.

Diamant, Neil J. 2000. *Revolutionizing the Family: Politics, Love, and Divorce in Urban and Rural China, 1949–1968*. Berkeley: University of California Press.

Ellenberger, Henri F. 1981. *Discovery of the Unconscious: The History and Evolution of Dynamic Psychiatry*. New York: Basic Books.

Epstein, Helen. 2010. "Cruelty in Ethiopia." *New York Review of Books*. April 22.

Fei Xiaotong. [1947] 1992. *From the Soil: The Foundations of Chinese Society*. Translated by Gary G. Hamilton and Wang Zheng. Berkeley: University of California Press.

Freud, Sigmund. 1989. "On the Unconscious." In *The Freud Reader*, edited by Peter Gay, 572–583. New York: W. W. Norton and Company.

Gold, Thomas. 1993. "Go With Your Feelings: Hong Kong and Taiwan Popular Culture in Greater China." *China Quarterly* 136:907–925.

Gries, Peter Hays. 2004. *China's New Nationalism: Pride, Politics, and Diplomacy*. Berkeley: University of California Press.

Hansen, Mette Halskov, and Cuiming Pang. 2008. "Me and My Family: Perceptions of Individual and Collective among Young Rural Chinese." *European Journal of East Asian Studies* 7, no. 1:75–99.

Hansen, Mette Halskov, and Rune Svarverud, eds. 2010. *iChina: The Rise of the Individual in Modern Chinese Society*. Copenhagen: NIAS Press.

Hanser, Amy. 2001. "The Chinese Enterprising Self: Young, Educated Urbanites and the Search for Work." In *Popular China: Unofficial Culture in a Globalizing Society*, edited by Perry Link, Richard P. Madsen, and Paul G. Pickowicz, 189–206. Lanham, MD: Rowman & Littlefield.

Harrell, Stevan. 1985. "Why Do the Chinese Work So Hard? Reflections on an Entrepreneurial Ethic." *Modern China* 11, no. 2:203–226.

Hoffman, Lisa. 2001. "Guiding College Graduates to Work: Social Constructions of Labor Markets in Dalian." In *China Urban: Ethnographies of Contemporary Culture*, edited by Nancy N. Chen, Constance D. Clark, Susanne Z. Gottschang, and Lyn Jeffery, 43–66. Durham, NC: Duke University Press.

———. 2010. *Patriotic Professionalism in Urban China: Fostering Talent*. Philadelphia: Temple University Press.

Hurst, William. 2009. *The Chinese Worker after Socialism*. Cambridge: Cambridge University Press.

James, William. [1902] 1985. "The Divided Self, and the Process of Its Unification." In *The Varieties of Religious Experience*, 139–156. Cambridge, MA: Harvard University Press.

Judt, Tony. 1998. *The Burden of Responsibility: Blum, Camus, Aron, and the French Twentieth Century.* Chicago: University of Chicago Press.

Kleinman, Arthur. 2006. *What Really Matters: Living a Moral Life Amidst Uncertainty and Danger.* Oxford: Oxford University Press.

Kraus, Richard C. 1981. *Class Conflict in Chinese Socialism.* New York: Columbia University Press.

Laing, Ellen Johnston. 1988. *The Winking Owl: Art in the People's Republic of China.* Berkeley: University of California Press.

Lee, Ching Kwan. 2007. *Against the Law: Labor Protests in China's Rustbelt and Sunbelt.* Berkeley: University of California Press.

Levenson, Joseph. 1959. *Liang Ch'i-ch'ao and the Mind of Modern China.* Cambridge, MA: Harvard University Press.

Levi, Primo. [1986] 1988. *The Drowned and the Saved.* Translated by Raymond Rosenthal. New York: Summit Books.

Liu, Xin. 2000. *In One's Own Shadow: An Ethnographic Account of the Condition of Post-Reform Rural China.* Berkeley: University of California Press.

————. 2002. *The Otherness of Self: A Genealogy of the Self in Contemporary China.* Ann Arbor: University of Michigan Press.

Liu Yanwu. 2009. "Cong hexin jiating benwei maixiang geti benwei: Guanyu nongcun fuqi guanxi yu jiating jiegou biandong de yanjiu" [From Nuclear Family–Based to Individual-Based: A Study of Rural Conjugal Relationship and the Changes in Family Structure]. *Xinan Shiyou Daxue xuebao* [Bulletin of the Southwestern University of Petroleum], no. 2.

Madsen, R. 1984. *Morality and Power in a Chinese Village.* Berkeley: University of California Press.

Mauss, Marcel. [1938] 1985. "A Category of the Human Mind: The Notion of Person; the Notion of Self." In *The Category of the Person*, edited by Michael Carrithers, Steven Collins, and Steven Lukes, 1–25. Cambridge: Cambridge University Press.

O'Brien, K. J., and L. Li. 2006. *Rightful Resistance in Rural China.* Cambridge: Cambridge University Press.

Ong, Aihwa, and Li Zhang. 2008. "Introduction." In *Privatizing China: Socialism from Afar*, edited by Li Zhang and Aihwa Ong, 1–19. Ithaca, NY: Cornell University Press.

Pan Suiming. 1995. *Zhongguo xing xianzhuang* [The Reality of Sexuality in China]. Beijing: Guangming ribao chubanshe.

————. 2006. *Zhongguo xinggeming zhonglun* [An Overview of the Sexual Revolution in China]. Gaoxiong: Wanyou chubanshe.

Peng Su and Ma Lingshan. 2009. "Weishenme qizi bu ai women le" [Why Our Wives

No Longer Love Us] . *Nanfang renwu zhoukan* [Southern Weekly of the People]. August 9.

Perry, Elizabeth. 2009. "A New Rights Consciousness?" In "China Since Tiananmen," special issue, *Journal of Democracy* 20, no. 3:17–20.

Pun, Ngai. 2005. *Made in China: Women Factory Workers in a Global Workplace.* Durham, NC: Duke University Press.

Read, Benjamin. 2008. "Property Rights and Homeowner Activism in New Neighborhoods." In *Privatizing China: Socialism from Afar,* edited by Li Zhang and Aihwa Ong, 41–56. Ithaca, NY: Cornell University Press.

Rivers, W. H. R. 1922. *History and Ethnology.* New York: Macmillan.

Rofel, Lisa. 2007. *Desiring China: Experiments in Neoliberalism, Sexuality, and Public Culture.* Durham, NC: Duke University Press.

Rolandsen, U. M. H. (2008). "A Collective of Their Own: Young Volunteers at the Fringes of the Party Realm." *European Journal of East Asian Studies* 7, no. 1:101–129.

Rose, Nikolas. 2007. *The Politics of Life Itself.* Princeton, NJ: Princeton University Press.

Saich, Tony. 2011. "Citizens' Perceptions of Adequate Governance." In *Governance of Life in Chinese Moral Experience: The Quest for an Adequate Life,* edited by Everett Zhang, Arthur Kleinman, and Wei-ming Tu, 199–214. New York: Routledge.

Scott, James C. 1990. *Domination and the Arts of Resistance: Hidden Transcripts.* New Haven, CT: Yale University Press.

Thaxton, Ralph. 2008. *Catastrophe and Contention in Rural China: Mao's Great Leap Forward Famine and the Origins of Righteous Resistance in Da Fo Village.* Cambridge: Cambridge University Press.

Tsai, Kellee S. 2007. *Capitalism without Democracy: The Private Sector in Contemporary China.* Ithaca, NY: Cornell University Press.

Wang, Eugene. "The Winking Owl: Visual Effect and Its Art Historical Thick Description." Critical Inquiry 26, no. 3:435–473.

Wedell-Wedellsborg, Anne. 2010. "Between Self and Community: The Individual in Contemporary Chinese Literature." In *iChina: The Rise of the Individual in Modern Chinese Society,* edited by Mette Halskov Hansen and Rune Svarverud, 164–192. Copenhagen: NIAS Press.

Xu, L. 2002. *Searching for Life's Meaning: Changes and Tensions in the Worldviews of Chinese Youth in the 1980s.* Ann Arbor: University of Michigan Press.

Yan, Yunxiang. 2009a. "The Good Samaritan's New Trouble: A Study of the Changing Moral Landscape in Contemporary China." *Social Anthropology* 17, no. 1:9–24.

———. 2009b. *The Individualization of Chinese Society.* Oxford: Berg.

———. 2010. "The Chinese Path to Individualization." *British Journal of Sociology* 61, no. 3:490–513.

Zhang, Li. 2004. "Forced from Home: Property Rights, Civic Activism, and the Politics of Relocation in China." *Urban Anthropology* 33, nos. 2–4:247–281.

———. 2010. *In Search of Paradise: Middle-Class Living in a Chinese Metropolis.* Ithaca, NY: Cornell University Press.

Zhang, Li, and Aihwa Ong, eds. 2008. *Privatizing China: Socialism from Afar.* Ithaca, NY: Cornell University Press.

Zheng, Tiantian. 2009. *Red Lights: The Lives of Sex Workers in Postsocialist China.* Minneapolis: University of Minnesota Press.

Zhou, Kate Xiao. 1996. How The Farmers Changed China: Power of the People. Boulder, CO: Westview.

CHAPTER ONE · The Changing Moral Landscape

Yunxiang Yan

This chapter depicts the changing moral landscape in contemporary China.[1] In nature, growing plants, blossoming flowers, flowing creeks, and floating clouds animate the earth and the sky. In a similar vein, the new ideas, ideals, and actions of individuals and the constant negotiations about their appropriateness bring life to the norms, values, and behavioral patterns in a society: this is the moral landscape. The regeneration of life bestows the unbounded beauty of nature; the remaking of the person—the moral person—makes the moral landscape into a limitless space of public reflection and intellectual exploration. Consider the following snapshots of everyday life.

In the summer of 2008, I conducted interviews with nine young people in Shanghai, all of whom went to Sichuan as volunteers after the May earthquake. I learned a great deal from them about the moral visions of Chinese youth, including some very interesting new developments that challenge the conventional understanding of Chinese ethics as collectively oriented. For example, when a twenty-five-year-old woman mentioned that she submits her salary to her mother, without thinking I praised her for being a filial daughter. She replied with a cunning smile: "You think I am filial because I give my income to Mom, right? But you probably don't understand the deal here."

It turned out that each month she gave her mother three thousand yuan out of her monthly salary of 3,500 yuan. But she lived with her parents, meaning free room and board, and received pocket money from her mother frequently, as she explained:

Whenever I want something, I just go to my mother. I did a rough calculation a few months ago and found out that I need at least five thousand yuan per month for basic expenditures. But I also need to change my cell phone every year and my parents pay for it; I often travel with friends to other parts of the country and my parents pay for it. And I need to drink Starbucks coffee every day and my parents pay for that too. I guess by now you would think I am not that filial anymore, right?

I finally admitted to her that, in my mind, an adult child should financially help parents, instead of relying on parental support. By this standard, she is probably not as filial as I thought in the first place. Quite intriguingly, she replied: "You are wrong again. I am quite filial. Why? Do you know what my parents' biggest hope is? My happiness! If I live a happy life, they will be happy. This is exactly what I am doing, and they are indeed very happy." At that moment, I felt like an idiot, but at the same time I was also excited by her new interpretation of filial piety, because it seemed to indicate an important ethical change. Two weeks later, I brought the issue up to a small group of young men in Xiajia Village, about 1,300 miles away from Shanghai, where I lived as an ordinary farmer from 1971 to 1978 and have returned to do fieldwork eleven times since 1989. Although these villagers were not as articulate as the young woman in Shanghai, they gave me similar answers: their happiness in life makes their parents happy and thus their pursuit of pleasure and comfort in life should be viewed as their way of fulfilling the duty of filial piety. Such an interpretation of filial piety in terms of one's own happiness is obviously quite different from the traditional definition in which one is expected to sacrifice one's time, labor, wealth, and even life to make parents happy.

In contemporary China, individual narratives about the pursuit of happiness typically include the elements of aspiration, determination, and hard work as well as the importance of personal connections *(guanxi)*. For most people the key point of departure is the revelation that their individualism is central to their moral obligations and practices. In her vivid and insightful portrait of factory girls who migrated from the countryside to work in the cities, Leslie T. Chang (2008) takes a closer look at the various efforts that these young women make to reinvent themselves, to become someone they long to be. Some underage girls used the identity cards of a cousin or a classmate and as time went by they became so closely identified with the fake name that they would not answer to their real names. Many others took commercial classes during their very limited spare time so that they could upgrade their work skills and move up to a higher level. As a seventeen-year-old girl states in an inspirational speech to fellow factory workers: "In a factory with one thousand or ten thousand people, to have the boss discover you is very hard. You must discover yourself. You must develop yourself. To jump out of the factory, you must study. You are here because you don't want to be an ordinary worker with a dull life. If you are waiting for your company to lift you up, you will grow old waiting" (Chang 2008: 174). By sitting in on a white-collar secretarial skills special training class, Chang observed and experienced what the young women were learning and how the knowledge was taught. The class ignored writing and never gave any exams; instead, it focused on instilling the confidence to speak up and providing knowledge of the white-collar work environment and proper etiquette and manners, ranging from the choice of color of one's clothing to the appropriate ways to sit and to walk. Individualism is one of the central messages, but it is promoted with a traditional appeal: by lifting yourself up, you will also lift up your whole family. Another key message is equally individualistic, but with a postmodern twist: if you look and act like someone of a higher class, you will become that person. This class, as well as many other classes, actually offers rural girls, most of whom are excluded from the formal education system for various reasons, a second chance to become the person they want to be. Many of them highly appreciate this opportunity. Work ethics, however, never came up as a subject in the class. As Chang observed, students learn how the office world functions so that they can use the knowledge to lie their way into jobs for which they are not qualified (white-collar jobs normally require a college diploma). Both teachers and students know the game and play it well, because they all accept the simple fact that the people who are too honest are those who will lose out (see Chang 2008: 171–189).

In contrast, ethics and the cultivation of virtues are the precise focal point for a group of affluent professionals and private entrepreneurs who live in a gated community of upscale high-rise apartments and low-rise villas in Beijing. During the summer of 2008 I participated in several study sessions in which I found the remaking of the moral person quite revealing. Once a week, a group of ten to fifteen gathered in the spacious living room in the home of the group leader, a freelance writer and community organizer. They studied ethical books used in kindergarten and primary schools in the United States and European countries, reading the texts aloud, doing the exercises related to each topic, and then holding soul-searching discussions that related the topic of the day—a particular virtue—to their life experiences at work and in the community.

On the day of my third visit, the virtue being studied was gentleness *(wenrou)*. Some male participants questioned the relevance of gentleness as a virtue since it is associated with femininity. Their perspective was criticized by some women who argued that the core of gentleness is to be sensitive to other people's feelings and not to hurt others, including nonhumans. Finally, the group reached an agreement that what makes gentleness a virtue is the underlying idea of equality—if one believes that people are all equal in moral worth, one will treat others with respect and sensitivity and thus will be gentle. Many of the participants then began to discuss the lack of gentleness in everyday life in Beijing, and some reflected on the rude ways of dealing with subordinates at work, a common phenomenon in their own life experiences. I must add that these people did not merely talk and reflect; they also actively participated in community and volunteer activities. One of their primary concerns was how to become a nicer person; yet, they all agreed that this is not easy in today's world as they all have had the experience of knowingly doing the wrong things. The study group thus also functions as a type of do-it-yourself psychological therapy for the participants.

It certainly would be wrong to assume that individual moral reflection and critique are positively correlated with one's social status or accumulated wealth. There is much evidence, in both officially published sources and public opinion, that shows how the rich and powerful violate basic moral principles and reap huge profits at the expense of the interest of others, such as the numerous cases of official corruption, money-power exchange scandals in real-estate development, and slave labor. Equally important are cases of rank-and-file individuals standing up to seek social justice, protect the weak, and cultivate the moral self. The most courageous are those individuals who fight valiantly for dignity, integrity, and decency from the margins of society. In a recent case, for example, a migrant worker-turned-small businessman turned himself in and confessed his counterfeiting and fraud. For more than two years, he had made money by purchasing inferior ice cream bars and frozen dumplings, repackaging them as high-quality brand-name products, and then selling them at a profit to lower-end retail stores. As his business took off, he began to suffer increasing guilt for cheating and damaging the health of consumers by selling low-quality frozen dumplings. It took him several months of intense self-questioning, interrogation with his conscience, and consideration of the cost of confession that could lead to several years in prison. The 2008 scandal of tainted milk powder and the prospect of becoming a father led to a breakthrough as he came to realize the responsibility of the individual to make a better society. Thereafter, he turned himself in and confessed (W. Zhang 2009).

What do these stories tell us about contemporary China? Most obviously, individuals making their own moral judgments and decisions is a common thread that runs through all these episodes; more often than not, by making moral judgments these individuals also redefine what it means to be a proper person in today's China and how to live up to it. "You must discover yourself. You must develop yourself," as the seventeen-year-old migrant worker whom I cited earlier proclaimed. The moral implications and consequences of the individual in self-discovery and self-development thus constitute the central theme of this chapter.

In the following pages, I will first examine the changing moral landscape at the level of ethical discourse on what is moral and how to be a moral person. Despite the continued insistence on socialist civilization and collective ethics in the official discourse, the most important change in popular discourse and moral practice has been a shift away from an authoritarian, collective ethics of responsibilities and self-sacrifice toward a new, optional, and individualistic ethics of rights and self-development. In the next section, I unpack the prevailing public perception of moral decline or moral crisis since the 1980s, and I identify three major ways through which such a perception is formed. In the third section, I take a closer look at the opposing trends at the level of moral practices: on the one side, the various sorts of immorality or morally disturbing behaviors that form the factual basis for the perception of moral crisis; on the other, the emerging new moral practices that are individual-centered yet tending toward more universal values. Together, these three sections lead to the conclusion that the moral landscape in post-Mao China has undergone a profound shake-up, and in many ways has been radically changed by the rise of the new ethics of individual rights and self-development. Yet, the collective ethics of duties and self-sacrifice remain deeply embedded in the everyday life of Chinese individuals. This contradiction causes not only the entanglement and confusion of different values and behavioral norms, but also tensions and conflicts in moral practice, making the moral landscape highly dynamic, complex, and uncertain.

THE ETHICAL SHIFT FROM RESPONSIBILITIES TO RIGHTS

In the early spring of 1980, a young female worker named Huang Xiaoju sent a long letter to *China Youth* *(Zhongguo qingnian)*, the official mouthpiece of the Communist Youth League. In the letter, she described her experiences during the Cultural Revolution, her disappointment with the existing collective ideals and beliefs, and her rethinking of the relationship between self and society. Her letter attracted the attention of the journal's editors because at the time party leaders had already noted worrisome changes in people's thoughts and sentiments, especially suspicion of socialist ideals and values and frustration in adapting to the rapid changes in society during economic reform. The editors (under instructions from party leaders, of course) helped Huang revise her letter and also included some ideas from another letter written by a college student, Pan Yi. The journal then published the letter under the pseudonym Pan Xiao, taking one character from each of the authors' names, under the title "Why Is Life's Road Becoming Narrower and Narrower?" in the May 1980 issue.

The published letter touched the heart and soul of millions of people, old and young alike. By the end of the year, *China Youth* had received some sixty thousand letters from readers, 111 of which were published in subsequent issues. On June 12, *China Youth Daily (Zhongguo qingnian bao)*, another mouthpiece of the Communist Youth League, began a special column to discuss the meaning of life and by the end of the year it had received more than seventy thousand contributions, two hundred of which the newspaper then published. At the same time, a large number of provincial and municipal newspapers and magazines, especially those targeting youth, also launched discussions along the same lines (for a detailed study, see Xu 2002: 51–71).

Two points in the Pan Xiao letter became the focus of debate. First, it describes the disillusionment with Communist ideals because of the gap between the ideals and reality; second, it demonstrates how through a journey of soul-searching many Chinese finally realized that selfishness is actually a part of human nature, and, in reality, everyone struggles to achieve her or his own goals, despite all the empty talk of selflessness and sacrifice for the collective interest.

At that time, both the disillusionment with collective moral values and the realization of selfishness as part of human nature were in direct conflict with the Party ideology and the Communist ethical discourse. The wide and enthusiastic responses from all over the country confirmed the Party leaders' worries that many people shared the opinions expressed in the Pan Xiao letter. This is why the debate on the meaning of life continued for so long and reached the entire nation, profoundly affecting millions of people. For example, the founder of the Lebaishi Group, one of the largest soft-drink companies in China, recalled the debate as a wake-up call. At the time, he was a branch leader of the Communist Youth League in rural Guangdong and was involved in serious discussions with a female colleague about the questions raised in the Pan Xiao letter. They concluded that self-development was the moral and best way to make a contribution to society. They later married and became nationally famous private entrepreneurs (see Wu 2007: 55). Many people whom I interviewed recalled that the debate was similar to a political campaign. Individuals were organized by the local youth league or other organizations to discuss both the letter and the meaning of life, debating whether or not people are selfish by nature and coming to a consensus point that the correct way to pursue self-interest is "subjectively for oneself, but objectively for all others" *(zhuguan wei ziji, keguan wei dajia)*.

The fact that after so many years people still remember their participation in the debate reveals its deep imprint on their moral experience. The most important impact that people remember is the beginning of a departure from a morality of collective responsibilities to the justification for self-interest, which, as the earlier quote shows, was packaged diplomatically so as to avoid offending Communist ethics.

The significance of the 1980 debate on the meaning of life is that it marked the first open departure from the dominance of a collective ethics that can be traced back to Confucian ethics in Chinese history. From Confucian ethics and traditional culture to the Chinese Communist Party (CCP) and the People's Republic, the emphasis on the absolute primacy and supremacy of the collective over the individual continued; what had changed was merely the replacement of the family, kinship groups, and the emperor with socialist collectives, the Communist Party, and Chairman Mao. The Communist ethical discourse went even further to deny the meaning and value of the self by promoting new values of complete impartiality and selflessness, "seeking no advantage for oneself, pursuing benefits only for others," and "being a rustless screw of the revolutionary machine." An awareness of the self was unhealthy because one was supposed to dedicate one's entire life to the Communist cause and to always follow the instructions of the CCP and Chairman Mao. Needless to say, it was immoral to pursue self-interest (see Madsen 1984).

There was, however, a gap between the Communist ethical discourse and the people's actual moral practices during both the Mao and post-Mao eras. Even during the radical years of the Cultural Revolution, many villagers still tended the crops in their private lots with greater care than those in the collective farms, and workers found various ways to advance their personal interests. Yet, because of the dominant influence of Communist ethics, the pursuit of self-interest not only lacked legitimacy in public but also could have negative effects on the individual. The psychological suffering and painful experience of battling against one's intuitive self-awareness, for example, are vividly described in the Pan Xiao letter:

> Having seen through life, I acquired a dual personality. On the one hand, I denounced this vulgar reality. On the other hand, I rode with the waves. Hegel once said: 'Whatever is realistic is rational, whatever is rational is realistic.' This has almost become a motto with which I comfort myself and soothe my

wounds. I am human. I am not a noble person, but I am a rational one, just like all other rational beings. I fight about wages; I calculate bonuses. I learn to flatter, to lie. . . . Doing such things, I feel terrible inside. Then I remember Hegel's words and I become calm.

It would be quite difficult for any Chinese individual in the twenty-first century to understand why the authors of the Pan Xiao letter felt guilty about their modest desires for bonuses and high wages, and many would not see anything wrong in their "riding with the waves." Yet, in the 1980s, considerations of personal interest were indeed regarded as immoral under Communist ethics, and the illegitimacy of self-interest made a morally sensitive person "feel terrible inside," as Pan Xiao put it.

Moreover, political campaigns, study groups, educational propaganda, and various mechanisms of awards and punishments created a rather oppressive environment for those who dared to put the self above the collective (Madsen 1984). For instance, moonlighting during spare time was considered immoral until the mid-1980s; as an employee of the state, one should not take up a second job elsewhere because, implicitly, one's spare time also belongs to the party-state. This was by no means mere rhetoric; serious punishment was a definite possibility. In 1985 an engineer named Zheng at a Shanghai textile factory was imprisoned for working at a private company during his spare time. Another engineer named Huang who had made six hundred yuan by moonlighting at a rural enterprise was sentenced to three hundred days imprisonment (Wu 2007: 86).

Despite the powerful constraints of Communist ethics and the associated regulations against individual interests, the trend of self-awareness and the emerging individual-centered morality of rights and self-realization seemed to be unstoppable. Throughout the 1980s, the official media and party propaganda outlets were filled with warnings about a moral crisis on the rise, known as the crisis of the three absences: the absence of moral values, beliefs, and confidence in Communist ideology. Interestingly, many people, especially the youth, seemed to care little about the officially defined moral crisis; instead, they embraced the accusations of lacking Communist/collective values and beliefs as a breakthrough in their search for the new self. This new moral experience was best expressed by Cui Jian, China's first rock star, in his famous song "I have nothing." As a Chinese scholar points out, the claim "I have nothing" actually represents an upbeat spirit of self-searching: "We live by seeking, searching for self, not because we have really lost ourselves, but because we have never really possessed our true selves. It is true, then, we have nothing" (Q. Liu 1988).

The collective morality of responsibility and self-sacrifice seemed to lose ground by the early 1990s, especially after Deng Xiaoping restored the market reforms in his south China tour. Thousands of scientists, artists, scholars, and government officials, including high-ranking party cadres, quit their jobs in the public sector, which formerly had been considered a symbol of their social achievement, and either joined or established their own private companies to make money by engaging in commercial activities. The large number of government officials involved in commercial activities quickly led to an upsurge of corruption among power holders, the moral implications of which will be explored later in this chapter. It is important here to note that the rush by the political and cultural elite to make money signaled the legitimacy of self-interest, profit-making, and a materialistic fetish. Consequently, the mentality and behavior among ordinary people began to change as well. As I note elsewhere (1994), being poor, which was regarded in the Communist ideology as an important marker of being part of the revolutionary force, came to be regarded as disgraceful. By the late 1990s the urge to make money had turned into a new fetish for monetary success. Moreover, individuals began to have a strong sense of competition; more and more people worked a second job in order to make extra money. Furthermore, the gradually emerging notion of a "Chinese dream" came to be shared by those who wished to become rich and successful, including many villagers who left their homes to seek better opportunities in the cities (Yan 1994).

The declining influence of collective values and Communist morality in everyday life does not mean that collective action disappeared. On the contrary, during the same period of shifting moral practices and ethical discourse, Chinese society began to witness the rise of new forms of public protests and social turbulence by which villagers, workers, and property owners took to the streets to protect their individual rights, such as the right to work, the right to have farm land, or the right to property (Lee 2007; O'Brien and Li 2006). Since the early 1990s, an increasing number of individuals have stood up to protect their interests against various predatory forces, such as developers, big companies, and local government agencies, and the number of public protests and the amount of social unrest have increased annually. The seemingly shocking number of more than one hundred cases of public protests in 1993 pales with that of more than seventy thousand in 2003, the year that was unofficially referred to as "the year of rights assertion" by the Chinese media, and eighty-seven thousand in 2005.

Focusing on villagers' actions, O'Brien and Li (2006) call these protests "rightful resistance" and highlight the following three features: operation near the boundary of an authorized channel, employment of the rhetoric and commitment of the powerful, and strategies to exploit divisions among the powerful. After carefully examining cases of public protests among workers in both the old industrial areas and the newly developed coastal cities, Lee (2007) wonders to what extent the protests might challenge the authority and legitimacy of the party-state, and whether in their protests against local authorities, these rights movements are actually seeking the intervention of the central government. What has been advanced by labor movements is social change instead of political change. Similar questions are raised by scholars studying the rights movements among urban homeowners, especially those initiated by displaced urban residents who were caught up in the rapid and often brutal process of urban development (Read 2008; Zhang 2010: 137–162). The most developed, however, is the assertion of consumer rights, which clearly and closely evolved around the rise of self-awareness and individual-centered ethics (Hooper 2005).

A similar ethical shift occurred in the sphere of private life. Based on longitudinal field research over a period of twelve years in a north China village, I charted the transformation of the private life sphere from the 1950s to the 1990s and discovered that the most salient feature of the individualization of rural families lies in the rise of the individual rather than in the changing family size or structure, and, consequently, the rise of a new ethics discourse that favors the individual. In everyday life, this is mostly reflected in the legitimization of individual desires for intimacy, privacy, freedom, and material comforts as well as in the actual pursuit of these desires. Unlike the traditional family, in which a person was nothing more than the personification of the family line, the contemporary individual is more interested in his or her personal happiness and the well-being of a narrowly defined private family (see Yan 2003). This is aptly illustrated, for example, by the changing nature of marriage transactions.

The practice of bridewealth was legally banned in China by the 1950 Marriage Law, although in reality it continued in various forms. The intriguing point is that by the 1980s urban and rural youth had gained power and independence in mate choice, marriage negotiations, and postmarital residence, yet the practice of marriage transactions remained intact and the standard value of bridewealth and dowry has continued to increase annually. For instance, in the village I studied, the standard cost of marital gifts increased from four to five thousand yuan in 1989 to sixty to seventy thousand yuan in 2008. In affluent metropolitan cities like Shanghai, the current standard is to receive at least a two-bedroom flat as bridewealth and a car as dowry, a quite firm demand that has contributed to the housing bubble in the new century.

Why has bridewealth survived radical socialist transformations and continued to get stronger? The key lies in a switch of the bridewealth recipients. Starting in the 1980s, the groom's family began to give bridewealth in both monetary and material forms directly to the bride who kept it for herself instead of giving it to her parents. Typically, after her wedding the bride uses bridewealth to fund her conjugal family, meaning that her husband benefits from the marital gifts as well. Consequently, young people are highly motivated to receive as much bridewealth and dowry as possible and they strategize in various ways to raise the standard payments, squeezing increasingly more money out of their parents.

To justify their demands for lavish bridewealth and dowry, Chinese youth resort to the notion of individual property rights and to the rhetoric of individualism, claiming that they should receive their share of the family property, while overlooking the fact that many parents must work extra hard and often have to borrow the funds to meet their children's marriage needs. Ironically, many youth have claimed that demanding financial support is a matter of personal freedom *(geren ziyou)* or of having individuality *(you gexing)*. When I discussed the same issue with college students in Shanghai in 2007 and 2008, I received answers essentially similar to those from the village youth, even though the college students could articulate their points in a much more sophisticated way (Yan 2009: 155–182).

Under the old collective system of ethics, the demand for excessive bridewealth and dowry for one's own interest would be regarded as selfish and absolutely immoral, because one was socialized to put family interest above self-interest and to respect the wishes of one's parents regarding these matters. The youth today—rural and urban alike—have gained freedom and independence from parental control when dealing with sex, mate choice, and marriage; yet they also make every effort to squeeze money out of their parents' pockets and they do not see anything morally unjustifiable in their behavior. When faced with criticism that they are being selfish, they simply shrug it off, arguing that selfishness is part of human nature. The point I want to emphasize here is that one's open claim of self-interest against that of the family may be accepted as legitimate by all those involved, which clearly indicates the shift of moral emphasis from family responsibilities and self-sacrifice to individual rights and self-realization. Similarly, the new interpretation of filial piety in terms of one's own happiness, as reflected in the opening story of this chapter, indicates such an ethical shift. In addition, the fact that the sanctioning power of accusing someone of being selfish has now become insignificant also shows how much the moral landscape in China has changed in comparison with the central issue in the debate over the Pan Xiao letter in 1980.

A notable study in this regard is Lisa Rofel's book *Desiring China* (2007), in which she examines a sea change that began to sweep through China in the 1990s. The Maoist culture of politics and associated socialist experiments were replaced by a state-initiated discovery of a universal human nature of individual desires and the various new forms of public culture that legitimize and promote both individual and national desires. Through a detailed and vivid description of television dramas, museum displays, legal cases, and other forms of public narrations of desires of various sorts in urban China, she argues that it is by constituting a subject who desires—a neoliberal practice of governance—that the party-state was able to regain its legitimacy of political monopoly in the post-1989 setting. By the same process, the Chinese individual was also able to create the link between the new self and the new cosmopolitan ethics of global neoliberalism and consumerism (Rofel 2007). Rofel does not explore, however, the ethical underpinnings and moral implications of this sea change, because her theoretical focus is set on the global trend of neoliberal governmentality and associated scholarly debates. Her ethnography, quite interestingly, also tells the story of the ethical shift from a collective system of responsibility and self-sacrifice to an individualistic system of rights and self-development, a point that was less emphasized. This ethical shift, in my opinion, may help us to better understand not only how but also why the rise of individual desires in post-1989 China is so important.

Moreover, I would argue that one cannot fully understand these rapid and radical changes in Chinese social life unless one takes into full consideration the shifting ethical discourse and moral practice. These cases reflect only the tip of the iceberg. The silent yet deep sexual revolution, the importance of romantic love, mutual understanding, and emotional attachment in personal relations, and the increase in depression, isolation, divorce, and suicide are all related to the shifting focus from responsibilities to rights, from self-sacrifice to self-realization, and ultimately from collectivity to individuality (see the chapters by Sing Lee, Wu Fei, and Everett Zhang in this volume for full discussions of these topics).

UNPACKING THE PUBLIC PERCEPTION OF MORAL CRISIS

Understandably, such a shift in ethics and moral practice is not easy, because it both challenges the existing order of the moral universe and also creates winners and losers, and sometimes even victims. The judgment on each specific change brought about by this moral shift to a great extent depends on the perspectives of different individuals: where some see moral decline and crisis, others may find the rise of a new ethics. Yet, more often than not, people tend to generalize about the changing moral landscape too quickly and vaguely, leaving out the specifics of the temporal, spatial, and social contexts as well as the concrete communications, negotiations, and engagements in moral practice.

For instance, in 2007 (after the abolition of the agricultural taxes and other levies in 2005) a Chinese scholar asserted that the earlier crisis of governance in rural China had been replaced by a new crisis of ethics that had developed to the dangerous level of undermining social stability (Shen 2007). His view was echoed strongly by many at the time, and his article was not only reprinted in several scholarly journals but also appeared in a number of popular magazines and newspapers. To demonstrate this crisis, he cited a moral decline in two areas: the increase in the divorce rate and the fetish for money in villages. According to his observations, the high divorce rate was caused mainly by young women's loose attitude toward sex and marriage and their yearning for a comfortable material life. As for the money fetish, the scholar found it puzzling that villagers did not look down upon those young women who made money as sex workers in cities. On the contrary, after returning home, these young women used their earnings to help their parents build new houses, to participate in normal gift exchanges, and to fulfill their moral duties like everyone else. In the absence of any stigma, these former sex workers were not only tolerated but even respected by the villagers (Shen 2007).

Is this a crisis of moral decline or a radical change in both ethical discourse and moral practices in rural China? By whose standard should these young women's attitudes toward sex and marriage be judged as loose? Why is the yearning for a comfortable life unethical? It turns out that the criticism of the young women's behavior came mainly from the older male villagers who still upheld the conventional ethics of collective responsibility. Thus, they disapproved of the women's pursuit of personal happiness and material comfort. Ironically, it is also by the same standard of collective responsibility that these elderly male villagers regarded financial contributions from the young women as evidence of their being filial, and therefore they did not discriminate against these former sex workers, whom they viewed as returning to the village to fulfill their family duties after making money in the cities. Here, the tension and conflict derive from the entanglement of individualistic and collectivistic ethics in real life across generational and gender lines. To what extent there is a moral crisis in this particular rural community, therefore, remains questionable. Yet, it is more important to ask why general statements of moral crisis like Shen's resonate so well with the public and why, since the late 1980s, a public perception of moral decay has circulated so widely in China.

To better understand the complexity of these issues, we need to make a distinction between the perception of a moral crisis and the reality of moral changes—good and bad alike. In an insightful analysis of the perception of a crisis in American values, Wayne Baker (2005) identifies three ways by which people perceive such a crisis. The first is to focus on the loss of traditional values by comparing the present with the past, the second is the unfavorable comparison of American society with other societies in terms of prevailing values, and the third derives from the division of American society into opposing groups with irreconcilable moral differences, that is, a culture war. With some modifications, Baker's approach can be applied to the Chinese case, as all three ways of thinking play a role in the making of a public perception of moral decline or crisis.

First, as far as values and moral practices are concerned, people from all walks of life tend to idealize the past and to use it to critique unsatisfying aspects of the present. Loss of traditional values is but one common complaint; another focuses on the moral decay of the younger generations who not only forget the traditional but also break the status quo by thinking and behaving differently from the older generations. The faster a society changes, the more complaints there are about the alleged lost paradise. This line of argument started in China more than 2,500 years ago with Confucius, who lamented the lost values and proprieties of the golden era of Duke Zhou. Similarly, the current complaints idealize social life under Mao as an era of high moral standards because all the major moral problems in the reform era, such as cadre corruption, commercial cheating, distrust of the public, and various forms of negative competition did not exist (at least to the same extent) in those egalitarian times. Moreover, the shift from collective ethics to individualistic ethics is not only rapid but also fundamental and thus only makes more acute the felt pain, confusion, and loss of direction among many Chinese individuals, especially those who prefer to have the protection of collectivism.

It is true that under Mao officials were much less corrupt in financial matters, yet the abuse of political power was more severe; commercial scams almost never existed under the planned economy, yet many more people suffered from the endless political battles. It is also true that public trust in the CCP, the government, and social institutions was high and trust in Mao was at the level of an irrational cult, yet nearly all people feared being reported on by others, including their closest family members and best friends. Under the Communist virtues of impartiality and selflessness, many individuals abused themselves mentally and others underwent brainwashing sessions and sometimes acted (such as during the Great Leap Forward and the Cultural Revolution) to expel the selfishness from their souls. Yet, recognition and rewards from the CCP and the government remained personal. Hence, the activists during the Mao era acted out of selfish motivations. The most fundamental difference is the dominance of the collective morality of responsibilities that was exalted during the Maoist era but quickly collapsed thereafter. The total denial of individual rights and of an individual identity by Maoist socialism, which was at least as unethical as any other vice, has been either forgotten or purposely neglected by the critics of contemporary moral practices, thus giving rise to a perception of moral decline. The same logic can be applied to those who have gone further in time to idealize Chinese ethics and moral practices during the pre-Communist, premodern, or even classical periods. For example, the divorce rate was low or even nonexistent in traditional China, but this was because of the unethical practice of subordinating women and denying their rights.

The unfavorable comparison approach contributes to the perception of a moral decline in China primarily in one area, that is, the cultivation of civility in public space. This was an issue at the turn of the last century, and leading Chinese intellectuals like Liang Qichao, Liang Shumin, Hu Shi, and Fei Xiaotong all regarded the absence of public morality as a serious problem in Chinese society. There were comparable discussions in Japan and the United States, commonly focusing on issues of clean governance, observation of public rules, awareness of public hygiene, public participation, and tolerance, honesty, and compassion toward strangers in public interactions. China ranked much lower in these comparisons, the main reason for which, as identified by the Chinese elite, was the selfishness of Chinese individuals.

Two points should be noted here. First, the unfavorable comparison approach has been used primarily to critique the lack of civility, or public morality *(gongde)* as it is commonly referred in Chinese. Second, this kind of moral comparison tended to be more frequent and attract more public attention when China's influence on the stage of international politics was perceived by the public as weak, such as during the turn of the last century or during the early stages of the post-Mao reform. Whenever nationalism and self-confidence were high, such as during the Mao era or during China's recent global rise, such unfavorable comparisons tended to decline. Thus, the unfavorable comparison approach contributes to a public perception of a moral crisis in a different way and at a different time from that of the lost-paradise approach.

Baker's third way of thinking about a moral crisis—as a culture war—is probably less relevant in China. First, Communist ethics remains the official discourse and the party-state still monopolizes power to determine the fate of any new public discourse. In order to survive, any new or renewed ethical discourse must win, often by fighting against other discourses, the tolerance and recognition of the official discourse. Thus, there is not yet any culture war among the legitimized ethical discourses. Second, the gap between ethical discourse and moral practice has constantly grown in the postreform era because of the politically sanctioned dominance of the Communist ethical discourse and its detachment from the moral practices of most Communist party members and officials (Wang 2002). As a result, people tend to treat the diversity of values like a supermarket option, justifying their moral practices with different values in different contexts.

Yet, at a deep level the diversification of values, including most notably the shift from collective ethics to individualistic ethics, indeed plays a crucial role in constituting a public perception of a moral decline or crisis. First, the personified and mystified moral authority, be it Confucius or Mao, no longer exists, and the dominance of a single version of collective ethics has ended. This has led to a national panic about a "moral vacuum." The so-called moral vacuum cannot be true in real life as people always make judgments about right or wrong in accordance with some values or beliefs, but it could be true in one's subjective experience, inasmuch as moral practices are observed that do not fit with any previously prevailing ethical standards. The collapse of traditional and Maoist moral authorities also led to widespread disillusion and cynicism among many people, and, when the pursuit for wealth seemed to be the only driving force in social life, the very foundation of the self appeared to crumble, resulting in the alienation and alteration of the self (Ci 1994; X. Liu 2002; Wang 2002).

This perceived moral vacuum is particularly true for the older generations who are more accustomed to a homogeneous, unified value system. "I don't know what to believe" and "I cannot understand why so-and-so thinks or behaves in this way" are among the typical reflections on the loss of an absolute moral authority. This sense of confusion with diverse and sometime conflicting values and moral practices has become stronger as Chinese society is rapidly becoming more open and heterogeneous, which also explains why the alarm about an impending moral crisis has been in the air since the 1980s. Although the content of the perceived crisis has changed, the perception of moral decline continues.

Second, although there is no culture war per se in China, the conflict of values and beliefs caused by radical social changes is something that Chinese individuals experience daily. Elsewhere, I took a close look at the changes in the social evaluation of the moral quality *laoshi*, which implies a cluster of personal attributes, such as honesty, frankness, good behavior, obedience, and simple-mindedness. Among these, obedience and honesty are emphasized more frequently in everyday life discourse. Until the early 1980s, being *laoshi* was a highly regarded merit in village society, and *laoshi* boys were normally welcomed as ideal mates and as trustworthy individuals in public life. But in the postreform era, *laoshi* has gradually become a negative term, and a male who is labeled as *laoshi* is looked down upon by ambitious young women for a number of reasons (Yan 2003: 77–78). According to Zhu Li's questionnaire survey of one thousand people in 2002 and 2003, for example, nearly 60 percent of the people surveyed regard *laoshi* as an outdated value that only hurt one's personal interest in today's China (Zhu 2006:343).

In my opinion, *laoshi* is a valuable moral quality adaptable for in-group social interactions associated with low mobility. When villagers were basically confined within the closely-knit local community and interacted only with people who were in the existing social networks, *laoshi* meant trustworthy and reliable, thus reducing transaction costs in social life. However, other merits of being *laoshi*, such as naïveté and honesty, turn out to be fatal shortcomings outside the local community, especially in the postreform era when villagers have had to deal with strangers in the unregulated market. Under these new circumstances, *laoshi* invites aggression and cheating; a *laoshi* husband can hardly provide the kind of safety and protection that a wife desires. Equally important, a nonvocal but hardworking young man may meet parental or in-law expectations from a familial perspective, but he does not necessarily fit the increasing demands for intimacy and companionship from young women as individuals. In other words, the existence or absence of social mobility, interactions with strangers, and individual choice determines whether being *laoshi* or not is a good moral quality at a given time.

In her insightful study of the sex industry in the northeastern city of Dalian, Zheng Tiantian (2009) examines both the everyday life and subjective world of a group of female sex workers. Contrary to the widely accepted view that sex workers are demoralized by the mainstream morality's negative view of prostitution, Zheng reveals how her informants gradually develop a new "moral vision" out of their experience of oppression and discrimination that rejects the dominant values regarding love, marriage, and family. By way of this moral vision, "commodification of the body and commodification of romance and intimacy are transformed from a denigration of female virtue into a route to empowerment" (Zheng 2009: 222). This new moral vision, needless to say, runs into a head-to-head collision with the traditional Confucian ethics and patriarchal definition of female virtue, contributing to the perception of moral decay or crisis among both scholars (see Shen 2007) and the populace.

In addition to the different ways of thinking about these moral changes, the emergence of new, unconventional social practices can also lead to a perception of moral decline by the majority in society. A good example in this connection is the sexual revolution that has silently yet forcefully pushed the envelope of sexual morality during the last three decades (see Zhang's chapter in this book). Premarital sex was taboo in the 1970s and a couple who intended to marry or even became engaged would be punished in various ways if they engaged in premarital sex. This taboo was widely challenged in the 1980s. A large number of high school and college students rapidly began to taste the forbidden fruit. By the turn of the twenty-first century, cohabitation had become a common practice among urban youth. Along this line of change, every step has caused a wave of perceived moral decline in sexual mores; yet, immoral behavior in one year became acceptable in the next year and then the standard thereafter.

Responding to the rapid social changes in China, individuals must often make moral decisions about their own behavior and moral judgments about others, many of which are both complicated, confusing, and, more often than not, are the result of entanglement of the old and new ethics. For example, a couple in Xiajia Village was regarded by their fellow villagers as unwise in the 1980s because they gave up trying to have a son after the birth of their second daughter. Against the widely shared wisdom about not investing too much in a daughter's education, the couple encouraged and supported their two daughters to attend the best local schools. The elder daughter graduated from a vocational school in 2003 and eventually landed a secretarial job in Beijing. The second daughter did even better, entering a good college in southern China in 2005. The elder daughter initially sent money home to help her parents buy an apartment in the provincial capital city of Harbin where they worked as street vendors. She then supported the college education of her younger sister who vowed to study even harder for a postgraduate degree and to earn more money to pay back her parents and elder sister in the future. The couple was widely admired until one day when a middle-aged woman from Beijing came to the village and accused the elder daughter of destroying the woman's marriage. It turned out that the elder daughter was living in an apartment with a regular stipend provided by her boss, a married man who was twice her age. It was only by becoming a mistress, the villagers told me, that the elder daughter had been able to send home so much money. Some regarded this as disgraceful and unacceptable, yet others praised the daughter for her devotion to her parents and her younger sister. How to make a fair moral judgment of her behavior became a highly controversial issue and was often debated among my informants during my interviews.

Finally, the ethical shift from responsibilities to rights that I describe should be viewed as a new, and, in my mind, the major trend in China's moral landscape. Yet, moral changes in the post-Mao era are certainly not unidirectional or one dimensional. While more and more Chinese individuals embrace the new ethics of individual rights and openly pursue various personal desires in both private and public life (Rofel 2007; Yan 2003), others lament the decline of collective ethics of responsibilities, especially the loss of the meaning of life that was previously defined by collective interests, and make the effort to preserve some collective values. The harmony and prosperity of the family remains the ultimate goal among the young migrant workers even though they have left their parents to pursue their dream of personal development in remote urban areas (Hansen and Pang 2008). The sense of cultural belonging has grown ever stronger since the 1990s as more and more individuals, especially the rising middle class, want to showcase their Chineseness through lifestyle and public discourse; nationalism and consumerism emerged together as the main threads to construct the world of meanings for most Chinese youth; and being patriotic is fashionable too among young urban professionals (Gries 2004; Hoffman 2010; Jankowiak 2004; Rofel 2007). Moreover, individuals can also claim rights by way of the old collective ethics. For example, most workers who engaged in a rights assertion movement when they were laid off and the enterprises where they used to work were sold out or dismantled did so in accordance with the socialist value of industrial workers being the leading class of the new society (see Lee 2007). The returned overseas Chinese in a state farm refused to privatize the collective farm because they did not see themselves fit for the market economy. Quite interestingly, they resorted to collective ethics and patriotism and eventually won their battle (Li 2010).

Furthermore, individuals apply different moral logics that seem to be the most appropriate to a given case in a particular time. In their study of inheritance disputes in Shanghai, Davis and Lu (2003) discovered that when fighting over family real estate, people first take into consideration the pathway by which the family obtained the property. If it is a privately owned family property or *sifang*, the logic of family estate will be applied; if it is a residential unit allocated by the work unit or rented from the city's real-estate bureau *(gongfang)*, a logic of the regulatory state will be emphasized; if it is a commercial flat purchased after the housing reform in China *(shangpinfang)*, the logic of the law and market overrules other systems. Interestingly, in divorce cases, the division of the family real estate not only involves the consideration of the pathway of property ownership but also more traditional moral reasoning, such as punishing the guilty party and allocating more to the needy. The conclusion that Davis draws from her study unmistakably illustrates the entanglement of the old and the new ethics and moral reasoning: "As a result, even as they demonstrated fluency with the legal rules for establishing ownership to property, ordinary citizens continue to use their own experience and draw on context-specific moral reasoning. And because divorce settlements after 2003 have most often been finalized by *xieyi* (agreements) drawn up without legal advice and outside the courts, the contextual and personal logics of ordinary citizens play a central role in the maturation of a post-socialist property regime as it incorporates expectations and practices rooted in pre-socialist, socialist, and market experiences" (Davis 2010: 482).

CONFLICTING TRENDS IN CHANGING MORAL PRACTICES

Turning to the practice dimension of the changing moral landscape, we find the situation is equally complex. Due to space limits, here I will only review the patterns of immorality as reflected in morally disturbing practices and the practices that reveal the trend of the new morality. The two trends, although diagonally opposite to each other at the surface level, are related to the deeper ethical shift from collective responsibilities to individual rights.

Morally disturbing experience, or immorality as perceived by local people, has been an understudied subject in anthropology. Most existing studies focus on the reproduction of the social order through coded norms of behavior, that is, concepts of the good and of ethics. Some recent efforts to renew the anthropology of morality turn to the other end, that is, the role of freedom and choice in ethical reflections among individuals (see Zigon 2008). Yet, looking at moral changes from the local people's perspective, I found immorality the most frequently addressed issue in daily conversations.

IMMORALITY AND MORAL CRISIS

The disturbing changes in old age security and the diminishing influence of the notion of filial piety also show that the public discourse on moral decline does not derive solely from ungrounded perceptions or differences in ethical values; instead, in most cases, the perceived moral decline or crisis has its base in social facts as well. If immorality is defined as an intentional violation of the prevailing ethical values and doing purposeful damage to other people's interests, there has indeed been a rise in individual acts that fall into these categories. Although the extent to which a violation of ethical values is immoral may sometimes depend on the larger context, as shown in the examples I have cited, deliberate harm to other people's interests through coercion, cheating, extortion, and abuse of power is widely viewed as immoral. Unfortunately, except for the political reporting and persecution that dominated the Maoist era, various other practices that benefit the actor at the expense of others have indeed been on the rise during the post-Mao reform era, clearly constituting the factual basis for the perception of a moral crisis.

Among all immoral behaviors, those that exceed the bottom line of morality—that is, those acts that violate the most basic and widely shared ethical values or intentionally hurt others in the most harmful of ways—have received a great deal of attention from both the popular media and academic circles. For example, it is considered to be crossing the bottom line of reciprocity when a distressed person who is helped by a stranger after an accident on the street turns around to accuse the Good Samaritan of being the original cause of the distress and attempts to extort money out of the Good Samaritan. And this has now become an established scam (for a detailed study, see Yan 2009). Unfortunately, it is by no means rare to find cases of extreme immoral behavior in today's China. Sociologist Sun Liping regards the lowering of the moral bottom line to be the most worrisome and potentially dangerous social problem in the rapidly changing moral landscape, because the constant assaults on the moral bottom line, the ethical bedrock of society, threaten the foundations of social life (Sun 2007, especially 1–9).

I would add that when extreme immoral behavior exceeds the level of isolated individual acts and involves a number of individuals in semiopen or open cooperation, the impact on the moral bottom line tends to be the greatest. This is because isolated individual acts, like the extortion of a Good Samaritan or commercial cheating, regardless of the frequency of their occurrence, do not shake ordinary people's trust in the society as a whole. In contrast, organized immoral behavior tends to involve institutions at various levels and thus develops into a kind of institutionalized immorality. Needless to say, the appearance of institutionalized immorality in any domain of social life will pose a serious challenge to the justice and fairness in society, and the cumulative result of an increasing number of acts of institutionalized immorality will indeed shake the basic ethical values and could potentially lead to a real moral crisis. The best illustration in this connection is the crisis of food safety and the ensuing national panic that it caused.

The production and distribution of fake and faulty goods have been a serious social problem since the mid-1980s, even before the rising tide of consumerism. To protect their rights, individual consumers have stood up in various ways to fight against fake and faulty goods. As early as 1985, the first consumer association was established in a county in Henan Province, and within a short period of time a nationwide network of consumer associations emerged. With financial support and semileadership from the state, the All-China Consumer Association quickly grew into the largest and strongest consumer organization, and a number of consumer protection laws were enacted. As a result, individual "consumer citizens," as Beverley Hooper puts it (2005), can fight against the market with the help of the state. It is fair to say that the awareness of individual rights among ordinary people began with an awareness of consumer rights, and in most cases the rights assertion movement in China has actually been a consumer movement.

Despite all the efforts for consumer protection, the problem of fake and faulty goods exacerbated over the years, culminating in the large-scale production and distribution of fake and contaminated foods and medicine that directly affected the health and lives of numerous consumers. One of the earliest safety scandals occurred in Jijiang County, Fujian Province. In 1980 local food processing factories began to produce fake medicines made of starch, sugar, and other common foodstuffs. Peasant producers managed to sell the fake medicine to state-owned hospitals and pharmacies by giving cash kick-backs to those in charge, thus making huge profits from the extremely low-cost fake products. By 1985, a total of fifty-seven factories in the county were specializing in the making of more than one hundred kinds of fake medicine and they quickly became a strong competitor to the state-owned pharmaceutical companies. Interestingly, it was the politically unhealthy development of rural industry challenging the state-owned enterprises, instead of the fake medicines hurting the consumers, that attracted the attention of the state. An explosive investigative report was published in the national *People's Daily* on June 16, 1985, exposing a large business scam and moral scandal that involved more than one thousand participants and various local government agencies. With more details revealed in other reports, the provincial party boss Xiang Nan, an important figure in promoting the economic reform in south China, resigned, becoming the highest-level political casualty of the food safety problem until 2008.

Unfortunately, the 1985 case of fake medicine was only the beginning of a nationwide wave of large-scale production and distribution of fake and faulty food products over the next twenty plus years. The contaminated baby formula produced by the Sanlu Group, a well-known joint-venture giant in the Chinese dairy business, is one of the latest that has caused a national public health and morality crisis. To artificially increase the amount of protein in inferior milk that was either diluted with water or spoiled, melamine, a chemical used to make plastic and to tan leather, was added, and the contaminated milk was used to produce baby formula, ice cream bars, and other products. By September 15, 2008, only Sanlu products had been found with melamine, and the company recalled seven hundred tons of baby formula. But on the following day a nationwide test conducted by the General Administration of Quality Supervision, Inspection, and Quarantine (AQSIQ) revealed that the milk products of twenty-two out of the 109 inspected firms were also contaminated with melamine, including products at the two top firms of Yili and Mengniu. Although most contaminated products were being sold on the domestic market, some were also exported to Hong Kong. The known number of children stricken by the contamination rose to more than fifty-three thousand in less than two weeks, among whom four died and nearly 12,892 were hospitalized with kidney problems.[2]

The most morally disturbing fact is that the production and distribution of these products also involved various government institutions. Moreover, a large number of people were actively participating, most of whom were ordinary people who were the direct producers, such as construction workers and dairy farmers. Others were economic or political elite at various levels, such as entrepreneurs, managers, professionals in quality-control agencies, and government officials. Regardless of their social status or the roles they played, they were all well aware of the consequences of the scam, that is, the potential harm to the lives and health of others. Another example is from Xianghe County, Hebei Province, where farmers soaked the roots of chives in a powerful pesticide called 3911 so that the plants would grow extremely large. From 1999 to 2004 the pesticide was used on thousands of acres of chive fields. This was an open collective action; when the pesticide was applied there was a very strong acrid odor in the entire area. Yet, no government agency bothered to question this harmful practice until outside journalists began to report it. Fortunately, investigative reporting has become stronger in the era of reform and has played a key role in the maturation of regulation, criminal justice, and ethical discourse. Moreover, in most cases of faulty food products, the producers and distributors have revealed indifferent attitudes toward the victims or have justified their behavior with a particularistic ethics. In a 2004 case, a reporter from the Chinese Central Television Station asked workers in a rural factory producing colloidal food additive out of leather waste, including old shoes, whether they knew that the contaminated products would end up in food to be consumed by people. The producers replied lightly: "So what? They are strangers, and we do not know them at all. In this region, no one would eat foods with colloidal additives because we all know the secret" (CCTV 2004).

As in most societies, food is regarded as an important part of life in China, and the truism "you are what you eat" fits Chinese culture very well as most Chinese individuals believe that their minds and bodies are shaped by the food they eat. Scandals and scams involving faulty, fake, contaminated, and in some cases simply poisonous foods have had an extremely negative impact on the moral experience of ordinary people. In the last few years, a long list of unsafe foods has circulated on the Internet, including as many as fifty items ranging from the most ordinary like salted eggs to health-enhancing luxury items, which are produced by small and big companies alike. "How could one do such harm to so many innocent people?" was the most common question posed after food scandals in the 1980s and 1990s; the initial shock and disbelief gradually developed into an extremely cautious psychology among many consumers. Outraged and morally disturbed, many lamented that they no longer knew what was safe to eat and who was worthy of trust. Beneath this widespread public panic regarding food safety, there emerged a much deeper crisis in the moral universe, that is, the decline of social trust.

In a highly mobile and open society, most social interactions occur among individuals who are not related to one another by any particularistic ties; thus, in many cases, people do not expect to interact with the other party again in the future. In such a society of strangers, social trust is more important than personal trust. Social trust is understood as the more generalized trust in social institutions, that they will behave in accordance with the stated rules, in experts who will guard the rules to make the institutions work well, and also in strangers who will engage in peaceful and nonharmful social interactions. In contrast, personal trust is only invested in people who are in one's social web, ranging from family, kinship, and local community, to a wider yet still well-defined network of friends. Personal trust derives from long-term interactions with the same group of people and thus is based on low mobility and a narrower scope of social interactions. In such a society of acquaintances, strangers are potential enemies, experts are not generally needed, and institutions are mostly unwelcome unless they are politically imposed upon people. The expansion of personal trust to social trust provides one of the key mechanisms in making a modern economy and society work and thus becomes a necessary condition of modernity (see Giddens 1990).

Based on an established network of interpersonal relations, traditional Chinese morality features low social trust. As Fei Xiaotong points out, traditional Chinese society is organized through a differentiated mode of association in which individuals are positioned in a hierarchy of various relations, such as that between parents and children, husband and wife, and friends and friends. Moral rights and duties are defined and fulfilled differently in accordance with one's position in a given relationship. Many of the behavioral norms and moral values do not apply to people who are outside one's network of social relationships (Fei [1947] 1992: 71–79). As the social distance increases, suspicion increases as well and may turn to hostility when dealing with total strangers. The distrust of strangers is an important piece of the cultural knowledge that is transmitted from one generation to the next through both formal and informal channels (see Chen 2006: 118–155). Consequently, treating an outsider poorly is normally taken lightly in Chinese communities, whereas abuse of one's own people is viewed as morally unacceptable. Although this particularistic morality was attacked during the heyday of Maoist socialism and the state made radical attempts to promote a new set of universalistic values of socialist morality (Madsen 1984), the divide between in-group and out-group members remained strong throughout the 1960s and 1970s. Moreover, in the name of the revolution and class struggle, hostility toward a political stranger—the people who were labeled as the "class enemy"—was actually encouraged by the state and developed to an extreme level of brutality and violence. By this logic of ethical thinking, the producers and distributors could justify their behavior because they did not know the victims of their products.

The promotion of social trust has thus become an urgent issue in contemporary Chinese society as it has rapidly become more open, modern, and highly mobile. It is puzzling that even though the market economy has developed quickly, social trust has declined. A Chinese sociologist describes the six kinds of distrust prevailing in contemporary China that contribute to the crisis of social trust: namely, distrust of the market due to faulty goods and bad service, distrust of service providers and strangers, distrust of friends and even relatives, distrust of law enforcement officers, distrust of the law and legal institutions, and distrust of basic moral values (Peng 2003: 292–295). The widespread production and distribution of fake and contaminated foods, as indicated earlier, has played an especially vicious role in spreading further distrust in strangers and social institutions.

The pursuit of individual interests and profit-making are the direct driving force behind the production and distribution of fake and faulty goods. Particularly noteworthy is the moral justification of pursuing one's self-interest at the expense of others. In the mid-1980s, a journalist once confronted the head of a township government by asking whether he knew that the production of fake and faulty goods was illegal and immoral. Pointing to the rows of new houses behind him, the government official proudly answered without hesitation: "I think that the highest morality under heaven is to let my poor hometown become rich" (see Wu 2007: 149). This utilitarian and self-centered logic of moral reasoning fits well with the party-state's strategy of prioritizing economic growth, the national obsession with modernity, and the pragmatic measurement of truth and good, which have dominated Chinese thinking—official and unofficial alike—since the late 1970s. At a deeper level, this cadre's utilitarian statement that shrugs off the basic ethical responsibility—not to purposely hurt other people—with the priority of economic growth reflects the dangers accompanied by the shift from a collective ethics of responsibility and self-sacrifice to an individual ethics of rights and self-realization: that is, who will be the moral authority and where is the social sanctioning system after faith in the truth is replaced by a sense of the truth?

Under the ethics of responsibilities, there is an external moral authority that demands obedience, making people fulfill their responsibilities even sometimes at their own expense. In many developed countries in the West, this omnipotent authority was God and, after the secularization movement, appeared under the guise of the nation-state, society, and so forth, with religion continuing to exert an important influence. In the Chinese context, before the revolution it was Heaven, the family, and community power and thereafter it was Chairman Mao and Communist morality. In either case, an external and absolute authority no longer existed after the shift from an ethics of responsibility to an ethics of rights. In the moral universe of a highly mobile society of strangers, the sole true master of the individual is no one but the individual herself. Yet, the independent and self-serving individual is more vulnerable than ever to encroachment and aggression by other equally self-serving individuals and thus must seek protection from social institutions. Modern social institutions only protect individuals well when social trust, rule of law, checks and balances of power, and freedom of speech are well developed. This is the paradox of institutionalized individualism and the individualization of society that has become a global trend in the contemporary world (see Beck and Beck-Gernsheim 2002; Lipovetsky 2005).

Unfortunately, the individual in contemporary China cannot count on social institutions for the much-needed protection in a society of increasing risk. As revealed in almost all the cases of fake and faulty goods (including unsafe construction), the institutions and experts who were responsible for quality control did not perform their basic duties; rather, in many cases they also became involved or actively participated in the illegal and immoral practices. In the 2008 case of contaminated milk products, it is outrageous that the government officially assured that the milk products provided for the Olympics and Paralympics were not contaminated, indicating the addition of melamine was indeed a deliberate act under effective control in the production and distribution processes. It has also been reported that the local government was informed of the health issues caused by the tainted milk products in early August; yet, to insure the success of the Beijing Olympics, the local government withheld the information for a month. During this time, tons of contaminated baby formula were distributed and sold to consumers nationwide.

I would like to reiterate that as far as the factual side of the moral decline is concerned, unethical or immoral acts that are carried out in a collective mode or structured in institutional ways are much more damaging to the society as a whole. The large-scale production and distribution of fake and faulty goods is only one of the major problems that pose real threats to China's moral landscape. The widespread corruption among power holders, which has developed over the years from individual corruption to collective and institutionalized corruption (see, e.g., Gong 2006), constitutes yet another major problem in the changing moral landscape, an important issue in its own right.[3] To address these problems, freedom of speech and independence of the judiciary seem to be necessary preconditions. Yet, the slow progress in political reform shows that China still has a long way to go to achieve these basic conditions. In this sense, we may say that the current moral crisis in China is actually also a political crisis, and the former cannot be resolved without successful political reforms.[4]

THE EMERGING NEW ETHICS AND MORAL PRACTICES

To obtain a complete picture of the changing moral landscape, one should not overlook the bright side that includes both the preservation of conventional ethics and the emergence of new ethics in social practice. For example, anthropologist Ellen Oxfeld (2004) cites countless examples of how residents in a south China village remember and remunerate the gifts and help that they previously received, considering them as both social and moral debts. The memory and the reciprocal acts play an equally important role in maintaining a social conscience, despite the impact of market instrumentality. William Jankowiak reveals the positive moral changes in urban settings, such as the increasing occupational prestige of lawyers because they are perceived as pursuing justice for other people in the form of rights assertion, the growing individual contributions in charity work and giving, and the rise of a broad sense of a shared community in what he calls "ethical nationalism" (2004).

Although both are important for our understanding of the moral world in Chinese people's everyday life, the moral changes presented by Jankowiak deserve special attention because these changes occurred in the volatile context of urban life and in most cases among strangers. Social interactions among acquaintances in a village setting are more likely bound by the conventional ethics of responsibility even under the conditions of the market economy, but the preservation of the old ethics does not necessarily equip the villagers with the appropriate ethics for dealing with strangers. As shown by numerous cases, the production of fake and faulty goods, including contaminated foods, has been mostly concentrated in rural areas and many villagers have willingly and actively participated in the production process. As noted, they tend to justify their behavior in terms of the particularistic morality that treats acquaintances and strangers differently from family members.

In contrast, the emerging trend of philanthropy and charity work in the urban areas represents a new ethic: the generalized notion of compassion and caring that applies equally to all. An exemplary individual is the pop singer Cong Fei. Like many rural youth, Cong left home to pursue his dreams in the city of Shenzhen, but he quickly became penniless. A friend helped Cong by giving him six hundred yuan to sign up for a pop-singing contest; after wining the contest, Cong became a professional singer and began to pay back society in his own way. From 1992 to 2002, the year he died, Cong had donated a major portion of his income for the education of 178 students from poor rural families who otherwise would have had to drop out of school, and he pledged to support these students from primary school all the way through college.

Cong's case deserves special attention for two reasons. First, as a local pop singer who never gained much fame and lived only on unreliable sources of income from his performances, Cong was not at all a rich person. His devotion to charity shows that ordinary people can be part of the newly emerging trend of individual philanthropy. Second, as an individual philanthropist without any background in government or any business connections, Cong was also vulnerable to social pressures, the influence of the media, and interference from the government. Shortly after his altruism was reported in the media, the local government made Cong into a Lei Feng-type model citizen who selflessly works for the people. (Lei Feng was one of the most prominent idealizations of a selfless Communist in the era of radical Maoism. His story was embellished and used for motivational purposes.) The government frequently called upon Cong for exemplary donations when it needed to raise funds from society. In return, Cong received various government certificates of recognition and honors, along with media coverage. Under pressure from these official and media expectations, Cong soon had no choice but to donate even more of his limited income, and by the time of his death from cancer in 2002, Cong had practically no property to leave to his wife. It was reported that, in his last hours, Cong described his life as a journey climbing up a ladder as high as heaven. "In the beginning I helped a few poor students out of a strong personal feeling of connectedness because I had earlier been in their situation. But once I received so much official recognition, I had more responsibilities and when I ran out of money, I felt crushed by the responsibilities. The ladder was just too high for me to climb."[5]

China has a long history of private charities that can be traced back to the Han dynasty (202 BCE–220 CE); by the end of nineteenth century, both the number and scale of private charities exceeded the official relief agencies of the imperial state. Although the Chinese charity tradition was also generally limited within the boundaries of kinship and local territory, goods and money were donated to address local needs such as building roads and bridges, constructing schools and hospitals, or for relief efforts during years of famine. It was rare for strangers in remote places to benefit from localized charities, and it was also rare for long-range goals promoting social change to be pursued.

The traditional philanthropy came to an end after 1949 as the party-state sought to monopolize the distribution of all resources in society. In the official discourse, private charities were viewed as the tools of the feudal and imperialist oppressors to deceive and beguile the Chinese people and thus they had to be eliminated. In practice, all private philanthropic organizations were either shut down or taken over by the government. The state was to take care of all of the needs of the people, and attempts to make donations were condemned as showing off individual wealth for ulterior motives.

Charity work was gradually rehabilitated in the 1980s and 1990s when the government realized its own limits in addressing all the new needs that the market economy created. The change started with government-sponsored foundations such as the China Red Cross Society, the China Youth Development Foundation, and the China Charity Foundation. Some successful projects, such as the Hope Project by the China Youth Development Foundation that focuses on improving education in China's poorest regions, demonstrated the importance of charities to the party-state, and, little by little, private philanthropy began to reemerge in China.

Since the late 1990s, an increasing number of private entrepreneurs have set up their own charitable organizations or have made donations to NGOs working for philanthropic causes, such as public health, education, and poverty relief. This new development attracted the attention of Rupert Hoogewerf, the founder of the monthly magazine the *Hurun Report*, which is best known for its annual "China's Rich List." In 2004, Hoogewerf made the first "Hurun Philanthropy List," featuring the top fifty most generous individuals in China who had donated millions of dollars in the previous year; the annual list has continued and since 2006 it has been expanded to include the top one hundred philanthropists.

Another development has been individual donations from ordinary citizens. These first appeared in 1998 when individual donations (as opposed to corporate donations that often include entrepreneur donations) were made by Chinese citizens who responded enthusiastically to the call to help the victims of the catastrophic floods that year. This new philanthropic spirit and practice among ordinary folk reached a high in 2008 in the nationwide relief efforts after the massive earthquake in Sichuan province. Within the first month, the amount of social donations, that is, donations from the private sector and individual citizens, reached a record high of more than eighty million dollars. In between these two events, numerous individuals made donations to various other charity projects, such as helping leukemia patients receive much-needed medical treatment or supporting students from poor regions to continue their education. A common feature of all these charitable donations from ordinary citizens is that they are made to help strangers instead of helping someone in one's kinship group or hometown. In this sense, a true spirit of philanthropy has sprouted in China during the postreform era.

Equally important is the more individualized trend in philanthropic developments. For years the Chinese government kept a tight hand over charity development and used its political power to reinforce its monopoly control. For example, the city government of Weihai in Shandong Province launched a charity month, asking public servants and state-owned enterprise employees to contribute to various government-sponsored charitable projects. Because the amount donated was used to judge the political performance and work achievements of the leadership of the organizations, the call for charitable donations turned out to be a forced collection of money from individuals. Such coerced donations, the outdated official discourse of collective responsibility, and the mismanagement of funds are common problems associated with government-sponsored charity campaigns and projects. These have discouraged Chinese individuals from philanthropic practices, or at least those run by government agencies. Thus, unlike in 1998 when individuals donated only to government-sponsored foundations, in 2008 most individuals preferred to make donations to Hong Kong charities or to give directly to the quake victims, and many gave as individuals in addition to giving at the office as government employees. A clerk with the Beijing special armed police said: "I wanted to separate the collective action from the individual action." He donated 120 yuan at his office and then six hundred yuan to a private foundation in his daughter's name. Mr. Zhao, the owner of a technology company, stated clearly: "I want to show that it's me who's donating. It's not connected to anybody else. I am donating in my own name" (Fan 2008).

These people's attempts to separate their spontaneous donations as individual acts from the required donations by the government clearly indicate the emergence of a new kind of ethics, that is, a generalized notion of compassion and charity that derives from individual choice and that is applied to unrelated individuals outside of one's own circle of acquaintances or local world. This effort at individualized charity also resists the official control of the old collective ethics of responsibility, or the "heavenly ladder" of selfless sacrifice that Cong Fei was forced to climb by the local government; consequently, a new foundation for private charity and philanthropy has been built whereby an optional individual ethics of rights and self-realization motivates individuals to give and to help. That is to say, pity for those in distress, compassion for their struggles, and responsibility for doing something to help are emotional and meaning-centered realities of individuals (not surprisingly, this resurgence of philanthropy at times relates to the resurgence of religious organizations).

A more radical example in this connection is Han Han, an independent-minded writer and car racer who became a national idol among the youth because of his highly individualistic behavior, including dropping out of high school to protest the examination system. Han Han openly doubted the capacity of the government-sponsored charitable foundations to properly manage public donations and stated on his personal blog that he would not make any donations to government foundations. But he was among the first to volunteer in the quake region to help find survivors.

This new individual-centered discourse of ethics can also be found among those rich whose names appear on the Hurun Philanthropic List. For example, Chen Guangbiao, who ranked number four on the 2008 list by donating 130 million yuan in 2007, is well known for seeking personal pleasure and for his sense of satisfaction from his philanthropic activities. Interestingly, Chen Guangbiao also took a cowboy approach to participating in the quake relief. In addition to making donations, Chen led a team of more than one hundred employees from his company who drove sixty bulldozers over one thousand miles nonstop to arrive at the quake zone before the army or any government-organized relief team (Xinhua News Agency 2008). Volunteerism is another highlight of the new ethics that suddenly appeared in China during the postquake relief efforts in 2008. It was estimated that by early July 2008 more than two hundred and fifty thousand volunteers had gone to Sichuan at their own expense and entirely of their own free will, the majority of whom were young people born in the 1980s. When asked why, many of them responded that they were moved by the suffering of the victims and thus they wanted to offer help, with a number of them specifically pointing out that helping others makes their personal lives more meaningful (Cha 2008). Such compassion toward strangers does not exist in traditional on-the-ground, locality-centered Chinese morality, even though it is part of institutionalized Buddhism. To a certain extent, it resembles the teachings of the Good Samaritan parable in the Bible: humanity's bonds in brotherhood should transcend geographical, racial, economic, and social boundaries. The altruistic behavior of these young volunteers was widely regarded as a pleasant surprise in Chinese society because most of the volunteers were singletons who are also widely known to be self-indulgent, self-centered, and irresponsible. It was difficult to make the link between the altruism and individualism of these youth.

Like private philanthropy, volunteerism also went through a long and winding process to reach this point in 2008. After the 1949 revolution, the party-state incorporated not only charity agencies but also all volunteer activities into its organizational framework, mostly through the work-unit system and other organizations such as the Communist Youth League. During the Mao era, citizens were mobilized to contribute to socialism through various forms of unpaid labor, known as *yiwu laodong* in Chinese, and there was a stigma to the term *volunteerism* due to its close association with church organizations such as the YMCA before the 1949 revolution. In the late 1980s, the government began to promote volunteerism and established a national Volunteers' Association, which, not surprisingly, is affiliated with the Communist Youth League.

The state sponsorship and collective nature of the association supports the conventional notion that volunteer activities must be organized by the government in one way or another. In a detailed ethnography of a group of young volunteers in a southern city, Rolandsen (2008) discovers that the motivations for engaging in volunteer work among the youth are highly individualistic, varying from efforts to expand one's social network, search for a meaningful life in a different domain, or train oneself with leadership skills to more opportunistic concerns such as the desire to obtain party membership. Yet they all must pursue their goals through the leadership and organization of the Volunteers' Association, which, in turn, has close links with the party-state apparatus. As a result, the young volunteers must go to study sessions, carry out party-state propaganda programs in their volunteer work, and organize activities on special days designated by the party-state apparatus, all of which constitute "a sign of performance for the state's agenda," as Rolandsen puts it.

For Chinese citizens, the first known act of volunteerism purely by individuals occurred in January 2008. After a heavy snowstorm paralyzed communications, transportation, and everyday life in south China, thirteen villagers from Tangshan rented a small bus and drove to Hunan Province where they stayed for weeks helping the local people. When asked about their motivations, the villagers simply replied that they all were child survivors of the 1976 Tangshan earthquake and had grown up hearing numerous stories about how people from other places had helped Tangshan after the quake. So they were motivated to reciprocate the help they had received earlier. Their story was broadcast on CCTV and in other official media, which for the first time showed Chinese citizens that volunteer work can be undertaken without the leadership and organization of the party or government. Ironically, the thirteen villager volunteers were later recognized and promoted by the local government as selfless heroes and were referred to as living Lei Feng models. On various occasions, they were invited to lecture on their values of selflessness and responsibility, and they even announced that they would form a permanent group of peasant volunteers. Like the pop singer Cong Fei, these villagers could not resist the government's efforts to reincorporate them into the framework of collective responsibility, thus they eventually abandoned the new volunteerism that they had pioneered in early 2008. Nevertheless, their original actions had a far-reaching impact on Chinese society and the official recognition also provided a sense of political safety. It is in this context that the wave of volunteerism surged after the earthquake in May 2008, which also changed the moral landscape of China.[6]

The list of new ethics and moral practices is long when we turn our attention to gradual and nondramatic changes in everyday life among ordinary people. The increasing awareness of environmentalism, animal protection, changing attitudes toward the handicapped and physically disabled, compassion and assistance toward disadvantaged groups, and the values of tolerance, choice, and diversity are all positive changes that have occurred in the post-Mao reform era. It is impossible to examine them all in this chapter; suffice it to point out that like the perceived and actual negative changes, they are also part of the changing moral landscape.

FINAL REMARKS

In conclusion, the prolonged public perception of a moral decline or crisis is by no means a mirage or ungrounded misunderstanding of social changes. However, to what extent and in what ways this perception of moral crisis reflects the changing social reality needs to be spelled out by well-grounded empirical research. As an initial effort, I have examined the important changes in both ethical discourse and moral practice, emphasizing that the ethical shift from a collective system of responsibility and self-sacrifice to an individualistic system of rights and development is the key to better understand the changing moral landscape in post-Mao China.[7]

Scholars disagree about how to evaluate the moral changes during the reform era, mostly because their respective studies focus on particular domains of social life or on a given group of people in a given time period. For example, focusing on value changes in moral discourse, Jiwei Ci and Xiaoying Wang emphasize the dissolution of the ethics of responsibility and the decline of collective values, while overlooking the rise of a new ethics of individual rights and freedom (Ci 1994; Wang 2002). In contrast, to highlight the development of a new rights morality in villagers' resistance struggles against real-estate developers and predatory local governments, Hok Bun Ku neglects the accompanying decline of a morality of responsibility (2003). In my own previous research, I paid more attention to the changing moral landscape in the domain of private life while rarely discussing parallel changes in public life (Yan 2003). As indicated earlier, both Oxfeld (2004) and Jankowiak (2004) focus on the bright side and argue for either the preservation of traditional ethics or the development of a new ethics. Yet, all these positive changes have occurred simultaneously and against the same background of a crisis of social trust (see Peng 2003).

How the transitional society at large shapes morality is also under debate. According to Xin Liu, in the 1990s "the lack of a moral economy in communal life in conjunction with the emergence of a moral space at large became a crucial condition of existence in post-reform rural China" (2000: 183). In this uncertain and highly contested moral landscape a person's character and the established sense of self could be easily challenged, changed, and twisted, leading to a discontinuity of the personhood or the otherness of the self as Liu put it (2002). Backed by longitudinal survey data and participant observations in the same city since the early 1980s, Jankowiak emphasizes the positive development of a "moral space at large" (in Liu's terms) and attributes the expansion of this new moral horizon mainly to the market economy and the expanded scope of social interactions (2004: 205). Concurring with these insightful arguments, I would add that the construction or expansion of this new moral space is likely multilayered, multidirectional, and with multiple consequences and meanings for different groups of people in China; but, at the same time, it has shown the tendency to be increasingly individualized. The shift toward a more individualistic ethical system and the individualization of the new moral space, in my mind, result directly from the ongoing process of the individualization of Chinese society itself.

As I argue elsewhere (Yan 2003, 2009b, 2010), the rise of the individual constitutes the most fundamental change in Chinese society. A central feature of post-Mao reform has been a process whereby the state first was forced and then took the initiative to make the Chinese individual more self-reliant, self-driven, and more competitive in a market economy. The direct result is the rise of the enterprising self and the individualization of society (see also the introduction of this volume). To cope with the challenges brought about by the market reforms and globalization, certain institutional reforms have been made to accommodate the rise of the individual, including the tolerance of the shift toward a more individualistic, pluralistic ethics and the encouragement of consumerism in the domain of ideology. Yet, both the rise of the individual and the individualization of society can be regarded as part of China's pressured and ever more rushed quest for modernity since the mid-nineteenth century, in which the individual has always been viewed as an instrument to a greater end, that is, the building of a strong, wealthy, and modern state. The call for the submission of the small self (the interest of the individual) to the great self (the interest of the nation-state) has been centrally influential in the ethical discourse on the self, morality, and meaning of life from the mid-nineteenth century to the present, albeit under different ideological and political disguises (Yan 2010). As a result, the two crucial social conditions for the individualization of society in the West (Beck and Beck-Gernsheim 2002), namely, a deeply rooted culture of democracy that promotes equality and liberal individualism and a welfare state that protects and supports the individuals, are missing in the Chinese process of individualization. The individual as the end, not the means to an end, still is an alien idea to the Chinese mind, and individualism has been understood merely as a way to claim individual rights and pursue personal interest. Overall, it is the party-state that actively manages the process of individualization and keeps the individual and the society under its shadow (Yan 2009b, 2010). Consequently, the individual turn of ethical discourse and moral practice has taken a rather different path and brought out quite a few new challenges in China.

First, the shift toward an individualistic ethics of rights and self-development stands in direct opposition to the outdated official ethics that calls for the complete submission of the individual to the party-state. It is difficult for the party-state to prescribe a different ethics without making serious political reforms; yet, in reality most people act in accordance with the newly emerged individualistic ethics. The disjunction between official and private ethics has resulted in a widespread trend toward cynicism, nihilism, and division of the moral self (Ci 1994; Wang 2002; see also the "divided self" discussions in the introduction and chapter 8 of this book).

Second, cynicism and nihilism, together with the weak development of social autonomy, prevent the development of public trust, one of the key elements for a healthy modern society (Giddens 1990: 79–124). Given that China is rapidly becoming a highly mobile and urbanized society where social interactions among strangers have replaced the in-group interactions among relatives and friends, how to build strong public trust stands out as an urgent and critical issue. Yet, the widespread immoral behaviors (including those illustrated earlier) and the continuing popularity of *guanxi* networks reveal only the importance of personal trust (see also Peng 2003). Moreover, the lack of public trust in post-Mao China has shown the alarming tendency to generate a disbelief in the good and in altruism, as shown in my research on the extortion of Good Samaritans and Jing Jun's insightful observation of the association between the government's doubts about altruism and the commercialization of blood donation (see his chapter in this volume).

Third, while most Chinese individuals have experienced an improvement in their living standard, all are aware of how rich some individuals have become. The flow of wealth is conspicuously visible among both individuals and government agencies, as is the widening disparity between rich and poor. How to deal with the sudden surge of wealth in particular and the irresistible trend of materialism in general poses another moral challenge to the Chinese individual and society. To a certain extent, China might be in a similar situation to what the Dutch individual and society faced in the seventeenth century: a challenge to come to terms with unprecedented wealth and to moralize materialism (see Schama 1987). Yet, unlike the Dutch case, most Chinese individuals are not equipped with a deeply rooted religion that emphasizes transcendent values. Nor do they reside in a world like modern Europe where the increasingly liberal context of political and moral philosophy has enabled the individual to enrich herself in both material and spiritual ways. Instead, the brutal attack on traditional culture, the collapse of Maoist morality, and the party-state's continuing suspicion about the autonomy of the individual and the independence of society seriously limit the possible sources by which the individual can reconstruct a new moral self to face today's unprecedented wealth and materialism. The increase of wealth per se cannot solve this moral issue; instead, it could and indeed has intensified the contradiction between the spiritual and the material and led to an increased sense of dissatisfaction and unhappiness amidst a booming economy (Brockmann et al. 2009).

The last challenge is the entanglement of old and new ethics, of collective and individualistic values, and of responsibility-centered and rights-centered moral practices in contemporary Chinese social life. Such an ethical entanglement actually derives from the entanglement of social conditions in China's quest for modernity. Chinese individuals have been allowed, and in some cases also pushed, by the party-state to pursue some goals in personal life that define industrial modernity in Europe and North America, such as the quest for a comfortable material life, accumulating wealth, searching for happiness, and seeking freedom and choice in private life. At the same time they also find themselves living and working in a postmodern environment where a fluid labour market, flexible employment, increasing personal risks and isolation, a culture of intimacy and self-expression, and a greater emphasis on individuality and self-reliance are created by the force of globalization. All of these things, we must not forget, have occurred in the context of the unchanging political authoritarianism of the Chinese party-state. In other words, the post-Mao society simultaneously demonstrates premodern, modern, and postmodern conditions, as does the changing moral landscape in both ethical discourse and moral practice. This double entanglement forces the Chinese individual into situations of difficult—and sometimes self-contradictory—moral reasoning and divided actions, which further animate the complexity of the changing moral landscape.

NOTES

1. The author would like to take the opportunity to express his gratitude to Joan Kleinman, who, while working closely with Arthur Kleinman, played a crucial role in his intellectual growth in general and his current research on moral changes in post-Mao China in particular. In addition, in connection with the writing for this volume during the last three years, he owes special thanks to Chen Yingfang, Li Tian, Lu Yang, Shen Yifei, Charles Stafford, James Watson, Xu Jilin, Zhang Letian, and all fellow authors of this volume for their advice, comments, and help.

2. The 2008 crisis of contaminated infant formula also reminded Chinese consumers of another milk crisis four years earlier. In 2004, dairy firms were found to be making fake infant formula out of flour that contained almost no protein and selling it in poor regions like Anhui Province in central China. This resulted in several dozen deaths and malnutrition among hundreds of babies.

3. The greatest negative impact of corruption for power holders in China is the collapse of the notion of rule by virtue *(de zhi)*, the core value that, historically, has legitimized rulers' claim to sovereignty. Rulers and officials, according to this Confucian dogma of political philosophy, must cultivate themselves as virtuous persons by enacting important values in their political careers. This may explain why the Chinese people reacted so strongly to the official corruption in the late 1980s, since much of the populace still believed at that time in the notion of rule by virtue. The intriguing point is that the current party leadership, under Hu Jintao, has picked up on this traditional notion as a way to combat corruption and increase the CCP's political legitimacy.

4. During the 2008 earthquake in Sichuan Province, hundreds of school buildings collapsed, causing the deaths of more than six thousand children. Most of these schools were built in the 1990s with inferior materials during a wave of expansion of educational facilities promoted by the state. A number of multifloor buildings were constructed without proper frames; in other cases, bamboo poles were used to replace steel wiring or steel frames. Parents who lost their children demanded from the government a full explanation for its decision to allow substandard schools to be built, but the government used various strategies, including providing statements from selected architects, to downplay the issue. This prevented angry parents from taking further public action. The 2008 case of contaminated infant formula created an unusually tense political crisis because the Chinese state had just improved its global image as a responsible member of the world community. It did this by effectively dealing with the catastrophe caused by the Sichuan earthquake in May and also by successfully hosting the Summer Olympics in August. The entire world was watching to see whether positive changes would take place in Chinese politics after the Olympics. It is clear that the production and distribution of hundreds of tons of contaminated milk powder would not have been possible without negligence and dereliction of duty on the part of a number of government agencies in charge of the safety and quality of dairy products, including the AQSIQ, the Bureau of Food and Drug Supervision, the Ministry of Health, and the Bureau of Industry and Commerce. Therefore, the moral and social implications of this food scandal were amplified by the timing of its occurrence.

5. The course of Cong Fei's life and death became the focus of public opinion in 2002, because some of the parents of the students whom he had supported requested money even after he became fatally ill. Although they knew that Cong was financially broke, they still urged him to go out and perform to earn more money to help their children. The lack of appreciation and aggressiveness on the part of these recipients of charitable assistance, known as *bi juan* in Chinese, constitutes another new phenomenon that parallels the development of private philanthropy in recent years. In 2007, for example, a number of people seeking help in Nanjing broke into the home of two individual philanthropists to demand monetary support after their charitable work had been reported in the media.

6. The thirteen volunteer villagers also went to Sichuan but did not receive as much media attention as the urban youth and private entrepreneurs, such as Han Han and Chen Guangbiao. Part of the reason for this was the semiofficial labeling of the "thirteen volunteer villagers" and the involvement of the local government in their second act of long-distance volunteerism, which in some respects is reminiscent of the organized volunteerism of *yiwu laodong*.

7. I am working on a book manuscript tentatively entitled *The Embarrassment of Virtues: The Individual and the Changing Moral Landscape in Post-Mao China*. The pri-

mary unit of analysis in this book is the Chinese individual, and the macro context is China's rushed quest for modernity under a strong and authoritarian state in the era of globalization. The central question is twofold: What are the impacts of the rise of the individual on the moral landscape of China, which is known to be a collective-oriented society? And, in turn, what are the impacts of the changing moral landscape on the Chinese moral self?

REFERENCES

Baker, W. 2005. *America's Crisis of Values: Reality and Perception*. Princeton, NJ: Princeton University Press.

Beck, U., and E. Beck-Gernsheim. 2002. *Individualization: Institutionalized Individualism and Its Social and Political Consequences*. London: Sage Publications.

Brockmann, H., J. Delhey, C. Welzel, and H. Yuan. 2009. "The China Puzzle: Falling Happiness in a Rising Economy. *Journal of Happiness Study* 10:387–405.

CCTV [Chinese Central Television Station]. 2004. *Shenghuo* [Life], June 17. For transcript see www.wanghai.net/article.aspx?articleid=3517. Accessed January 6, 2008.

Cha, A. E. 2008. "Young Volunteers in Quake Zone Ultimately Find a Modest Mission." *Washington Post*, May 22.

Chang, L. T. 2008. *Factory Girls: From Village to City in a Changing China*. New York: Spiegel & Grau.

Chen R. 2006. *Gonggong yishi yu Zhongguo wenhua* [Awareness of the Public and Chinese Culture]. Beijing: Xinxing chubanshe.

Ci, J. 1994. *Dialectic of the Chinese Revolution: From Utopianism to Hedonism*. Stanford, CA: Stanford University Press.

Davis, D. 2010. "Who Gets the House? Renegotiating Property Rights in Post-Socialist Urban China." *Modern China* 36, no. 5:463–492.

Davis, D., and H. Lu. 2003. "Talking about Property in the New Chinese Domestic Property Regime." In *The New Economic Sociology*, edited by F. Dobbin, 288–307. New York: Russell Sage Foundation.

Fan, M. 2008. "Chinese Open Wallets for Quake Aid." *Washington Post*. May 16.

Fei X. [1947] 1992. *From the Soil: The Foundations of Chinese Society*. Translated by G. G. Hamilton and Wang Zheng. Berkeley: University of California Press.

Giddens, A. 1990. *The Consequences of Modernity*. Stanford, CA: Stanford University Press.

Gong, T. 2006. "New Trends in China's Corruption: Change amid Continuity." In *China's Deep Reform: Domestic Politics in Transition*, edited by L. Dittmer and G. Liu, 451–469. Lanham, MD: Rowman & Littlefield.

Gries, P. H. 2004. *China's New Nationalism: Pride, Politics, and Diplomacy.* Berkeley: University of California Press.

Hansen, M. H., and C. Pang. 2008. "Me and My Family: Perceptions of Individual and Collective among Young Rural Chinese." *European Journal of East Asian Studies* 7, no. 1:75–99.

Hoffman, L. 2010. *Patriotic Professionalism in Urban China: Fostering Talent.* Philadelphia: Temple University Press.

Hooper, B. 2005. "The Consumer Citizen in Contemporary China." Working Paper no. 12, Center for East and South-East Asian Studies, Lund University, Sweden.

Jankowiak, W. 2004. "Market Reforms, Nationalism and the Expansion of Urban China's Moral Horizon." *Urban Anthropology* 33, nos. 2–3:167–210.

Ku, H. B. 2003. *Moral Politics in a South Chinese Village: Responsibility, Reciprocity, and Resistance.* Lanham: Rowman & Littlefield.

Lee, C. K. 2007. *Against the Law: Labor Protests in China's Rustbelt and Sunbelt.* Berkeley: University of California Press.

Li, M. 2010. "Collective Symbols and Individual Options: Life on a State Farm for Returned Overseas Chinese after Decollectivization." In *iChina: The Rise of the Individual in Modern Chinese Society,* edited by M. Hansen and R. Svarverud, 250–270. Copenhagen: NIAS Press.

Lipovetsky, G. 2005. *Hypermodern Times.* Translated by A. Brown. Cambridge: Polity Press.

Liu Q. 1988. "Cong 'wo bu xiangxin' dao 'yiwu suoyou': Xinshengdai wenhua de yanjiu beiwanglu" [From "I Do Not Believe" to "I Have Nothing": A Research Note on the Culture of a New Generation]. *Dangdai qingnian yanjiu* [Contemporary Youth Studies], no. 8:5–6.

Liu, X. 2000. *In One's Own Shadow: An Ethnographic Account of the Condition of Post-Reform Rural China.* Berkeley: University of California Press.

———. 2002. *The Otherness of Self: A Genealogy of the Self in Contemporary China.* Ann Arbor: University of Michigan Press.

Madsen, R. 1984. *Morality and Power in a Chinese Village.* Berkeley: University of California Press.

O'Brien, K. J., and L. Li. 2006. *Rightful Resistance in Rural China.* Cambridge: Cambridge University Press.

Oxfeld, E. 2004. " 'When You Drink Water, Think of Its Source': Morality, Status, and Reinvention in Rural Chinese Funerals." *Journal of Asian Studies* 63:961–90.

Peng S. 2003. "Wo ping shenme xinren ni?" [By What Should I Trust You?] In *Zhong-*

guo shehui zhong de xinren [Trust in Chinese Society], edited by Zheng Yefu and Peng Siqing, 292–301. Beijing: Zhongguo chengshi chubanshe.

Read, B. 2008. "Property Rights and Homeowner Activism in New Neighborhoods." In *Privatizing China: Socialism from Afar*, edited by Li Zhang and Aihwa Ong, 41–56. Ithaca, NY: Cornell University Press.

Rofel, L. 2007. *Desiring China: Experiments in Neoliberalism, Sexuality, and Public Culture*. Durham, NC: Duke University Press.

Rolandsen, U. M. H. 2008. "A Collective of Their Own: Young Volunteers at the Fringes of the Party Realm." *European Journal of East Asian Studies* 7, no. 1:101–129.

Schama, S. 1987. *The Embarrassment of Riches: An Interpretation of Dutch Culture in the Golden Age*. New York: Vintage Books.

Shen D. 2007. "Zhongguo nongcun chuxian lunli weiji" [Ethical Crisis Emerged in Rural China]. *Zhongguo pinglun* [China Review], no. 3.

Sun L. 2007. *Shouwei dixian: Zhuanxing shehui shenghuo de jichu zhixu* [Defending the Bottom Line: The Basic Order of Life in Transitional China]. Beijing: Shehui kexue wenxian chubanshe.

Wang, X. 2002. "The Post-Communist Personality: The Spectre of China's Capitalist Market Reforms." *China Journal*, no. 47:1–17.

Wu, X. 2007. *Jidang sanshinian: Zhongguo qiye 1978–2008* [The Vibrant Thirty Years: Enterprises in China, 1978–2008], vol. 1. Hangzhou: Zhongxin chubanshe and Zhejiang renmin chubanshe.

Xinhua News Agency. 2008. "Chinese Entrepreneur Moves Quake Debris." June 4.

Xu, L. 2002. *Searching for Life's Meaning: Changes and Tensions in the Worldviews of Chinese Youth in the 1980s*. Ann Arbor: University of Michigan Press.

Yan, Y. 1994. "Dislocation, Reposition and Restratification: Structural Changes in Chinese Society." In *China Review 1994*, edited by M. Brosseau and Lo Chi Kin, 15.1–24. Hong Kong: Chinese University Press.

———. 2003. *Private Life under Socialism: Love, Intimacy, and Family Change in a Chinese Village, 1949–1999*. Stanford, CA: Stanford University Press.

———. 2009a. "The Good Samaritan's New Trouble: A Study of the Changing Moral Landscape in Contemporary China." *Social Anthropology* 17, no. 1:9–24.

———. 2009b. *The Individualization of Chinese Society*. Oxford: Berg.

———. 2010. "The Chinese Path to Individualization." *British Journal of Sociology* 61, no. 3:490–513.

Zhang, L. 2010. *In Search of Paradise: Middle-Class Living in a Chinese Metropolis*. Ithaca, NY: Cornell University Press.

Zhang W. 2009. "Shu zui" [Redemption]. *Zhongguo qingnian bao* [China Youth Daily], February 18.

Zheng, T. 2009. *Red Lights: The Lives of Sex Workers in Postsocialist China.* Minneapolis: University of Minnesota Press.

Zhu L. 2006. *Bianqian zhi tong: Zhuanxinqi de shehui shifan yanjiu* [The Pain of Change: A Study of Social Anomie in China's Transition Period]. Beijing: Shehui wenxian chubanshe.

Zigon, J. 2008. *Morality: An Anthropological Perspective.* Oxford: Berg.

CHAPTER TWO · From Commodity of Death
to Gift of Life

Jing Jun

In this chapter, as a further illustration of the transformation in subjectivity and moral experience that *Deep China* explores, I focus on the relationship between an HIV/AIDS outbreak in China and the country's collection of human blood for medical purposes. First, I will discuss the warning of a British scholar from four decades ago about the perils of blood trade. Then, I will review how trade in blood and plasma in central China contributed to the spread of HIV among blood sellers and recipients in the 1990s. My central argument in this chapter is that the Chinese government made several disastrous policy decisions rooted in its assumption that Chinese cultural concepts concerning blood, health, and the human body posed an insurmountable barrier to voluntary blood donations. This perception resulted in a tacit acceptance of underground blood sales from the founding of the People's Republic in 1949 to the late 1980s. Because of a government ban on imported blood products after some were found to be contaminated with HIV, domestic pharmaceutical enterprises trying to make a handsome profit off of blood products contributed to a thriving blood and plasma market in the early 1990s. The drive for profit through blood and plasma laid the ground for the HIV/AIDS outbreak in central China, as human blood, a potential gift of life, was transformed into a commodity of death. By 1998, in response to the blood-driven epidemic, the country's first blood donation law was promulgated, marking the beginning of official decisions to rely on the combination of voluntarism and altruism as a safeguard of public health.

In writing this chapter, I relied on four sources of information. The first consists of the findings from my own research, including a four-village study I conducted in Henan Province in 2002, three research trips I made to Anhui Province from 2002 to 2005, and an AIDS patient oral history project that I led at Tsinghua University from 2003 to 2008. The second is a body of mostly unpublished writings by Chinese social activists working on AIDS, including Gao Yaojie (2005), Wan Yanhai (2003), Zhang Ke (2005), Liu Wei (2004), and He Aifang (2001). The third includes government documents, news articles, corporate reports, and industry reviews. The fourth consists of works by scholars, notably Richard Titmuss ([1970] 1997), Arthur Kleinman (1988), Shao Jing (2006), Kathleen Erwin (2006), and Ann Anagnost (2006).

A WARNING BY RICHARD TITMUSS

Richard Titmuss (1907–73) taught social policy at the London School of Economics and Political Science. His writings such as *Problems of Social Policy* (1950), *Essays on the Welfare State* (1958), and *Commitment to Welfare* (1968) established him as a leading voice on Britain's welfare policies in the post–World War II period. In 1970, Titmuss published *The Gift Relationship: From Human Blood to Social Policy*, a work that remains strikingly prescient in the concerns it raises about the commercialization of blood and other human tissues for medical usages.

The Gift Relationship criticizes those economists who reflexively take self-interest as the starting point of their analyses. In the afterword to a later edition, Julian Le Grand recalls: "I was one of a group of Ph.D. students in the United States at the time, studying economics and being fed an exclusive diet of neo-classical microeconomic theory. Suddenly this book appeared. It seemed to challenge all the received wisdom concerning the universal superiority of markets—or at least the wisdom as we were receiving it. We devoured it hungrily, reveling in its iconoclasm; even our mentors were impressed, no doubt partly because economics guru and Nobel-Laureate-to-be, Kenneth Arrow, gave it respectful attention in the lead review of the *New York Times*" (1997: 333).

The central argument of *The Gift Relationship* is that based on the experience of Britain, Japan, and the United States in the 1950s and 1960s, an unpaid donation system would produce a safer blood supply with less waste and lower cost than a market-based system. Each of these countries approached the issues of blood supply differently. Britain relied on unpaid donations, stemming from the practice during World War II. Japan had a free donation system before World War II and yet shifted to predominantly commercialized collections after the war. In the United States, paid and donated blood coexisted.

Titmuss found that the British system produced a larger supply of blood at lower cost and that the blood was less likely to be contaminated than in the United States or Japan. For example, hepatitis was a serious problem in Japan's blood supply in the 1960s. And in the United States, the rate of hepatitis contamination in the same period was four times higher than in Britain. These problems in Japan and the United States were, said Titmuss, direct consequences of commercialized blood. He argued that when blood is freely given, the donor is motivated by a wish to share his own good health with others (Titmuss 1997: 3–9, 124–126, 277–280). By contrast, he wrote, when blood is paid for, the provider is motivated primarily by financial gain and has incentives to downplay any ailments that might prevent him from making the sale. The possibility of contaminants entering the blood supply thus increases. The commercial models found in Japan and the United States, if widely adopted, Titmuss warned, could lead to deadly epidemics.

In 1981, the first AIDS case was reported in the United States. As the number of AIDS cases increased not only in the United States but also in other parts of the world, it became apparent that blood collected and used for the purpose of transfusion and making blood products was one of the epidemic's main drivers. From the mid-1980s to the mid-1990s, for example, thousands of people in the United States, Japan, Canada, and France contracted HIV through contaminated blood supplies (see Feldman and Bayer 1999; Keshavjee, Weiser, and Kleinman 2001). Hemophiliacs who had been using clotting Factor VIII to control their condition were particularly affected.[1] As time went on, it was estimated that 10 percent of all HIV cases could be traced to unsafe blood supplies (World Health Organization 2005). The warning by Titmuss about the threat to blood supplies has been borne out on a global scale.

THE CENTRAL CHINA AIDS EPIDEMIC

Safe blood transfusions and safe blood products all depend on safe blood collection procedures, which are hinge on how governments regulate blood supplies. In developed countries such as the United States, Canada, France, and Japan, the safety of blood supplies came to be ensured only in the mid-1990s, following a series of blood scandals that led to public investigations and even the removal of government officials from office. In many developing countries, in contrast, there is still no centrally organized blood bank. Patients who need blood are dependent on donations from family members. When the blood type of family members is not suitable, purchases from strangers have to be used (World Health Organization 2006).

Purchases from strangers create blood markets, and this was especially the case in China from the late 1940s to the late 1990s. The blood market in China was sustained in part by authorities' belief that a donation-based collection model would not generate sufficient levels of blood to meet medical needs. Authorities assumed that Chinese citizens would be reluctant to donate owing to a widely held set of beliefs—a cultural model—that construed blood as being central to the body's vitality; hence, any loss of blood would have negative health effects. Therefore, they concluded that Chinese citizens would be unwilling to imperil their health by contributing blood to the banking system without additional incentive, and relied on a combination of compulsion and financial compensation to provide that incentive. Authorities did not curb blood sales until 1998, when they promulgated the country's Blood Donation Law. This law was put into effect largely in response to an AIDS outbreak in central China, where a blood market had existed since the early twentieth century when blood transfusion technology was introduced by missionary hospitals, and then thrived in the early 1990s. The epicenter of the AIDS outbreak in central China, which affected seven adjacent provinces in total, was the province of Henan. The AIDS outbreak in Henan was discovered in 1995 when doctors in the Zhoukou District tested blood sellers living in rural areas and found the majority to be HIV positive. But this finding was suppressed by local officials out of embarrassment and fear of punishment by higher authorities (He 2001).

The blood market in Henan and six of its neighboring provinces involved both whole blood and plasma. Whole blood was bought exclusively for blood transfusions. Plasma, the liquid in which red blood cells are suspended, was bought to extract albumin, globulin, platelets, and coagulants (including Factor VIII). To separate the plasma from the blood cells, a high-speed centrifuge was used. It had twelve compartments, each containing two four-hundred-milliliter bags of blood. As it spun, the red cells, being heavier, were pulled down while the plasma flowed up. The merchants then reinjected the sellers with the unwanted red blood cells on the spot. However, this process was riddled with unsafe procedures: The blood was seldom tested. Needles and syringes were not sterilized. Above all, the blood from multiple sellers was pooled into one centrifuge and the extracted red cells were reinjected into many people (Gao 2005; Shao 2006). Thus, if one person had HIV, the virus was transmitted to all the others.[2]

Local officials were especially culpable for not intervening responsibly. There was no shortage of early warnings of hepatitis contamination in the whole blood being received by hospitals and in plasma received by pharmaceutical corporations. And yet, doctors who informed local authorities of the presence of hepatitis viruses in the blood supply were silenced by officials who not only feared punishment by higher government agencies but were also concerned that news of diseases associated with the blood trade would scare away Chinese and foreign investors (Anagnost 2006; Irwin 2006; Z. Yu 2005).

The unsafe blood-collecting procedures gave rise to HIV infections in three main groups by the mid-1990s: the patients who received blood transfusions, plasma sellers who received injections of pooled red blood cells, and hemophiliacs who received blood-clotting medication. Normally, in the production of blood products such as albumin, globulin, and blood platelets, the use of high temperature kills HIV. But the manufacturing of Factor VIII, a blood-clotting medicine, required at the time a lower temperature. Those who relied on regular transfusions of the clotting factor were especially vulnerable.

That the blood trade in central China boomed in the early 1990s had a lot to do with corporate interest. As late as 1990, China simply did not have the capability to produce albumin, globulin, platelets, or Factor VIII on a large scale (see, e.g., China's Hematological Products Market Annual Report 2004). Although China had begun producing some of these products in the 1960s, the scale was so small that plasma-based medications had to be imported. But the discovery of HIV in imported plasma products in the late 1980s prompted the Chinese government to impose a ban on imports. This created a tremendous business opportunity for domestic pharmaceutical companies. After several years of accumulating investment, importing equipment, and building blood collection networks, these companies started a major campaign to buy plasma. The campaign to make money out of human blood attracted thousands of individuals and hundreds of institutions. Most companies that entered the blood business were not registered for this purpose.

GIVING BLOOD VERSUS SELLING BLOOD

Regardless of how blood is obtained, its application to save lives developed out of several important scientific breakthroughs. In 1628, the English physician William Harvey published his work on the circulation of blood. This was followed by many experiments in Europe in transfusing blood between animals and between humans. The experiments on human blood transfusions experienced many failures, until the Austrian-born medical researcher Karl Landsteiner discovered the variation of blood types in 1901. Before this, blood transfusions usually entailed taking blood from one person and immediately injecting into another, without regard to incompatibility. A separate problem entailed storing blood for future use, since blood solidified so quickly. It was only in World War I that scientists found a solution by freezing the collected blood for storage, thus making possible the establishment of blood banks.

Western medical institutions and missionaries introduced blood-transfusion technology to China in the late nineteenth and early twentieth centuries. One of these institutions, the teaching hospital of Peking Union Medical College, has transfusion records dating to 1925, which show that payments for blood were the norm. By 1932, the hospital had employed 1,265 paid blood providers. Among these were regular blood sellers who were housed and fed by the hospital (Q. Wang 2002). During the Sino-Japanese War (1937–45), the Canadian surgeon Norman Bethune moved to north China to help the Communist resistance. Drawing on his experience in 1936–37 assisting the Republican fighters during the Spanish Civil War (1936–39), Bethune persuaded commanders in the Eighth Route Army (Ba Lu Jun) under the Communist leadership to establish a mobile blood bank which was sustained by four thousand civilian volunteers (Gordon 1974). During the Korean War (1950–53), the Chinese government launched a blood donation campaign to help treat wounded soldiers. College students were mobilized into blood donation teams, and the Communist Youth League (Gong Qing Tuan) designated donating blood as a political task (Li 2006).

But apart from these wartime exceptions, blood transfusions in China depended almost entirely on purchases from strangers and occasionally on donations by relatives. During the Cultural Revolution (1966–76), blood donations were organized by the Communist Party, with the Communist Youth League and the military playing a major role. Students and soldiers donated blood under political pressure or out of the realization that it was a demonstration of loyalty to the Party. Even during the Cultural Revolution, campus-based blood donations were paid for, although the payment was small (Liang 2007).

It was not until the late 1970s that the government called for free and voluntary blood donations. However, because the government was convinced that most Chinese citizens were afraid to donate blood and unwilling to give blood to strangers, it continued to rely on mobilization campaigns to generate the nominally free donations. In practice, urban work units that had been assigned an annual blood supply quota *(xian xue zhi biao)* often paid their employees to give blood.

One could argue that voluntary donations were not possible in the Maoist era when central authorities dictated so much of social life and individual contributions to the general welfare were seen as inescapable political obligations. Thus, the state made blood donations compulsory for individuals, whose donated blood was paid for by their work units. The blood collected from such work units went mostly to large urban hospitals. But the compulsory blood donations from soldiers, students, and members of urban work units during the Maoist era still fell short of the overall demand. Smaller urban hospitals and rural hospitals had to generate their own blood supplies, and so it is hardly surprising to learn that blood sales continued even under the Maoist command economy.

This underground market is well described in Yu Hua's novel *Chronicle of a Blood Merchant*, published in China in 1996 and in English in 2004. The story focuses on Xu Sanguan, a cart pusher at a rural silk factory who repeatedly sold blood throughout his life as a way of coping with financial difficulties. Xu curried favor with a blood chief *(xue tou)* so that he could sell blood more frequently than hospitals would normally allow. Over the course of four decades, Xu tried to overcome every family calamity he met with by selling his blood. The author, who was trained as a dentist and is the son of two doctors, recounts the tricks poor farmers employed in order to disguise their ill health and sell their blood as often as possible to earn money for food and medicine and to pay off debts.

By the early 1990s, the formerly underground blood market received the blessings and encouragement of local government agencies, as the striving of pharmaceutical corporations for profits became entwined with local officials' hopes of boosting their districts' economies. Central authorities made economic performance a criterion for promotion, which only fueled local officials' eagerness to generate money through the blood trade.

That the city of Zhumadian, in southern Henan Province, was to become a focus for some of the most horrific consequences of the blood trade is perhaps easy to comprehend. Zhumadian is encircled by rural areas characterized by severe poverty and environmental degradation. With some of the poorest farmers in China, these were ideal sites for pharmaceutical companies to procure blood at low cost. As China's domestic blood industry's need for supplies increased, the Zhumadian-centered blood market extended its reach to other parts of Henan and eventually to six nearby provinces.

The blood trade was abetted by official corruption. In early 1992, Liu Quanxi became the director of Henan's provincial department of health. He proposed a way for the department to make money by using the department's powers of inspection and approval to build networks for whole blood and plasma collection. Liu's brother-in-law oversaw a small army of blood contractors financed and even staffed by government-controlled institutions and businesses that had no obvious connection to public health, such as police departments, factories, and coal mines. In 1994, Liu visited the United States twice, trying to strike a deal with a pharmaceutical company to invest in Henan. According to Need a Hand, a Chinese nongovernmental organization that monitors the consequences of the Henan blood trade, when the American company detected HIV in three of the fifteen blood samples Liu delivered, the deal was called off (Need a Hand 2004).

The Chinese government began cracking down on the blood trade in Henan in 1995, but blood sales persisted elsewhere because donations could not meet demand. Recognizing this, the 1998 Blood Donation Law did not completely outlaw the blood trade for fear of a sudden shortage of blood supplies and the government continued to require urban work units to meet an annual blood quota. In 2004, the government admitted that 15 percent of the country's blood supplies still came through paid sources. Instead of shutting down the blood trade, the government emphasized a set of procedures to safeguard the blood supplies and stipulated that any violation of these procedures would be illegal. For instance, in October 2004 the Ministry of Health released information about ten illegal cases of blood collection (China News Service 2004). An examination of two of these cases sheds light on why and how the blood trade continued.

The first case involved the arrest of two farmers in Zhejiang Province. These farmers had an arrangement with several work units in the city of Shanghai to organize migrant workers from rural areas in order to help the work units meet their annual blood quotas. The work units paid the two farmers one thousand yuan for every four hundred milliliters of blood they helped obtain. The migrant workers who were recruited under this scheme passed themselves off to the collection centers as members of Shanghai work units by using counterfeit identification cards provided by blood merchants. The contractors paid the migrant workers 380 yuan for four hundred milliliters of blood. In this case, however, Shanghai municipal government's continued imposition of annual blood quotas was not questioned by the Ministry of Health. Nor was the continued reliance by work units to use cash incentives to meet blood quotas. Thus many work units continued to find it easier and cheaper to use blood contractors to meet their annual obligation rather than attempting to mobilize their own employees for donations.

The second case involved a blood center run by a pharmaceutical company in the city of Xi'an. In this case, 4,500 farmers were recruited to provide blood on a monthly basis. A serious degree of exploitation in monetary terms and especially the fact that some of these farmers had hepatitis made this case notorious once the ministry exposed it. The company had been willing to risk punishment for not screening the blood partly because the screening process could be complicated and partly because the potential for profit was huge. In 2003, the global market for plasma products was valued at US$25 billion (Jianda Pharmaceutical Group 2004). China became a new player in this market in the early 1990s during the boom of the central China blood trade. But in the 1980s, the Chinese government had to spend an average of US$1.2 million a year to import plasma-based medications, as the country at that time had little capacity to produce these medicines itself.

The opportunity for Chinese medical companies to profit from blood came with the discovery of HIV in imported blood products in 1984. That year, Dr. Zeng Yi, president of the Chinese Academy of Preventive Medicine and leader of Chinese researchers working on AIDS, reported that HIV had been detected in imported Factor VIII. In response, the Ministry of Health, the Ministry of Foreign Trade, and the Chinese Customs Bureau issued an urgent notice to prevent the import of contaminated blood products. In August, 1985, the China Customs Bureau simply banned the importation of plasma, albumin, globulin, platelets, and coagulants.

This government ban was a turning point for China's own pharmaceutical industry. Instantly, the Chinese plasma market became completely domestic with no overseas competition. Seven institutions under the Ministry of Health that specialized in blood research led the way in the rapid creation of China's own lucrative plasma industry, followed by military hospitals and pharmaceutical companies. As the potential for profits became even more apparent, investors with little experience in medicine also entered the plasma industry. At the grassroots level, local officials transferred public funds originally designated for other purposes into the blood market by establishing their own companies and building their own networks of blood contractors (He 2001). By the time the central government intervened in 1995 to discipline the plasma industry and clean up the blood market, 579 unregistered blood collection businesses were operating throughout China. Another 738 blood collection centers, although registered, were found to be using unsafe collecting practices. This means there were at least 1,300 enterprises nationwide that entered the blood trade.

TRADE AND AIDS

In a proposal the Chinese government submitted to the Global Fund in 2003, it said that the blood trade had extended to fifty-six rural counties in seven provinces, employing 1.5 million rural blood sellers. The government also estimated in this proposal for funding that two hundred and fifty thousand of these blood sellers had contracted HIV (Global Fund China Office 2003). One year later, the central office of the State Council AIDS Working Committee teamed up with the World Health Organization and the Joint United Nation Program on HIV/AIDS to issue "A Joint

Assessment of HIV/AIDS Prevention, Treatment and Care in China, 2004," which stated that in 2004 nearly one-quarter of all the people in China with HIV were blood sellers. In 2007, however, the Chinese government drastically revised this figure downward by declaring that only fifty-seven thousand people who were living with HIV had contracted the virus through the blood trade. The new and revised figure was recognized by the World Health Organization and UNAIDS (State Council AIDS Working Committee Office and UN Theme Group on AIDS in China 2007).

But according to Dr. Zhang Ke (2005), who worked in Henan Province for years tracking the spread of HIV, the number of people in Henan who sold blood and plasma in 1992 and 1993 alone is staggering: six hundred thousand sold whole blood and another two hundred and forty thousand sold plasma. He also found that the infection rate among plasma sellers in Henan was 30 percent. If this is correct, Henan would have at least seventy thousand blood sellers who had contracted HIV by 2005. And yet, following what purported to be a village-by-village survey, the Henan provincial government insisted in 2005 that there were only twenty-five thousand former blood sellers living with HIV/AIDS in the province. Leading AIDS experts in China continue to regard the Henan provincial government's figure as unrealistically low and believe that it contributed significantly to the Chinese central government's downward revision of infections via the blood trade.

But even if we accept the Chinese central government's new figure of fifty-seven thousand individuals infected with HIV through the blood trade, that number still constituted more than 8 percent of the country's official estimate of seven hundred thousand people living with HIV/AIDS between the end of 2006 and the end of 2007. It is also important to note that this number does not include those who have died. During the first wave of full-blown AIDS cases in rural China, in 2000 and 2001, HIV tests were not available at local hospitals. Only about four hundred patients from the rural provinces of Henan, Anhui, and Hebei who came to Beijing for treatment received HIV tests. In other words, those who had died of AIDS in rural China because of the blood trade but never had HIV tests were not included in the revised official estimate.

THE SUFFERING OF BLOOD SELLERS

What motivated Chinese farmers to sell blood? How was the central China blood trade organized? And what happened to the blood sellers and the recipients of tainted blood who were infected with HIV? The voice of the affected individuals provides some answers. In 2003, I initiated a research project at Tsinghua University collecting the oral histories of people living with HIV/AIDS. I was inspired in this by *The Illness Narratives* (Kleinman 1988), a work that deals with individuals' attempts to make sense of their illness. This work reminds us that personal narratives reveal far more than the disease as a medical problem; they are in fact personal interpretations of social suffering caused by illness and by the sociocultural environment in which illness takes place. Such interpretations are embedded in morality, the force of public opinion, and patterns of human understanding of illness and suffering typical of a given society or culture (see Kleinman 1988: 31–55). By 2006, the oral history project had accumulated interviews with fifty people who contracted HIV by all means—ranging from sex work and drug abuse to contaminated blood—and came from across China, including the provinces of Henan, Hubei, and Anhui as well the cities of Beijing, Wuhan, and Xi'an. But the majority were connected to the blood trade: one had received tainted Factor VIII, eleven had received blood transfusions, and eighteen had sold blood.[3]

Many of the narratives we have collected touch on government responsibility. The story told by a rural Anhui woman is a case in point. Age thirty when interviewed, she had begun selling blood at eighteen. At the time of the interview, her parents, her uncle, and her aunt all had died of AIDS. She described her experience of selling blood this way: "The government began to vigorously support the sales of blood in 1990 or 1991. In the special economic development zone in the city of Fuyang, a huge horizontal banner was raised to glorify selling blood. At first, many people went to sell blood at collection centers. But later, local blood contractors showed up at our doorsteps." This part of her story tells us that the city government of Fuyang approved the sale of blood by allowing a publicity drive to be launched. It also tells us that the blood trade was not short of its grassroots collaborators as the so-called blood contractors were not government officials or company staff but ordinary farmers and townspeople who used their local knowledge to find the poor and the needy who might be tempted to sell blood.

Her story also reveals a process of collecting blood that was mostly an act of cruelty. "It was a horrible experience. Drawing too much blood in too short a time made people's feet numb. Selling blood excessively made it difficult to draw more blood. So the blood contractors would hang people upside down by their feet against a wall to make the blood flow down into the arms. The most terrible years were 1993 and 1994, when the blood contractors brought high-speed spinners to the villages. We stretched out our arms, got fifty yuan each time, and were given something to eat and drink on the spot."

Above all, the combined force of rural poverty and official corruption was at play. As this woman put it,

> We sold blood because we were poor. Wang Huaizhong was in power at that time and the government under him demanded that each farmer pay an extra agricultural tax. If you failed to pay, the officials would take away your pigs, corn, and grain. So the harvest was only good enough for a basic living. But keeping children at school was expensive. Giving out gifts every year cost a family nearly ten thousand yuan. Building rooms to bring in a wife cost thirty thousand to forty thousand yuan. But if the government did not encourage blood selling, we would not have sold blood to make money.

In talking about her experience, she referred to Wang Huaizhong as someone responsible for depriving local farmers of a good life and encouraging them to sell blood. This Wang Huaizhong was the mayor of Fuyang in the early 1990s and later became deputy governor of Anhui Province. He was sentenced to death in 2003 for official corruption and abuse of power. Under his rein, official corruption was rampant in Fuyang and the city eventually became bankrupt. Using blood to generate local revenues was one of Wang's policies. By 2004, a year after Wang received his death sentence, an epidemiological survey was conducted in Fuyang and found that at least three thousand local farmers had acquired HIV through the blood trade.

The combination of dire poverty and corrupt officials was, however, only one of the many factors that laid the foundation of China's blood trade. For example, blood had long been bought and sold in places like Zhumadian and Fuyang, but the introduction of high-speed centrifuges to separate blood into red cells and plasma turned the process of blood collection into a highly dangerous one in rural China. Under the health ministry regulations, these machines, which local farmers called "high-speed spinners" *(kuaisu fenxue ji)*, could be operated only by properly trained health workers; they should not have fallen into the hands of local blood contractors. Furthermore, the widespread practice by the contractors of reinjecting the unwanted red blood cells back into the sellers, on the grounds that this enhanced donors' health and allowed them to give blood more frequently, was a special hazard as well.

We should also note what Chinese doctors describe as "clustered infections," which means that certain families in a community were infected while other families were not. According to older people I interviewed in Henan and Anhui, before the 1990s blood selling was a shameful matter and blood sellers were regarded as too lazy to make an honest living. Selling blood was then something done secretly that one would not brag about in front of other villagers. But by the late 1980s and early 1990s, the deepening of China's market reforms was accompanied by fierce competition in many rural communities to show off household wealth by building new houses, staging extravagant wedding banquets, and buying electronic goods like televisions and washing machines. Selling blood thus became a quick way to accumulate family wealth.

This is how local villagers described this new way of making money: "Stretch out your arm, blue veins stand out. Make a fist, get fifty yuan." But in village after village, it was predominantly the poor who sold blood as part of collective action. By that I mean the coming together of the poor to sell blood in order to avoid stigma. Since selling blood had been widely viewed as the behavior of the gluttonous and lazy *(haochi lanzuo)*, people averse to farm labor, the poor tried to justify their action by asserting that they were selling blood for reasons of patriotism and in the interest of their own health.

The first part of their justification was supported by local officials who described blood selling as "glorious" and set up companies themselves to collect blood. The second part of their justification found its echo in the blood contractors' story that repeatedly selling blood and injecting red cells back into the donor's body would lead to better health. Once blood sales were encased in these explanations, the number of sellers increased. And with the increasing number of blood sellers, the payment for each transaction fell.

A woman in Henan described the fluctuating blood price in these terms: "Our family had nothing valuable, not even enough food to feed three children. So my husband and I resorted to selling blood. Each time, we could make fifty yuan. Later on, however, many people tried to sell blood and we had to use personal connections to have our blood sold. The payment for each transaction dropped to thirty yuan, but local farmers continued to ride on a large horse-drawn cart every day to a nearby blood center. We used the blood money to buy a television and a sewing machine, and we also built a small three-room house." Soon in her village, HIV infections were clustered among those who once rode on the horse-drawn cart. Their immediate benefits were described by local villagers in the following popular saying: "Needle goes in with a fizz, and you get two bags of food and two kilograms of meat. Then you walk on the street to drink beer and eat preserved eggs."

There was another kind of infection cluster. Namely, some communities in a region were hit badly by the AIDS epidemic while other communities in the same region were not. Social geography—the distance between rural communities and blood centers as well as the state of the connecting roads—made the difference. A woman in Henan explained:

> My husband and I both have HIV because we sold blood. We sold blood more than thirty times from 1992 to 1995. At that time, we went to a hospital to sell blood and we had to stand in a long line to do so. Sometimes, we could not make the appointment to sell blood as there were too many people waiting to sell blood. By 2000, I felt sick, had a high fever, and lost strength throughout my body. In my birth village, there are also people who have become sick like me. But that village is farther away from the county seat and so there are fewer sick people there. You see, we had more people selling blood here because we had a hospital nearby where we learned about our blood types and we became so used to following one another to sell blood at the hospital.

This woman's contrast of her birth village and the village she married into points to the contribution of a hospital to the clustered HIV infections. It reminds me of what three researchers and I discovered in 2002 in Shangcai County, Henan Province.[4] In Shangcai that summer, we conducted a study of four villages badly affected by AIDS. We noticed that all four of these villages were located along a paved road connecting them to the local county seat. We asked county officials to give us a list of other villages that they thought were hard hit by AIDS. We checked the list against a local map and found that all the so-called AIDS villages *(Aizi cun)* were either near the county seat or had easy road access to the county seat. Further interviews revealed that a large blood collection center was located inside the county seat and blood collection vans were sent out seeking donors along a handful of paved roads all connected to the county seat. We realized that there were even poorer villages in Shangcai County, but they avoided the epidemic because they were far from the county seat or had not been served by the road system.

It was precisely because of the participation by state agencies such as county hospitals that local officials ignored the potential peril of buying and selling blood despite a series of warning signs. The earliest signal was a local antiepidemic station's discovery of malaria among Henan blood sellers in 1992. The next warning signal came with the discovery in 1994 of HIV in the plasma received by a biomedical research institution with an affiliated pharmaceutical company. The third warning signal came also in 1994 when a Shanghai biological research institute notified the Shangcai County Hospital that plasma it had collected and sent to Shanghai was contaminated with HIV.

In 1996, a doctor in Hekou Prefecture in Henan discovered, for the first time, that local blood sellers had contracted HIV. Unlike the previous incidents, this one pinpointed the location of an HIV-positive population. The doctor quickly reported her discovery to the Chinese Academy of Preventive Medicine, and was later forced by local officials to quit her job. In all these cases, bad news was covered up by local officials. But by 2001, the death rate in the AIDS epidemic in Henan had risen sharply, and *The New York Times* published an investigative report about the devastating impact of the blood market. Local officials in Henan immediately imposed a news blackout. By the summer of 2002, when our research team arrived in Shangcai, the reality of the devastation caused by AIDS had become impossible to cover up. Funerals and wailing for the fallen victims were daily events in local villages. In one village, I saw a ten-year-old girl holding the hand of her sick grandmother lying in bed. Upon inquiry, I learned that her parents and her grandfather had already died of AIDS. In another village, I heard from a village doctor who had graduated from a nursing school that the most profitable business in the village was a small workshop that produced paper offerings for the dead.

THE SUFFERING OF BLOOD RECIPIENTS

As discussed in the previous section, the blood trade in central China involved both whole blood and plasma. Whole blood was used for transfusions while plasma was used to manufacture a variety of blood products. Plasma collections primarily damaged the health of the sellers. In the case of contaminated whole blood, it was the receivers who were the victims.

This was especially so at rural hospitals and at smaller urban hospitals that were not supported by state-controlled blood banks and therefore had to find their own blood supplies. There are still no reliable statistics on how many people were infected by HIV via blood transfusions in central China or in the country as a whole. But the following court cases suggest that such infections are hardly rare.

In 2001, a Mr. Shen sued two hospitals, two blood centers, and a pharmacy in the city court of Wuxian, Jiangsu Province. Mr. Shen said that his wife underwent four blood transfusions in Wuxian Second Hospital during labor in 1989. Two years later, his wife and their daughter both tested positive for HIV. Mr. Shen won the lawsuit and compensation of thirteen million yuan because the court determined that the blood used in the transfusion came from a blood seller even though the hospital did not have a government permit to buy blood.

In 2004, a Ms. Li sued a local hospital in the intermediate court of Pingdingshan,

Henan Province. According to Ms. Li, she had received a blood transfusion during surgery at the hospital in 1994. When she developed a high fever in May 2004, she was given a blood test and found to be HIV positive. The court determined that the hospital bought the blood for the transfusion but did not have a government permit to do so. Ms. Li won compensation of ninety thousand yuan.

In 2005, a Ms. Sun sued the People's Hospital in the city of Gongyi, Henan Province. Ms. Sun said that she was given a blood transfusion during an abortion at the hospital in 1995. In 2003, she tested HIV positive. The court found the blood she received had come from an unidentified blood seller. Ms. Sun won compensation of ninety-eight thousand yuan as the court found that the hospital did not have a government permit to collect blood.

In 2006, a Mr. Li appeared in the city court of Yangzhou, Jiangsu Province. A migrant worker from Henan who had found a job in Yangzhou, Mr. Li said he wanted to sue a hospital in Zhumadian in Henan on behalf of his dead grandson. Mr. Li said that his grandson received a blood transfusion during treatment for a burn in 1996. Mr. Li claimed that his grandson died of AIDS in 2005 and that this was contracted from contaminated blood. Mr. Li lost his case, primarily because the court required a new HIV test as part of the evidence even though Mr. Li's grandson had died long before the trial.

Also in 2006, a group of sixteen people with HIV sued a hospital in Heilongjiang Province, claiming that the hospital had resorted to illegal blood collections and caused HIV infections among nineteen people working at the same state farm. The court found the hospital guilty of negligence but significantly reduced the compensation the victims demanded.

There have been many similar cases in China in the last decade. They point to a geographic distribution of tainted blood transfusions that goes well beyond central China. An important factor in the outcome of these lawsuits is whether the blood transfusion took place before 1995 or after, because the Chinese government shut down the blood trade in central China in 1995 and began a certification system for collecting blood for clinical use. But since many small hospitals were not supported by state-controlled blood banks, they secretly bought blood supplies without certification. They usually were found guilty in court.

Winning a lawsuit claiming a contaminated blood transfusion takes a long time, and hospitals are powerful local institutions with multiple layers of protection. Quite often, people with HIV are reluctant to go through the ordeal of a court case, fearing that they don't have enough evidence to win it. Adding to their physical suffering and their frustrations with the courts, AIDS carries a powerful stigma in China (see chapter 7 in this volume), even for those "innocent" victims who became infected by blood transfusions. In collecting the oral histories, we found that every individual we interviewed has been stigmatized and that the most powerful sources of stigma were the family and the work unit. One woman who was infected through a blood transfusion during surgery said:

> At first I thought AIDS would kill me quickly and I decided not to take any medication. I was persuaded by a good-hearted doctor to join an antiretroviral treatment program, but then my husband became fearful of my condition. He took our son away and arranged for him to live separated from me. And when my work unit heard about my illness, I was told not to come to work but could receive two hundred yuan a month. I insisted on going to work anyway, but the leader of my work unit then said that if I did so I would be fired.

A similar story was told by a forty-year-old nurse who was infected by a blood transfusion during labor:

> I am now receiving antiretroviral treatment and physically feeling quite well. But the pressure from within my family is unbearable. My mother-in-law is mentally ill and an alcoholic. She insults me by cursing me and saying that I have AIDS because I am a slut and got AIDS from men I slept with in the past. My husband was an honest and good man before. Since I became sick, he has avoided me. He will not touch things I have touched. He does not allow my child to eat fruit I have bought. I want a divorce and he says no, but he continues to avoid me. I don't dare bring the medical bills to the hospital where I work for reimbursement. I don't dare sue. If I do so, my colleagues will know I have HIV and I'll have no means of making a living any more.

This nurse dwelt upon the social aspects of her life as someone with HIV rather than her physical condition. She emphasized that she already knew that her condition would remain stable if she had access to antiretroviral medicine. But at home, she felt like a prisoner, and at work she constantly worried that her HIV-positive status would be exposed. She could, she said, win a handsome compensation if she sued the hospital responsible for her infection and yet she worried that the lawsuit would expose her identity and the compensation might not be enough to support her if she lost her job. When we asked how the hospital where she worked as a nurse would discriminate against people with HIV, she said medical professionals were as capable of fear and bias regarding AIDS as other people, and that the hospitals she was familiar with were quick to turn away people with AIDS seeking treatment for opportunistic infections.

During a training course for health reporters in 2005, I relayed what the nurse had said. One of the journalists decided to test the assertion that hospitals discriminated against AIDS patients. A few days before that year's International AIDS Day (December 1), this journalist pretended to be an HIV-positive person seeking treatment for flu. He went to six hospitals in Beijing and was told by each that he would have to go to a hospital specializing in treatment of AIDS. He tried to explain to the doctors that he was merely seeking treatment for flu, not trying to enter an antiretroviral treatment program. He was told, politely but firmly, that he must leave immediately. The journalist promptly published a story about his experience on International AIDS Day.

Unlike the situation in 2001, when the Chinese government first admitted that the country had a serious AIDS epidemic, discrimination by Chinese medical personnel in 2005 was no longer based on the fear-driven belief that doctors or nurses might be easily infected through contact with HIV-positive patients. Rather, the new fear was that a hospital providing treatment for people with HIV/AIDS might frighten away other patients and therefore hurt its revenues. This fear was at the core of an unspoken agreement between hospital administrators and ordinary health workers in turning such people away.

FLAWED JUDGMENTS

In dealing with the history of China's blood market and the consequences of its convergence with AIDS, one must confront the question of government responsibility in three quite different eras. In the first, which can be called the central planning era, the Chinese government tolerated an underground blood trade. In the second, the market reform era, the government gave the blood trade a green light to operate in the open. In the third, which can be characterized as the AIDS era, the government issued a law that favored free and voluntary donations but allowed compulsory, paid, and incentive-based donations to continue for fear of a sudden shortage of blood supplies. Apparently, the blood trade was treated very differently by government authorities over time. One could argue, however, that government decisions in all the three eras consistently embodied a mistrustful judgment of humanity in general and distrust of Chinese citizens in particular. As indicated in the previous section, this attitude was encased in a cultural model.

A cultural model is a set of shared beliefs, perceptions, expectations, and behavioral reference points in a given society about a given issue of collective concern. A cultural model can influence everyday social life as well as major political decisions. Chinese authorities consistently behaved in a manner suggesting a mistrust of the willingness of Chinese citizens to give blood voluntarily and especially to give blood to strangers. Part of this mistrust came from the reluctance of authorities themselves to give blood because they shared the cultural concepts regarding blood found among many ordinary Chinese.

The following two cases illustrate this point. In 1987, the Beijing Blood Bank and the Chinese Red Cross tried to persuade municipal officials and younger central government authorities to set an example for voluntary blood donations. Only two—Chen Haosu, deputy mayor of Beijing, and Chen Minchang, the minister of health—came forward to donate blood. Some local officials outside Beijing also tried to encourage voluntary blood donations. Wang Xilong, mayor of Xuzhou in Jiangsu Province, donated blood in 1988, and it was reported that his example was followed by five hundred officials in the city's government and Party organizations. But the Xuzhou case was an exception, not the norm among government officials at this time (Chen 1993: 18).

One could argue that even the passage of the 1998 blood donation law did not represent an entire breakthrough in official attitudes. The law was proposed by a top AIDS researcher who was a member of the National People's Congress. He warned fellow delegates of the perils of an AIDS epidemic, emphasizing that it could ruin the country's economic achievements in the market reform era. The law was finally passed after it was presented to the congress three times, and yet the Chinese government continued to allow paid, compulsory, and incentive-based blood donations. So, even when faced with the alarming news about AIDS within the country, the government failed to make a complete breakthrough in its attitude toward giving blood. This was a blunder that had its roots in cultural perceptions of blood that shaped expectations of the human willingness to do good deeds.

Institutional arrangements mattered a lot too. When individual voluntarism to perform good deeds was habitually regarded by political elites and ordinary people as a demonstration of loyalty to the Party in the central-planning era, donating blood was a political action, not simply altruism or voluntarism. Like any action demonstrating loyalty to a political institution, it expected reciprocity from the receiving institution. So, political activists were encouraged to donate blood in the name of voluntarism and yet they were rewarded with career promotions, holidays, extra pay, better jobs, and material incentives. College students would receive extra credit and better grades after donating blood. Student leaders who refused to give blood would be disciplined. Their willingness to give blood as required by the campus Communist Youth League would be taken into account during job assignments at graduation. In the market-reform era, political corruption, corporate greed, the government's focus on rapid economic growth, and the long-frustrated eagerness among the rural poor to make money all helped create an environment in which the blood trade thrived.

Now, I will push my discussion of the role of the cultural model further by revisiting Richard Titmuss. I opened this chapter by mentioning *The Gift Relationship,* in which Titmuss argued that the commercialization of blood is inferior to free donations for four reasons. First, it creates waste and is inefficient. Second, it encourages sloppy practices and leads to the contamination of blood supplies. Third, it exacerbates social inequality by the transfer of blood from the poor to the rich. Fourth, turning human blood into a commodity damages the moral fabric of a society by encouraging the expectation of profits and by creating justifications for exploitation.

Strictly speaking, the first three points can all be challenged. For example, if a blood market is well regulated and pays attention to cost and benefit, the problem of inefficiency and waste can be avoided. And if a blood market is grounded in fair competition, the poor could also profit from it by becoming receivers of paid blood at a reasonable cost. But the last point made by Titmuss about the damage to the moral fabric of a society remains salient. Let me explain.

Titmuss addressed the moral dimensions of giving blood by referring to anthropological literature on gift exchange and communal ethics in primitive societies. He paid special attention to the works of Marcel Mauss and Claude Lévi-Strauss, French scholars whose research on gift giving has remained influential among social anthropologists to this day. Mauss in particular believed that the evolution of humans could not have been possible without cooperation, and that the most common form of cooperation was the building of social networks of reciprocal relationships. Gift giving was the epitome of human reciprocity. For instance, a hunter who came back to camp with a wild boar would share the meat with other families who might not have caught anything recently. The next time this hunter's family was without meat, another family in the group would share their catch with his family and others. Without giving and sharing, this group could not survive. Human survival so depended on reciprocity that it served as a social contract as well as the moral foundation of primitive societies. According to Mauss, the gift was regarded as if it had a soul that perpetuated a continuous circle of gift giving. Because human survival hinged so heavily on giving, being human meant giving to other humans.

But Titmuss went far beyond this interpretation of gift giving. He realized that the gift of blood to other people in modern society does not necessarily involve the return of the gift, as the majority of unpaid blood donors will never have a blood transfusion. And this is exactly where Titmuss understood the spirit of gift exchange better than many anthropologists. Whereas the anthropological literature on gift exchange places an emphasis on reciprocity, Titmuss was fascinated by the idea that the very spirit of gift giving was the moral foundation of human society to begin with. This idea enabled him to see giving blood as something leading not to the return of blood, but to a greatly enhanced level of civility and altruism in a given society. This is why Titmuss used the term "gift of life" to characterize unpaid and voluntary blood donations. Altruism, the selfless concern for the welfare of others, is a virtue in many cultures and central to many religious traditions. It can be distinguished from a sense of duty. Altruism focuses on a motivation to help others or to do good without reward, while duty focuses on an obligation toward a specific individual, an organization, or an abstract concept (for example, patriotism). To Titmuss, the altruism behind donating blood is central to a society's morality.

Returning to our analysis of China's blood trade with this in mind, we can address in detail the question of whether the Chinese government misjudged its citizens' willingness to give blood without compulsion or compensation. In a document issued in 1978, the Ministry of Health appealed to the State Council to tighten up regulations on blood transfusions at hospitals. The ministry proposed the establishment of a voluntary blood donation system and various procedures for testing blood collections. The document was a reaction to a rapid increase in hepatitis infections in China, which contributed to a prevalence of more than 10 percent of Chinese carrying hepatitis, most commonly blood-borne hepatitis C. The proposal did not receive serious attention by the State Council, which was preoccupied by the political struggles that brought Deng Xiaoping to power.

For some years after this, the Ministry of Health set aside any appeal for free and voluntary blood donations. For example, in 1985 the ministry issued a document on the discovery of HIV in imported blood products. But the peril of the domestic blood trade was ignored, whereas the earlier appeal by the Ministry of Health for free and voluntary blood giving was not mentioned at all. In the 1998 blood donation law, free and voluntary blood donations finally received state endorsement but there was no mention of how the issue of paid blood should be handled. The law emphasized legal procedures for collecting blood and punishment of irregularities, but it did not say if paid blood should be discontinued.

The government's reluctance to push for a blood donation system based on voluntarism was culturally grounded in the longstanding Chinese belief that any loss of blood damages the vitality of the human body and can cause fatigue, poor appetite, or loss of sleep. Another widespread fear was that the needles used to draw blood might not be properly sterilized and might cause infections. A third concern involved public cynicism regarding the new market-based health system. With the withdrawal of state subsidies and the increasing reliance of hospitals on generating revenue, many Chinese assumed that blood donations would be used by hospitals to make money and therefore they should not donate blood anymore.

Faced with these obstacles and worried about a shortage of blood, Chinese legislators and policymakers allowed paid blood and compulsory donations to continue. Until 2004, urban work units were awarding blood donors with bonuses, extra holidays, Communist Party memberships, or career promotions. Also in 2004, for example, Beijing Normal University was forcing students to give blood or jeopardize their degrees or entry to postgraduate programs (Hu 2004). An especially outrageous case of compulsory blood donations involved three thousand residents of Chongqing who were dependent on the municipality's welfare provisions. They were told that if they refused to donate blood, they would be denied welfare payments (Sanjiu Health 2004a). China has yet to eliminate paid, compulsory, or incentive-based blood donations.

TURNING TO THE GIFT OF LIFE

Would voluntary blood donation be impossible to institute in China? This is actually a question about whether altruism and voluntarism can manifest themselves in a country where so many scholars bemoan what they see as a collapse in public morality. One way to answer the question is to examine the shifting sources of China's blood supply for clinical usage. Until 1998, China relied on compulsory and paid blood supplies. When the blood donation law was promulgated in 1998 and took effect in 1999, the country's blood supply was primarily from paid sources. What happened in the few years following the passage of the blood donation law was a marked increase of voluntary donations every year with the exception of 2003, when everyday life was interrupted by the SARS epidemic. Some statistics may demonstrate that voluntary donations are indeed winning. Specifically, the share of voluntary donations in the country's blood supply went up from only 5.5 percent in 1998 to 84 percent in 2005. Meanwhile, the share of compulsory donations to China's blood supply was 16.5 percent in 1998, increased dramatically to 37.5 percent in 2000, and then sharply declined to 11 percent in 2005. The steady increase of voluntary donations and the eventual decline of compulsory donations have the following implications. First, voluntary donations became the norm. Second, compulsory donations—although contributing to one-third of China's blood supply for three years following the passage of the blood donation law—became much less significant by 2005, only 11 percent of the total annual blood supply. Third, the drop of paid blood from 78 percent in 1998 to 5 percent in 2005 was so significant that one could finally say the country's blood trade was losing out.

With this encouraging change, the Chinese government put a greater emphasis on voluntary donations (Xinhua News Agency 2005; M. Wang and Liu, 2006). In Beijing, home to the country's leading hospitals, the city government decided in April 2006 to totally revoke its previous regulations on compulsory donations and made a complete shift to voluntary donations (China Youth Daily 2006).

In Shenzhen—a city of immigrants, no less—compulsory blood giving was replaced by a voluntary system before most cities in China. But in 1993, the city had only fifty-three voluntary blood donors. The number increased to 249 in 1994. Responding to a blood shortage, in 1995 the city government launched a major media effort to encourage free donations. That year, the city had more than six thousand voluntary donors, and by 2004, the city was easily meeting its blood needs (Sanjiu Health 2004b). In an interview I had in 2006, an official at Shenzhen's Center for Disease Control recalled that people panicked when the city's blood bank was exhausted in 1995. "But the next morning, hundreds of people who had watched the news on television showed up to donate blood before going to work. So the city made it a habit to call for blood donations on television whenever reserves were running low. Instead of panic and chaos, this city experienced the gradual growth of blood donation clubs organized by volunteers."

Other cities discovered the advantage of free and voluntary blood donations by accident. For example, during the SARS crisis of 2003, the city of Chengdu experienced a shortage of blood. As part of the effort to curb the spread of SARS, universities, military units, and other work units had imposed quarantine measures that made it difficult for the government to mobilize them for compulsory blood drives. So city officials ordered mobile blood-collecting stations to be set up at street corners and in front of department stores. They were surprised to see many people coming forward to donate blood, and even more surprised when their calculations at the end of 2003 showed that more than 70 percent of the city's monthly blood supply during the SARS crisis from April to July came from voluntary donations. So the city government also decided to shift entirely to voluntary donations (Cheng and Zhao, 2005).

The national statistics and the experiences in Beijing, Shenzhen, and Chengdu show that it is indeed possible for China to rely on voluntary donations to ensure a safe and adequate blood supply. There are two key factors involved here. The first is the government's recognition of ordinary citizens' capacity for altruism. The second is the use of innovative ways in promoting blood donations, through public health education programs, convenient sites for blood donations, and the use of celebrities as role models for giving blood. The first factor determines the second, as it involves how a state sees its citizens and how an existing cultural model can be modified by state power that is adapted to serve the purpose of social and cultural innovations without using coercive measures and top-down approaches.

The steady shift from paid and compulsory blood supplies to nonrenumerated and voluntary blood donations in the People's Republic during the last decade is a powerful example of the great potential among Chinese citizens to engage in voluntarism and perform acts of altruism. This kind of citizen action has proved to be crucial not only for the general supply of blood for medical usages but also during times of great crisis. A case in point was the Wenchuan earthquake on May 12, 2008, which killed close to seventy thousand people in Sichuan and Gansu provinces. In just ten days after the earthquake, six hundred thousand Chinese citizens rushed to hospitals to give blood. Many more ordinary people donated money to the relief effort. The monetary donations from nongovernment sources eventually amounted to a total of RMB 60 billion (US$9 billion), which put great pressures on the Chinese government to keep allocating more resources to the relief effort. This outpouring of public spirit in reaction to the Wenchuan earthquake formed a sharp contrast with the Tangshan earthquake in 1976 which killed more than two hundred and forty thousand people. One of the great tragedies of the Tangshan earthquake was the severe shortage of blood to save the wounded. Many people in Tangshang who died of injuries could have been saved if given a blood transfusion. By contrast, the rescue effort in Sichuan and Gansu in 2008 had an ample supply of blood, as thousands and thousands of donors stood by throughout China to provide the much needed blood. The rush to give blood in the Wenchuan case was consistent with a growing public spirit to view blood giving as a gift of life, a spirit that promises to override the longstanding Chinese cultural model regarding human blood and blood donations. One ramification of this spirit is that China does not lack citizens who are willing to go out of their way to help other people. By the same token, cultural traditions regarding blood are not an insurmountable barrier. Taken together, these things stand for the transformation in subjectivity and moral experience that *Deep China* discusses, and also illustrate why this transformation is important to the state and its processes of government. From a time when human blood was turned into a commodity of death, China has finally moved to embrace the notion of voluntary blood donations as a gift of life.

NOTES

1. In the United States, about ten thousand hemophiliacs and twelve thousand recipients of transfusions contracted HIV. In Japan, more than two thousand hemophiliacs were found to be HIV positive because they had used blood products imported from the United States. In Canada, 1,400 people got HIV through contaminated whole blood and plasma. In France, 1,783 hemophiliacs and more than six thousand recipients of blood transfusions got HIV (Asia Catalyst 2007).

2. The technology of plasmapheresis was introduced into China by a medical scientist named Liu Junxiang. He had worked with scientists at Harvard University to invent an easy-to-operate plasma separator. In 1987, the Ministry of Health in China adopted a handbook he wrote as a technical guide for collecting plasma in China. Sensitive to safety issues, Liu emphasized in his book the importance to test plasma donors for infectious diseases and procedures to avoid blood contamination. Unfortunately, both of these recommendations were ignored by many blood banks at the height of the plasma trade (Su Chunyan 2010: 101–116).

3. This oral history project has led to two PhD dissertations, one addressing the sales of blood in Henan Province and one concerned with HIV-related stigma. These oral histories were also used as teaching cases in six training workshops for Chinese medical workers and journalists to understand and find ways to deal with HIV-related stigma.

4. Local officials at the time tried to cover up the HIV epidemic in the county of Shangcai by forbidding researchers and journalists from visiting the local villages. We were able to visit four villages in Shangcai because we were commissioned by a national poverty alleviation agency operating under the Chinese State Council. A senior official at this agency thought that the sales of blood in Henan had a lot to do with rural poverty and therefore his agency had a special role to play in combating the HIV epidemic in Henan. Following our investigation in Shangcai, this national agency provided special funds to Shangcai to refurbish run-down village clinics.

REFERENCES

Allan, Ted, and Sydney Gordon. 1952. *The Scalpel, The Sword: The Story of Dr. Norman Bethune*. New York: Little, Brown.

Anagnost, Ann. 2006. "Strange Circulations: The Blood Economy in Rural China." *Economy and Society* 35, no. 4:509–529.

Asia Catalyst. 2007. "AIDS Blood Scandals: What China Can Learn from the World's Mistakes." Research report.

Chen Weiyuan. 1993. "Gongmin xianxue mianmian guan" [Various Aspects of Blood Donation by Citizens]. *Guoji rencai jiaoliu* [International Talent Exchange] no. 9:15–18.

Cheng Qinzhen and Zhao Xiaojia. 2005. "Dui sanzhong xianxue moshi de fenxi bijiao" [Comparative Analysis of Three Blood Donation Models]. *Xiandai linchuang yixue* [Journal of Modern Clinical Medicine] 31, no. 3:185–186.

China News Service [Zhongguo xinwen she]. 2004. "Weishengbu gongbu shida feifa caixue an chachu qingkuang" [Update by Ministry of Health in Handling Ten Serious Cases of Illegal Blood Collection]. Oct. 20.

China Youth Daily [Zhongguo qingnian bao]. 2006. "Beijing feizhi xingzheng xianxue zhibiao" [Beijing Abolishes Regulations on Government Organized Blood Donations]. March 3.

China's Hematological Products Market Annual Report [Zhongguo xueye shichang hangye diaoyan baogao]. 2004.

Erwin, Kathleen. 2006. "The Circulatory System: Blood Procurement, AIDS, and the Social Body in China." *Medical Anthropology Quarterly*, n.s., 20, no. 2:39–159.

Feldman, Eric. 2000. "Blood Justice: Courts, Conflict, and Compensation in Japan, France, and the United States." *Law and Society Review* 34, no. 3:651–701.

Feldman, Eric, and Ronald Bayer. 1999. *Blood Feuds: AIDS, Blood, and the Politics of Medical Disaster.* New York: Oxford University Press.

Gao Yaojie. 2005. *Zhongguo aizibing diaocha* [China AIDS Investigation]. Nanning: Guangxi Normal University Press.

Global Fund China Office. 2003. "Round 3 Proposal from China to the Global Fund."

He Aifang. 2001. "Jiekai Henan sheng chuanbo aizibing de xuejia" [To Open the Blood Sores of Henan AIDS Epidemic]. Unpublished manuscript.

Hu Zhentu. 2004. "Xuesheng xianxue de beihou zhushi" [Principal Instigator of Student Blood Donations]. *Zhongguo daxuesheng jiuye* [China University Students Career Guide] no. 21:10.

Jianda Pharmaceutical Group. 2004. "Xueyebing zhiliao shichang yuji zai 2008 nian jiangda 350 yi meiyuan" [Market for Treating Blood Diseases Set to Reach 35 Billion U.S. Dollars by 2008]. April 27.

Jing Jun and Heather Worth, eds. 2010. *HIV in China: Understanding the Social Aspects of the Pandemic.* Sydney: University of New South Wales Press.

Keshavjee, Salmaan, Sheri Weiser, and Arthur Kleinman. 2001. "Medicine Betrayed: Hemophilia Patients and HIV in the US." *Social Science and Medicine* 53, no. 8:1081–1094.

Kleinman, Arthur. 1988. *The Illness Narratives: Suffering, Healing, and the Human Condition.* New York: Basic Books.

Le Grand, Julian. 1997. "Afterword." In *The Gift Relationship: From Human Blood to*

Social Policy, rev. ed., edited by Ann Oakley and John Ashton, 333–341. New York: New Press.

Li Xianfu. 2006. "Kangmei yuanchao zhong de xianxue" [Donating Blood to Help Korea Fight against the American Invasion]. August 23. http://bbs.tiexue.net/post_2612460_1.html. Accessed February 22, 2011.

Liang Xiaomin. 2007. "Wenge goushu ji" [Purchasing Books in the Cultural Revolution]. *Dushu wenzhai* [Digests for Reading] no.11:58–62.

Liu Jun. 2005. "Zhongguo yiwu renyuan aizibing xiangguan taidu ji peixun xuqiu diaocha xianzhuang" [Attitudes about AIDS among Chinese Medical Professionals and Their Needs for Training]. *Zhongguo aizibing xingbing* [Chinese Journal of AIDS & STD] 11, no. 6:479–480.

Liu Wei. 2004. "Yiqi shuxue ganran aizibing peichang anli wenji" [Collected Writings on an AIDS Compensation Lawsuit]. Unpublished manuscript.

Meier, Barry. 1996. "Blood, Money and AIDS." *New York Times*, July 11.

Need a Hand [Xieshou Xingdong]. 2004. "Henan aizibing shijian de zong genzi" [Ultimate Source of Henan AIDS Incidents]. December 13. www.needahand.org/intro/aids/zxbd/1213–3.htm. Accessed February 22 2011.

Sanjiu Health. 2004a. "Sanqian dibao renyuan zao qiangzhi xianxue" [Three Thousand People Living on Welfare Benefits Experience Forcible Blood Donation]. Oct.14. www.39.net/HotSpecial/xianxue/huifang/68627.html. Accessed February 22, 2011.

―――. 2004b. "Quxiao jihua xianxue zhibao" [Abolish Planned Blood Quotas Now]. Oct. 15. www.39.net/HotSpecial/xianxue/baodao/68772.html. Accessed February 22, 2011.

Shao Jing. 2006. "Fluid Labor and Blood Money: The Economy of HIV/AIDS in Rural Central China." *Cultural Anthropology* 21, no. 4:535–569.

State Council AIDS Working Committee Office and UN Theme Group on AIDS in China. 2004. *Joint Assessment of HIV/AIDS Prevention, Treatment and Care in China.*

―――. 2007. *Joint Assessment of HIV/AIDS Prevention, Treatment and Care in China.*

Su Chunyan. 2010. "Red Oil: The Role of a Machine in the HIV Outbreak in Central China." In *HIV in China: Understanding the Social Aspects of the Pandemic*, edited by Jing Jun and Heather Worth, 101–116. Sydney: University of New South Wales Press.

Titmuss, Richard. 1950. *Problems of Social Policy*. London: H. M. Stationery Office.

―――. 1958. *Essays on the Welfare State*. London: Allen & Unwen.

―――. 1968. *Commitment to Welfare*. London: Allen & Unwen.

―――. [1970] 1997. *The Gift Relationship: From Human Blood to Social Policy*, rev. ed., edited by Ann Oakley and John Ashton. New York: New Press.

Wan Yanhai. 2003. "Henan aizibing de liuxing he yingxiang" [AIDS in Henan and the Epidemic's Impact]. Unpublished manuscript.

Wang Minghao and Liu Xin. 2006. "Linchuang yongxue 95.5% laizi wuchang xianxue" [95.5 Percent of Clinical Blood Supply Comes from Unpaid Donations]. *People's Daily*, March 6.

Wang Qiaoling. 2002. "Zhongguo xueye anquan wenti de zhidu fenxi" [Institutional Analyses of Blood Supply Safety in China]. MA thesis, Chinese People's University.

World Health Organization. 2005. "Blood Safety and Donation." Press release.

———. 2006. "World Blood Donation Day." Press release.

Xinhua News Agency. 2005. "Weishengbu jiang jianli wuchang xianxue gongshi jizhi sannian nei xiaomie youchang gongxue" [Ministry of Health Makes Notifications on Public Blood Donations in Effort to Eliminate Paid Blood]. February 6.

Yu Hua. 2004. *Chronicle of a Blood Merchant*. New York: Anchor.

Yu, Zhiyuan. 2005. "Dying for Growth: The Blood Trade Associated AIDS Crisis in Central China." PhD dissertation, Department of Sociology, University of Chicago.

Zhang Ke. 2005. "Henan aizibing wunian diaocha baogao" [Five Years of Study on AIDS in Henan]. Unpublished manuscript.

CHAPTER THREE· China's Sexual Revolution

Everett Yuehong Zhang

In October 2005, an academic event marked a turning point in the study of Chinese sexuality. During a conference organized by the Institute for Research on Sexuality and Gender at Renmin University of China in Beijing, participants raised the following question: what is the Chinese translation of the English term *sexuality?* This discussion was the result of the efforts of many Chinese scholars who, since the early 1980s, had attempted to distinguish between the English words *sex* and *sexuality* in Chinese translation (Peng 2005).

In fact, even *xing*, the Chinese word commonly used today to translate the English word *sex*, did not have the connotation of sex until the 1920s (Ruan 2005). It was not until the post-Mao reform that the need to differentiate *sexuality* from *sex* in translation emerged. During a lecture given in the 1980s, a professor at Beijing Medical College pointed out the lack of a Chinese translation of the term *sexuality* and tentatively suggested that *xing xing* might be a solution.

This choice of words did not gain currency, because the phrase was awkward and confusing and therefore failed to lend clarity or precision to the English term in translation. For example, in translating Foucault's *History of Sexuality, Xingxing shi* simply made no sense to Chinese readers; therefore, it was not used. Instead, each of the three Chinese translations of *History of Sexuality* carries a different title: *Xing jing-yan shi (History of Sexual Experience), Xing yishi shi (History of Sexual Awareness),* and *Xing shi (History of Sex)*. The failure of translators to forge a consensus around how best to render the title of Foucault's influential work exposes the difficulty of articulating the term *sexuality* in the Chinese language.

Scholars studying Chinese sexuality were under increasing pressure to figure this out simply because the rapid growth of interest in the topic created an urgent need for a precise term to describe its central concept. In the 1990s, Pan Suiming, a renowned sociologist specializing in Chinese sexuality, proposed *xing cunzai* (sexual existence), but he later withdrew it because it was easily confused with existentialism as well as being awkward (Peng 2005). Finally, during the 2005 Institute for Research on Gender and Sexuality conference, the problem was tentatively resolved by putting quotation marks around *"xing"* to refer to *sexuality*, as opposed to *xing* without quotations marks to refer to *sex*.

The significance of this choice goes beyond linguistics or an intellectual history of the emergence of gender and sexuality studies in China. The effort to find a proper Chinese term reflects increasing self-consciousness among Chinese of the need to define properly the domain of Chinese sexuality (from sensibility through identity to practices) in response to drastic transformations in Chinese subjectivity over the past few decades. It is a response to the need to find a proper place for the study of Chinese sexuality in the transnational scholarly field of the history and social study of sexuality. That said, the unsmooth process of finding a solution cautions against simply importing theoretical and historical models developed outside the Chinese context. On the one hand, over the past few decades a new experiential awareness of subjective sexual identity has emerged in China—so new that a proper Chinese term for describing it remains to be agreed upon. So fundamental is this change in sexual subjectivity, it might be said that a sexual revolution has taken place in China. On the other hand, despite the enormous flow across languages in the study of sexuality over the past decades, the difficulties scholars encountered in translating *sexuality* into Chinese caution against simplistic or reductive equations of the sexual revolution and emergent subjectivities in China with those recorded in Western history (e.g., the sexual revolution in the United States in the 1960s and 1970s). If no other expression than the phrase "sexual revolution" is accurate in capturing the enormousness of the changes in sexuality in China over the past decades, my view is that this sexual revolution has to be understood as "China's sexual revolution."

In this chapter, instead of offering a comprehensive account of China's sexual revolution, I will address two questions, primarily by making use of ethnographic accounts, including my own and other empirical studies. To contextualize these questions, I will first give an account of the important dimensions of this revolution. Then, I will inquire into its unique driving forces, in order to shed light on their implications for China's transforming social and cultural milieux. Finally, I will raise the question as to whether or not the increasing importance and prominence of sexual life in post-Mao China have contributed to the well-being and happiness of Chinese people. My focus, in keeping with the other chapters in *Deep China*, is on the lived experience of Chinese; in this instance, their sexual experience, which includes their desires and practices.

DESIRE JUSTIFIED ON ITS OWN TERMS

No one would deny that, overall, China is a "sexier" place than it was thirty years ago. Unlike in the Maoist period, girls no longer try to hide their figures in public. Even *luguzhuang*, a type of shorts that show a part of the buttocks, have started to become fashionable among some young women. In May 1979, *Popular Films (Dazhong dianying)*, a popular magazine, ran a back-cover photo of a scene from the movie *The Slipper and the Rose* in which Cinderella and the prince kiss. This editorial choice triggered outrage among some readers. In a letter to the magazine, one reader scolded: "I can't help but ask: What are you doing???... Does our socialist China most urgently need hugging and kissing? ... By doing this, you show your ill-intention, that is to utterly poison our young generation. Where do you want to lead our youth? ... I heard the masses of workers, peasants, and soldiers condemning you for being so shameless!" (Wen 1979). Now, in parks or even in city streets, open expressions of affection, such as kissing or embracing, no longer shock people as they might have three decades ago. As trite as it might seem, on Qixi (the seventh day of the seventh month of the lunar calendar, the so-called Chinese Valentine's Day, which, according to Chinese mythology, is the only time of the year when the legendary cowherding boy and weaving girl may cross the Magpie Bridge to meet) in 2008, a county in Sichuan Province even organized a challenge in which couples competed for the longest kiss.

Navigating the Internet, one can hardly encounter a popular Chinese website without seeing erotic images. Even on the website of the *People's Daily*, the mouthpiece of the Chinese Communist Party (CCP), images of near-nude female bodies pop up on the screen, only inches away from articles reporting on serious topics such as the relief efforts for the earthquake in Sichuan or the meeting of the Central Disciplinary Committee of the CCP. In the streets of some cities, it is common for men to be stopped by someone handing out colorful picture cards, no larger than a playing card, detailing sexual escort services and contact information. In almost any Chinese city or county seat accessible to travelers, a taxi driver can take you, without hesitation, to places where prostitutes are available. Sex workers often collaborate with hotel staff to solicit clients. Upon checking into a hotel room, it is not unusual to be bombarded with phone calls selling sex services under the name of massage: "Sir, do you want a massage?" One joke, which turns out to be a helpful tip, is that in order to stop such phone calls, it is necessary to say: "I already have someone massaging me right now!"

One day in 2006, on a website hosting the virtual board game *weiqi* (known in English as *go*), which I often visit from the United States, a click led me into the *shequ* (community) where a couple more clicks brought up information about girls who were selling sex. One of the girls claimed to be a college graduate from the city of Qingdao. She listed information about her body size, the prices of different sexual services she offered (e.g., one-time and overnight services were priced differently), her cell phone number, and QQ number (which enables instant message exchange via a popular website), an alleged webcam photo of herself, and the name of the street in Shanghai where she currently lived. She stated she did not prefer to *chutai* (go with the client to his place) but preferred to guide the client to her residency by phone once the client arrived at the cross street. I dialed the cell phone number she listed from the United States to see if the advertisement was legitimate. It was early morning in China. A girl picked up the phone and answered: "Hello, sir, do you want to come over?"

The Chinese landscape—in its material and virtual, as well as geographical and social dimensions—is increasingly a sexually charged space. A survey confirms that sexual desire is not going to corrupt society or youth as the condemnatory letter written in 1979 to the editors of *Popular Films* assumed. In the following section, I compare popular and political reactions to two erotic novellas, produced more than thirty years apart, to illustrate several dimensions of the expanding domain of Chinese sexuality.

FROM *THE HEART OF A YOUNG GIRL* TO *THE LEFT BEHIND LOVE LETTERS*

In the mid 1970s, an anonymously authored, hand-copied novel titled *The Heart of a Young Girl* was secretly circulated throughout middle school campuses. It was said that this novel contained explicit descriptions of sex. To many who knew of it, *The Heart of a Young Girl* represented danger. An investigation was launched on many middle school campuses to find out who had read it; those accused were socially stigmatized and punished by authorities. Punishment ranged from repudiation to detention. In some criminal cases, the novel was blamed for inducing crimes.

I didn't have the opportunity to read *The Heart of a Young Girl* until 1999, when a friend gave me a copy while I was conducting fieldwork in China. To me, the story of the book's purchase is as revealing as its contents are of the changes that social values regarding sexuality in China have undergone since the beginning of the reform era. My friend bought it from a book vendor in the Confucian Forest near the Confucian Temple in Shandong Province. He intended to purchase only a copy of *The Portable Analects*, but as he paid for it, the vendor asked him if he wanted something else, and produced a copy of *The Heart of a Young Girl* from underneath the counter.

The little book was simply printed out without a binding by a factory in Shenzhen and sold illegally. The narrative does indeed contain very graphic accounts of sexual organs and sexual intercourse. Manna, the young heroine, narrates in the first person her experience of falling in love with her cousin and having sexual intercourse with him. What's more, the overarching theme revolves around demonstrating how lust and sex could be sources of pleasure for women. However, this book is not the original *The Heart of a Young Girl* at all. According to those who read it, the original story is about a female middle school student's relationship with two young men. It follows her progression from having no sexual experience at all to her being trapped in a love triangle with two men, and ends with the deaths of her two lovers (Wang 2004). According to one account, the story in the original derived from a confession written by a young girl in prison, who became the model for the central character of the novel, and whose confession forced by the police became the source of the detailed description of sexual scenes (Li and Sun 2008). Even though far less erotic than its Shenzhen version, the original book's depiction of sexual contact stood in such stark contrast to the desexualized world of the Cultural Revolution that the text became a political threat. The novel's implication is that individual sexual desire, rather than collective enthusiasm for class struggle, could become one's passion, and this was probably feared to have the potential to awaken the reader's awareness of the lack of discursive and material space for articulating individual needs and desires. The forbidden nature of this novel and the criminalization of its readers reveal the logic of the late 1970s state—because lust endangered the foundation of the socialist country, it should be resolutely repressed.

Today, decades after *The Heart of a Young Girl* was first circulated, lust is no longer considered to be a danger to the foundation of the Chinese state, because what constitutes that foundation has largely changed from collective dedication to class struggle to private passion for financial profit; in this changed context, self-interested pursuits and the expression of personal desires are more acceptable in part because collectivism is no longer the dominant socioeconomic ethos. During the Cultural

Revolution, *xingyu* (sexual desire) was most often articulated euphemistically as *shengli xuyao* (biological need). Not until the free market reforms of the post-Maoist era could it be spoken of literally and explicitly without the connotation of being *diji xialiu* (low and base). Following the onset of these reforms, seeking sexual pleasure was no longer seen as an impediment to achieving success; rather, it became fused with success as both means and end. This confluence of individual financial aspiration and sexual desire is illustrated by business transactions known as *goudui*— a practice in which businessmen build relationships with government officials or industry associates by socializing with them in night clubs where sex workers stoke and even fulfill fantasies (E. Zhang 2001; Zheng 2009; Uretsky 2007; Osburg 2008). *Goudui* is one example of the lustful "heart" that has emerged out of the underground world into the public realm.

The best-known example of changing social attitudes regarding the open expression and fulfillment of sexual desire was the publication of *The Left Behind Love Letters (Yiqing Shu)* on the web in 2003. *The Left Behind Love Letters* began as a blog written by Muzi Mei, a magazine staff writer in her mid-twenties living in the city of Guangzhou. Muzi Mei used the blog to chronicle her sexual encounters with numerous male partners—both acquaintances whose telephone numbers she chose from the long list in her address book, as well as men she picked up in bars or other public settings. In her blog entries, Muzi Mei describes in detail the bodily sensations she felt during her exploratory sexual experiences, in an equally experimental writing style. For a time, *The Left Behind Love Letters* generated such a high volume of online traffic that Muzi Mei's website temporarily crashed. She later added an audio component to enhance the blog by uploading digitally recorded sounds of her sensual screaming during sex; once again, this generated so much interest that the site temporarily crashed. Popular opinion of her project was split: many commentators hated it, and many others loved it. To me, its fate says much about the transformation of sexuality in post-Mao China.

First, despite the negative responses from some outraged readers, Muzi Mei's writing continued to circulate among the Chinese public. Even though the state banned publication of her diaries in print media, it did not criminalize their online production or consumption. The motivation behind this decision is unclear, though several things may have contributed to the state's tolerance of Muzi Mei's blog. Compared to the numerous websites hosting erotic and pornographic materials that were then available, *The Left Behind Love Letters* was of some literary value. It also appealed to a huge number of netizens, including many white collar professionals with growing economic and political clout. Its popularity among this group of netizens, as well as the acrimonious debate it gave rise to among the broader Internet-browsing Chinese public, may have made the state realize that laws and regulations against personal lifestyle choices, following free-market reforms, were increasingly untenable owing to their growing incompatibility with the lived experience of ordinary Chinese.

Second, *The Left Behind Love Letters*, notorious for its positive depiction of the pursuit of sexual gratification, which critics condemned as unethical, nevertheless promoted strongly Muzi Mei's alternative ethical position: that seeking sexual pleasure was not shameful but a celebration of life, so long as the persons involved were willing participants in the encounter. This individualistic, self-deterministic position may have resonated with some of her readers' social and moral experiences as consumers in the brave new world of the free market. Indeed, their interest in, and implicit support of, Muzi Mei's pursuit of sexual gratification might reflect the development of the notion of "sexual citizenship" among some Chinese (Farrer 2007), meaning that sexuality was slowly but seemingly inexorably becoming part of what citizenship in China included. It also reveals the unique way in which the open expression and fulfillment of sexual desire has become increasingly permissible in China owing to the sexual revolution.

Muzi Mei still updates her blog occasionally, but cannot create as shocking an effect as she did in 2003. In this sense, it fulfilled the function of a writing left behind and dedicated to bygone love, like *qingchun yishu* (letters left behind from a bygone youth), as she claimed in its introduction. It is said that China's GDP has roughly doubled every five years since the beginning of the post-Mao reform era; every three months, many Chinese cities update their maps to account for urban development. In short, China has undergone—and continues to undergo—rapid change since economic reforms were first initiated, and anything that might have been shocking to ordinary Chinese five years ago is likely no longer shocking today. What's more, China has entered the age of digital erotica. The proliferation of pornographic websites has created space for an unprecedented national erotic gaze. The state never officially annulled its policy outlawing pornography, but in practice, it has grown hesitant to enforce that policy, where once it was not. This change is evident from its drastically different responses to *The Heart of a Young Girl* and *The Left Behind Love Letters*.

That erotica and pornography are easily accessible has become a de facto reality for many ordinary Chinese today. For most of the 1980s, watching pornography was a privilege of the few who had access to a VCR. This included governmental employees who had the opportunity to travel abroad to places where they could purchase VCRs and erotic videos, and public security officers who had access to pornography through confiscation. As opportunities to travel increased, media technologies (particularly digitalization) improved, and a transnational pornography production network flourished, access to pornography was "democratized." In an anthropological field trip I made in the mid-1990s, a friend of mine, who was quite immersed in writing, asked me to read *Lady Chatterley's Lover* by D. H. Lawrence aloud to him while simultaneously translating it into Chinese. This was a notoriously controversial novel that the U.S. Postal Service had prohibited from being mailed even in the 1950s. It took lawsuits to win the right to circulate it in the United States. I did not read this novel to my friend at the time; today, he no longer needs my assistance as translator, for a Chinese version was recently published.

In the 1990s, VCD (video compact diskette), the first generation of DVD technology, came into being and lowered the cost for watching movies. VCD show rooms spread from the cities, where they were first available, to rural areas. Many show rooms attracted audiences simply by advertising erotic or pornographic movies. At the turn of the millennium, as digital technology became more advanced and more affordable, and online entertainment became a national pastime, the consumption of pornography reached new record highs. A viewer of pornography could easily buy *dieẓi* (DVD discs) from vendors in the streets, or simply download pornography from the Internet. This technologically mediated, visualized form of sexual pleasure provided many, many people entry to a sensual world at a rapid speed not seen in the history of sexual liberation in the West (China had the largest population of netizens in the world in 2008).

In the late 1990s, vendors selling pornography often concealed their activity to protect themselves from becoming targets of police raids; for example, the book vendor who sold my friend a copy of *The Heart of a Young Girl* in the Confucian Forest used legal transactions as an opportunity to peddle banned books secretly. One day in 1999, a pregnant woman, perhaps in her third trimester, was selling illegal VCDs outside the Haidian Book City in Beijing, a complex which contains many bookstores. She approached passers-by with the discs, some of which were pirated copies of new movies. Those who expressed interest in purchasing pornography were asked to follow her into a back alley so that she could produce a collection of erotic and pornographic films she had tucked into the waistband of her pants, where they were hidden by her jacket and protruding belly. In this sense, perhaps she relied on the reproductive symbolism of her body to protect her from the accusation of being involved in the sex industry. But what she was really selling via the digital products could not be further from the business of having a baby.

During my fieldwork in Beijing, I ran into pregnant women selling pornography twice after this first encounter, and was unsure of how to interpret the relationship between the contrastive forms of sexuality—procreative and nonprocreative—they represented. It seems to me that in the 2000s there is no longer a need to feign an air of reproduction as in the 1990s. The consumption of pornography has become more common than ever. A student at a vocational school in Beijing said that he possessed a lot of *maopianr* ("uncut movies," meaning porn DVDs), which he stored in his drawer. His father had a collection of porn as well. "My father likes to watch them by himself in the night." He also said that he had gradually gotten into the habit of visiting pornographic websites and sometimes downloaded porn movies (Song 2006). Pan Suiming and his colleagues found in their survey that 43 percent of men and 19 percent of women between the ages of eighteen and sixty-one had watched pornography in 2006. Those with more education were more likely to watch than those who had less education. For example, 68.8 percent of college students had watched porn, in comparison with only 3.4 percent of those without any education. Similarly, those with higher incomes were more likely to watch pornography. What is also interesting is that across different groups of people—from CCP members to the religiously active—the percentage of pornographic viewing remains the same (Pan 2008). In broader terms, viewing sexual erotica has become an activity in which more than two-fifths of men and about one-fifth of women who are sexually active engage. These statistics give a sense of the extent to which Chinese citizens have embraced information technology and visual media as means and ends for personal sexual gratification.

As the consumption of pornography began to rise in China, the state took measures to prevent people from viewing it in Internet cafes by requiring owners to install software on their computers that restricted online browsing to government-sanctioned sites. However it has not prevented people from watching in their homes. Perhaps its relaxed regulation of individual consumption of pornographic media in private spaces reflected the state's primary concern with respect to regulating new IT-enabled personal freedoms: to prevent the use of technology as a social-networking and information-dissemination tool that could generate popular awareness of and support for political reform and social justice movements. These, it was feared, would challenge the state to cede some control over its citizens by granting them greater personal freedoms as inalienable political rights. Though viewing pornography constitutes an exercise of individual freedom and self-expression, it does so in a way that prefigures that freedom as a consumer choice rather than a political right, and transforms self-expression into the monologic demand for personal gratification, rather than a dialogic demand for social and/or political recognition of the legitimacy of one's subjective sense of self. Hence, because it constitutes an apolitical and privatized means by which to exercise choice and self-expression, the consumption of pornographic media arguably does not engender the civic consciousness and interpersonal networks that may be required to build powerful social and political reform movements for the democratization of China's political sphere. In fact, it may impede the emergence of such movements by isolating the act of self-expression and relegating it to the consumer realm. If the increasing size of China's pornographic media audience provides evidence that the country is undergoing a sexual revolution, then it does not necessarily follow that this revolution has or will be an impetus to political and social activism.

Inasmuch as it has not been politicized, in what sense has this growing desire for freedom to consume pornography generated new experiential dimensions of sexuality and sexual identity in China? In my fieldwork, a well-known urologist in Beijing in his seventies recalled that in the Maoist period and even early in the reform period he often gave consultations to married couples who could not successfully conceive because they did not know how to have sex. Nobody doubts the decline in the demand for such a consultation today, as the increased availability of erotica and pornography has played a big role in imparting some kind of sexual know-how (albeit often misleading and exaggerated). A number of middle-aged men recalled learning about the physical exigencies of sexual intercourse by reading the illicit *The Heart of a Young Girl* underneath their quilts by flashlight during the Cultural Revolution. As emphasized earlier, in contemporary China when people sit down to watch erotic DVDs at home, they do not need to worry about being targeted by the government as criminals; this, presumably, is one reason why more people are willing to view them. Thus, a growing percentage of adults in contemporary China have access to materials that teach them, in however limited a sense, how to develop their capacity to give and derive physical pleasure though sex acts.

"THE EPIDEMIC OF IMPOTENCE" AND THE RISE OF WOMEN'S DESIRE

When I started to do fieldwork on this topic in the 1990s, one could not help but notice the cultural phenomenon of "the epidemic of impotence" (Farquhar 2002; E. Zhang 2007b). Recent developments in the domains of clinical care, pharmaceutical marketing, and popular media seemed to support this characterization. For example, in the ten years prior to my arrival, a new clinical specialty had emerged for the treatment of impotence. This specialty, *nanke* (men's medicine) was beginning to emerge as a new field of clinical care as early as 1983, when the first *nanke* clinic was established in Hunan Province. From that point, clinics began to crop up across the country; today, it is a flourishing field. Many hospitals practicing traditional Chinese medicine host a *nanke* clinic, as do some biomedical hospitals. The development of *nanke* in clinical care was accompanied by the emergence of aggressive advertising campaigns for *zhuangyang* herbal tonics, a popular category of medicinal used to strengthen men's potency.[1] New brands of these herbal tonics— patent pills or liquids—appeared frequently on pharmacy shelves. In addition to these indicators of China's "impotence epidemic," a final indicator emerged in the realm of commercial entertainment, as radio talk shows and Internet forums dealing with the topics of sexuality and sex education began to feature discussions about treating impotence.

A commonsense explanation for the emergence of medical, commercial, and media practices organized around the treatment of impotence since early 1980s is that these things developed in response to a spike in the incidence of impotence in China that occurred around that time. Many of the people I interviewed during my fieldwork implicitly suggested this was the case by linking the impotence epidemic to the social and economic reforms of the post-Maoist era. A woman said, "Look, the whole scene of the commercials for *zhuangyang* herbal tonics in the street is making fun of men: you are impotent!" Many of the *nanke* doctors I spoke with suggested that free-market reforms had improved the standard of living for a considerable number of Chinese men, enabling them to make lifestyle choices that deleteriously affected their health. For example, some doctors noted that indulgence in high calorie and fatty foods, such as meat, sweets, fried foods, and so forth, had become more common in China. They surmised that the potential health effects of this change in diet, which include high blood pressure and diabetes, could contribute to the onset of impotence. Some psychologists offered an alternative interpretation: that male potency fluctuated as men felt more or less pressure to succeed in market competition.

But the emergence of an "impotence epidemic" in post-Mao China may not necessarily indicate that the number of cases of impotence is on the rise. Based on observation and interviews with patients, their spouses, or sexual partners, and doctors of *nanke* and urology in clinics in Beijing and Chengdu, my research shows that in the Maoist period not only was there no *nanke*, but also that within the general field of clinical medicine certain institutional practices and attitudes discouraged men from seeking treatment for impotence unless they did so in order to procreate (E. Zhang 2007b). In the post-Moa era, as medical practitioners and affiliates began to encourage men to seek treatment for impotence regardless of procreative intent, the increase in patients seeking medication for impotence could mean that more men than before were willing to seek treatment, rather than that more men were actually suffering from impotence.

How were impotent patients encouraged to see doctors? Some doctors who treated impotence were also frequent guest speakers on radio or television talk shows such as *Whispering, Whispering Tonight,* and *TV Clinic.* It was common for them to use their appearances to encourage men to take medication for impotence without suggesting that they do so for procreative ends; thereby, these doctors implicitly justified sexual desire on its own terms, and generated flows of patients from talk show audiences to their clinics. The movement from media virtuality to medical actuality constituted a prominent front of what Deleuze and Guattari called "desiring-production" in the social landscape of post-Mao China (E. Zhang, forthcoming) and facilitated the shift in public sentiment from an ethos repressive of sexual desire and pleasure-seeking to one that encouraged enjoyment of sex.

Changes to the standard way of reporting positive results for impotence medication testify to a widespread change in moral sentiment regarding the pursuit of sexual gratification. In the Maoist period, impregnation of the patient's wife must have followed treatment for impotence if the treatment was to be considered successful. In contrast, by the 1990s, the evidence for the effectiveness of impotence medication was a subsequent increase in "the satisfaction of [patients'] sexual life." Hence, sexual gratification became an acceptable reason to seek treatment for medical conditions that prevented persons from achieving it. This shift did not just occur among the young and the middle aged, but also among old people. *Nanke* doctors with whom I spoke during my fieldwork reported an increase in the upper limit to the age range of patients seeking medication for impotence. After one doctor reported, with an air of exuberance, that he had just seen an impotent patient who was seventy-nine years old, another doctor quickly retorted that he had treated an eighty-one-year-old man for impotence. Hence, satisfying sexual desire was no longer shameful by the 1990s; instead, it had become a valued end of sexual practice. It is no wonder, then, that more impotent men were willing to see doctors in post-Mao China.

One counterintuitive experiential change that contributed to the emergence of China's "impotence epidemic" is women's heightened awareness of their own sexual desires. One day, Beijing Television Station's program "Television Clinic" ran a show on sexual dysfunction that featured urologists answering callers' questions. Many callers were women who asked about their husbands' potency, signaling a strong desire to gain their own sexual pleasure. Equally revealing was the attention women callers paid to the issue of premature ejaculation. Many women confessed to Dr. Ma Xiaonian, an expert on sexual dysfunction, that they had not known about premature ejaculation until they heard about it from him on his radio talk show. Thus, the heightened concern over, and discussion of, impotence and sexual satisfaction in popular medicine and commercial media in the 1990s provided Chinese women with new ways of reflecting on and elaborating their own sexual desires; in turn, women's participation in this discussion helped to sustain it.

Hence, it might be said that the discourses and practices organized around the treatment of impotence and other forms of sexual dysfunction in medicine and popular media contributed to the construction of personal gratification as a legitimate object of sexual intercourse in post-Mao China and enabled new intersubjective modes of experiencing and expressing sexual desire for both men and women. That said, it would be mistaken to conclude that these changes have simply increased individuals' sexual pleasure; they also may have led to the establishment of excessive, unrealistic, or rigid norms for individual sexual desire and practice that, ironically, could curtail pleasure for some (Farquhar 2002). This rigid normalization or excessive sexualization of social bodies may be fostered by the formation of new kinds of expertise—for example, such as that claimed by sexologists—that bolster "normal" desires and expectations for sexual pleasure. However, new discourses of sexual expertise, such as those associated with *nanke* and talk-radio doctors, did benefit people who were groping in the dark. My fieldwork experience shows that many people—men as well as women—who were suffering from real problems in sexual life greatly appreciated the medical help they received from doctors like Dr. Ma. Some women welcomed the opportunity for consultation with him, especially because they could not turn to the specialty of obstetrics and gynecology, which deals only with the reproductive body (E. Zhang, forthcoming). Similarly, though masturbation may have always been common, many men were plagued by a resulting sense of guilt. Dr. Ma was one of the pioneers in advocating the "reversal of the verdict on masturbation" in the media, which helped alleviate men of the psychological and moral burden associated with it. In the final analysis, the heightened attention to premature ejaculation was an increase in women's awareness of their own potential and entitlement to have orgasms. It went hand-in-hand with increased curiosity about bodily processes, including how to achieve orgasm.

A study conducted by Pan Suiming and colleagues (2008) of changing sexual education levels among Chinese men and women suggests that women did indeed grow more knowledgeable about the physiological basics of sexual pleasure. Pan et al. found that more people in 2006 than in 2000 had knowledge of the male orgasm, female orgasm, and location of the clitoris, which are considered to be the three most important indicators of the level of sophistication of a person's sexual knowledge. Notably, the increase in knowledge among women during this period was greater than among men. In 2006, 91.6 percent of women were familiar in some way with the concept of the female orgasm, up 16.8 percent from 2000; men's knowledge level remained almost the same. Women who knew the exact location of the clitoris increased from 22 to 32 percent, and women who roughly knew the location of the clitoris increased from 39 to 50 percent. On average, women's increase in knowledge about the clitoris was four times greater than men's (Pan et al. 2008). This change is even more pronounced when situated within a broader historical perspective: For example, during my field research, a doctor recalled to me how big the contrast was between the present day and the 1960s when he was a medical school student intern. On medical rounds, while examining a woman, he was asked by a senior doctor not to touch the clitoris. He did not know what that meant until many years later. Medical school only taught students about the reproductive body, and there was very limited access to sexual knowledge even about one's own bodily experience at that time, leaving the other part of the body—the sexual body—unaccounted for.

In the early 1990s, sex shops selling vibrators, oils, lubricants, and other related items started to emerge (McMillan 2006). In 1995, when I was conducting fieldwork in a sex shop located in the bustling Yu Yuan shopping area in Shanghai, the vibrators standing on the shelves presented a rather grotesque scene. I was the only customer in the shop when an employee dressed in a white medical coat approached me. Nevertheless, she spoke in hushed tones: "Do you need anything?" Her tone was calm and discreet, as if she wanted to assure me that I should not feel embarrassed making an inquiry about the items on display. Her discretion spoke to the newness of sex shops at that time, and their slightly transgressive reputation. By the late 1990s, such shops were commonplace: more than two hundred sex shops had opened in Beijing alone. Unlike the United States, where such shops are often located in rundown areas, some of the shops in China opened right on the busiest commercial streets. The transgressiveness and discretion associated with them were gone. They had been replaced by open curiosity on the part of customers, and on the part of store clerks, the typical eagerness of salespeople in other kinds of shops.

The sex shops I visited reinforced the notion of sexual pleasure in that most of their products were designed to enhance gratification; the few products that did allude to the reproductive end of sexual intercourse—all prophylactics—construed reproduction as something to be prevented. Most products sold in them, moreover, were designed specifically to enhance women's pleasure during intercourse. That said, the profusion of women's products in sex shops does not necessarily imply that they were marketed in response to increasing sensitivity to women's desires or to meet women's demand for sexual gratification. In The Adam and Eve Healthcare Center, the first shop of this type in China (it opened in 1993) and probably the largest at the time of my fieldwork, the most prominent display featured vibrators. Despite the fact that vibrators were presumably designed to enhance women's pleasure, according to my observation, shop customers were predominantly male. A man who had worked in such a shop for years told me that this observation was not unusual: men were more likely than women to purchase vibrators—either for a female lover, spouse, or spouses of superiors. The relative absence of women from this kind of public space sheds light on the gendered landscape of post-Mao China. It suggests that the sexualized female body, as represented in the consumer sex products market, may not necessarily resonate with women's desires and sexual self-fashioning, though perhaps women's sense of shame prevented them from articulating their desire. The most shocking articulation of sexual desire has come from women such as Muzi Mei; yet, more often, in the public domain, it is men who articulate demands for sexual pleasure on behalf of women. Hence, sex shops are places where both the profusion of desire—in the form of products designed for the sexualized female body—and the poverty of desire—indicated by the relative absence of female customers—are displayed.

AN INCREASING TOLERANCE OF HOMOSEXUALITY

Homosexuality was mostly repressed during the Maoist period. As late as the 1980s, homosexuals were reportedly rounded up by the police in their gathering places such as public toilets or parks, and were often charged with "hooliganism." There was no law against homosexuality in China, but the crime of hooliganism offered legal means to stigmatize and punish homosexual behavior. People were disciplined for homosexual behaviors in work units. In addition, homosexuality was pathologized through biomedicine—psychiatry classified it as a mental disorder.

The repression of homosexuality through state and biomedical institutions began to change in the 1990s, and the rate of that change increased in the new millennium. In 1998, a taxi driver was likely unable to tell you where to go if you wanted to meet homosexuals, but on the Internet a map of gay bar locations in major cities was already available. In my fieldwork, I went to several such bars in Shanghai and Beijing, gaining an extraordinary sense of entering a different world. Several gay men in one bar were drinking; a few of them were eager to talk and others reserved—

not all that different from other bars. Only when a pair of gay men started to dance with their hands around the other's waist was the underground atmosphere of "otherness" brought into relief. After talking to two travelers—one from Hong Kong and another from Japan—I talked to a twenty-six-year-old gay man, a native Shanghainese. Subdued, he said that he had known that he was gay for some time, because in retrospect he had fallen in love with his physical education teacher when he was in elementary school. However, he did not consciously recognize this orientation until high school. When I spoke to him, he had not "come out," but thought people were able to infer that he was homosexual. He used to work for a hotel and now spent time learning English. He lived with his parents, who were putting pressure on him to find a girl and get married. Because they could not accept their son's homosexuality, he simply dodged them by saying that he was not yet ready to be married. At the same time, he was looking for an older gay partner. He believed that a conflict with his parents would inevitably erupt in the end. Solutions vary from person to person in response to situations similar to the one this man described to me. Some homosexuals with whom I spoke chose to go abroad with their foreign lovers. A second group married, but saw gay friends secretly; yet a third group lived openly as gay or lesbian (Engebretsen 2009; Rofel 2007). Each solution engendered different joys and difficulties.

Because of his own sense of vulnerability, this gay man perhaps underestimated the hiddenness of his identity. A male friend went with me one day to the bar described in the preceding paragraph and acknowledged that he had not realized his blindness to such a different world until then. Afterward, he related his experience at the gay bar to some of his colleagues, and was surprised to be told by those who were better informed that several of their coworkers seemed to be gay. In general, homosexuals seemed to be more tolerated in culturally and educationally refined institutions. A hostess and anchor of the show "Half the Sky" on China Central Television said that in professional circles, people liked to spread word about who was gay and who was a lesbian. She said, "It was fashionable to do this" (Kim 1999). A female journalist told me that once she was misidentified as a lesbian by a famous female singer she was interviewing. The singer simply told her: "I am really very sympathetic with you homosexuals."

However, homosexuals in China aren't necessarily seeking sympathetic understanding from heterosexuals. One gay man told me, "We don't need sympathy." He said this as we dined with HIV/AIDS activists in Beijing in 2000. This statement reflected both the man's confidence in the broad ethicality of the principle of sexual equality animating his activism and his contempt for any condescension from voyeuristic sympathizers who would reinforce the "otherness" of the gay and lesbian community. I had been invited to the dinner by a sexologist who wanted to introduce me to a new circle of friends. The dinner was arranged by Zhang Beichuan, a professor of medicine from Qingdao, Shandong Province. Zhang Beichuan was also the editor of *The Friends*, a bimonthly *tongzhi* (a communist term meaning "comrades" that was appropriated by the homosexual community) publication funded by the Ford Foundation to raise the awareness of HIV/AIDS in China. *The Friends* celebrated its tenth anniversary in 2008.

Things have changed a lot since *The Friends* was first circulated in 1998 as a small newsletter; it was probably the only publication for homosexuals in China at the time of its inception. Ten years later, numerous websites devoted to homosexuals were operating in China, where, according to one study, thirty-nine to fifty million individuals are or will become gays or lesbians (B. Zhang 2004). Awareness of the rights of homosexuals has been rising among the young educated population, and the effects of this can be seen in mainstream public spaces. When Fudan University began an undergraduate course on homosexuality in 2005, the classroom was packed. When a reporter asked the course's professor whether she would be supportive if her daughter chose to be a lesbian, the professor answered affirmatively and without hesitation: "I [would] help her find a partner if she [had] difficulty" (Chengshi ribao 2005).

Despite the growing acknowledgement and acceptance of homosexuality in some parts of Chinese society, including popular discourse, the long-term effects of stigmatization and repression during the Maoist period continue to influence homosexuals' experiences. Indeed, even during dinner with the HIV/AIDS activist group, I was reminded that the gay community is still, to some degree, an underground community. I gave my name card to every person present at the dinner, yet received no name cards in return from gay attendees. Also, most gay attendees used a nickname or pseudonym, and did not reveal their work units' or companies' names when, at the dinner table, we went around introducing ourselves. I realized that when the worlds of sexuality and political activism intersected, the gay community felt strong pressure to protect itself. Even though the Chinese state dropped the crime of "hooliganism" from the Criminal Code in 1997 and the authoritative *Diagnostic Manual of Psychiatric Disorders* dropped homosexuality from the list of mental disorders in 2001 (but still lists it as contributing to symptoms of problematic self-identity), in everyday life there is still a very long way to go before gays can live openly without the risk of being labeled "other."

The state does not interfere with the gay and lesbian world, even though the police in some cities still launch sweeps of homosexual hangouts popular among those same-sex couples who cannot afford to go to gay bars. Yet, when a confrontation between gay men and the police occurred recently during such a sweep in People's Park in Guangzhou, those who eventually retreated were not the gay men, but the police (Foreman 2009). Popular sentiment has become more tolerant of homosexuality, but tolerance does not mean full understanding and acceptance. More importantly, the Chinese state is far from realizing equal citizen's rights on specific issues such as marriage, housing, and so on. The gap between the world of gays and lesbians and the heterosexual world remains wide. In 1998, the owner of a gay bar in Beijing told me that the police station was nearby, but that officers did not interfere with his business. "We are on good terms, and once in a while we invite them to have dinner," the owner said. Later that evening, I walked out of the bar, along the alley, and finally into the main street, where I got into a taxi. The taxi driver said that he often came here to pick up customers. He did not know who they were and only guessed that inside the alley there might be a bowling place. I told him there was a gay bar. The driver made a grimace and said, "Huh, what a lack of fun! Isn't the affair between men and women the thing that matters in life?!" These two anecdotes exemplify the growing tolerance and persistent lack of understanding that are becoming more typical of attitudes toward homosexual lifestyles in local government and heteronormative society. Few people in the mainstream heterosexual world know that China's gays and lesbians celebrated the first national gay and lesbian festival on December 16, 2005. Since the beginning of the millennium, Li Yinhe, a scholar of Chinese sexuality and gender from the Chinese Academy of Social Sciences, has continued to submit a proposal for legalizing same-sex marriage to the People's Congress, and plans to carry on this struggle until the proposal passes. How far Li's movement can go and how soon the goal will be reached in legal terms remain to be seen; obstacles to its success may remain embedded in popular moral sentiments regarding homosexuality among a broad swath of Chinese society. For example, as the chapter by Guo and Kleinman in this volume reveals, stigma in families of gays with HIV/AIDS is still strong.

On February 14, 2009, dressed in wedding attire, two couples had wedding photos taken under Zhengyang Gate in the bustling Qianmen area near Tiananmen Square in Beijing. This is a common scene on Valentine's Day in contemporary Beijing. What distinguished these two couples was that they were same-sex lovers—one gay couple and one lesbian couple. It was cold outdoors, but the smiles on their faces seemed capable of thawing ice. This was a courageous "coming out" near the symbolic center of the Chinese nation. Judging from the photos, the passers-by looking on did not seem any uneasier with the couples than the taxi driver mentioned earlier. Things indeed have changed. This scene resonates with the irreversible change in Chinese sexuality and symbolizes a gradual routinization of sexual lifestyles and practices that would in the past have been morally shocking and even unacceptable.

"ONE BIG RED LIGHT ZONE"

The description of sex workers at the beginning of this chapter may leave the impression that China is "one big red light zone." There are two ways to evaluate this impression. It is true that the illegal sex industry has flourished in post-Mao China. By contrast, the Chinese socialist state claimed in early 1964 to have successfully eradicated prostitution and venereal disease. Nevertheless, regardless of whether sex work was ever completely eradicated in Maoist China, few would contest the observation that it burgeoned as consumer culture rose in the 1990s and that it shows no sign of disappearing from contemporary Chinese society. Moreover, venereal disease rates have become epidemic.

However, the characterization of contemporary China as a "big red light zone" is reminiscent of the tendency to frame the social problems that take root in the sex industry in moralistic terms. A simplified moralistic analysis primarily condemns prostitution as a social vice, and those involved in sex work are marked as vicious or immoral persons. Hence, those who engage in this sort of analysis tend to disregard the social, political, and economic conditions that foster the efflorescence of sex work; rather, they simply brand it immoral and advocate its eradication. A more analytically sophisticated alternative is to view sex work through the lens of moral economy. This perspective situates the growth of the sex industry in its unique historical context, especially the rise of the market economy and consumer ideology, which encourage the pursuit of individual desire—including sexual lust, a primary manifestation and catalyst of desire—as an important practice in everyday life. Moreover, sex work is examined as an activity in the political economy of the reform era with an imperative and moral valence reflective, in part, of contemporary consumer demand. Thus, advocates of this perspective do not deny the moral nature of such economic activity; rather, they recognize its complexity by acknowledging the economic, social, and personal stakes it carries for those involved, and stress the need to regulate it to prevent exploitation, disease transmission, and other harmful consequences. However, those who hold this view disagree over how to assess the moral impact of the sex industry on traditional social institutions and practices such as family, marriage, and gender dynamics, and therefore over how to regulate it. Since the 1980s, and especially over the past decade in China, viewing the sex industry as part of the post-Mao state's moral economy has become an acceptable alternative to the moralistic view outlined earlier. This is especially true in scholarly circles, a point to which the growing body of systematic empirical studies of the moral economy of China's sex industry attests (Hershatter 1997; Pan et al. 2005a, 2005b).

A number of conclusions can be drawn from a survey of the sex industry about sex work and the nature of its moral economy in contemporary China. To begin, a considerable number of men see prostitutes, but the number is not as high as imagined. Pan Suiming et al. (2008) discovered that in 2006, about 7 percent of men between the ages of eighteen and sixty-one saw sex workers for vaginal intercourse or anal sex. This does not include those men who received erotic services such as massage, *da feiji* (literally, to "shoot an airplane," meaning to receive manual stimulation), and *chuixiao* (to "blow a vertical bamboo flute," referring to fellatio).

Moreover, Pan and his colleagues found that this percentage remained the same from 2000 to 2006. In other words, the number of men soliciting sex from prostitutes ceased to grow, despite the fact that the reforms that enabled the sex industry to flourish continued to transform the lives of an ever-broadening swath of the Chinese populace. Why, then, did the percentage of men seeing sex workers fail to increase in the new millennium? Pan's interpretation was that not everyone who wanted to see sex workers actually did so. Among men surveyed, 35 percent wanted to see sex workers, but only 7 percent actually did so. Evidence that fewer men saw prostitutes than desired to prompted Pan to suggest that soliciting sex entails more than simply desiring to do so (Pan et al. 2008). Pan concluded that, owing to other limiting factors and despite its recent historical growth, the sex industry would simply remain at the level it reached at the turn of the millennium.

Nevertheless, because it is covered extensively in popular media and is present nationwide, the sex industry has become an iconic representation of the change in sexuality in China over the past three decades. Despite containing some elements of truth, this representation threatens to obscure a more important change in sexuality that has had a much more profound effect on ordinary people's sexual relationships. This change is an increase in sexual intimacy in dating and conjugal love, which is visible in the quest for privacy, the increase in premarital sex, and so forth. Yan's 2003 study of sexual practices in a village in Heilongjiang Province is a good example of how, for so many Chinese, this increase in sexual intimacy has been realized in and through the ordinary rhythms and relations of everyday life, even as it has transformed them. Overall, this change has generated new forms of sexual relationship beyond those that may be forged through traditional heterosexual and marriage practices. These new forms include relationships organized around premarital and extramarital sex of all sorts, such as: *bao ernai* ("having a second pair of breasts"), which means to have a regularly paid mistress or concubine; *yang xiaomi* ("having a small sweetie"), which means to have a female subordinate as a mistress; *yiye qing* ("one night stand"), a one-time sexual liaison, with emphasis on sentiment; *jieban bu jiehun* or *tongju* ("to keep sexual company without getting married or cohabiting"); *hunwailian* ("love outside marriage"); and so forth. At the same time, those involved in sexual relationships established within the traditional context of heterosexual marriage have become more open and more attentive to sexual satisfaction. Indicators of this change include an increase in the overall divorce rate in China, as well as the growing importance accorded to discontent with the sexual aspects of marital relationships (Woo 2006). These emerging means of expressing and achieving sexual intimacy in the domestic sphere arguably drive down the percentage of men seeking prostitutes in China. As people become accustomed to communicating sexual attitudes and desires to their spouses, and it becomes more permissible, or at least feasible, to establish sexual relationships that do not conform to the traditional, family-oriented model, fewer men are inclined to patronize sex workers.

It is not controversial to argue that the most profound effects of China's sexual revolution are seen within the domestic realm and in responses to the tension that obtains between the normative modes of sexuality encompassed within traditional family structures and sexual desires authorized by an emerging individualistic ethos. An incident that occurred in 2010, dubbed "The Bureau Chief's Erotic Diaries" or "Diarygate," is a good example of this tension. The bureau chief, who was employed by a government agency in a city in Guangxi Zhuang Autonomous Region, had saved on his work computer personal diaries cataloguing his primarily consensual sexual relationships with female coworkers, including some subordinates. The files were somehow uploaded to the Internet and circulated widely to become an internet sensation in 2010. According to the diaries, the bureau chief had sexual liaisons with six female coworkers, married and unmarried alike. At the same time, he maintained his reputation as a supportive husband who took good care of his family. Unlike the common practice of seeing *xiaojie* (bar hostesses or sex workers), his extramarital affairs in the office became an integral part of his enjoyment of life (Xinmin zhoukan 2010). Following the publication of the diaries and the identification of the author, the bureau chief lost his job and membership in the CCP. Nevertheless, despite his sexual exploits being the most sensational aspect of the diaries, they were not the reason given for his dismissal. Instead, punitive action was taken because he had accepted bribes when acting in a professional capacity, which was also recorded in the diaries (B. Li 2010). The offense cited as grounds for his dismissal is relevant to the project of charting shifting attitudes toward sexuality in China; under the Maoist regime, the bureau chief likely would have been punished for *shenghuo zuofeng wenti* ("the problem of sexual behavior"), a notoriously common charge levied against disgraced persons at that time.

It has taken a while for a consensus to develop among scholars of Chinese sexuality regarding the implausibility of eradicating the sex industry. Based on the moralistic view discussed earlier, the judgment was made early in the post-Mao period that prostitution could be eradicated in China, free-market reforms notwithstanding. This judgment has served as the basis for *saohuang* political campaigns (literally, "sweeping yellow"), which involve dismantling the sex industry through authoritarian means. But these campaigns have consistently fallen short of their goal. The numbers testify to the futility of *saohuang:* in 1994, 288,000 people involved in the sex industry, including those who saw sex workers, were punished (arrested, detained, or otherwise disciplined). This number generally rose over the next four years: to 362,000 in 1995, 416,000 in 1996, 429,000 in 1997, 398,000 in 1998, and 450,000 in 1999. Over a period of ten years, from 1984 to 1993, approximately 1.03 million people were disciplined; over the following six years, from 1994 to 1999, about 2.3 million people were disciplined (Liu 2007). In other words, compared to the preceding ten years, the number of people caught in government crackdowns on the sex industry doubled in the six year period between 1994 and 2000. This increase reflects the dramatic expansion of the sex industry during those years. Hence, instead of eradicating the sex industry, the state has found itself facing a trend toward the routinization of that industry.

The reason why the state's *saohuang* campaigns have been largely ineffective is quite simple: in the Maoist period even food was rationed, and the flow of cash between individuals was very limited under the central planning economy. The rise of consumption, as well as the march toward consumer society, provided the conditions necessary for the large-scale consumption of sex. Taking a close look at over two decades of *saohuang* campaigns against the sex industry, one sees that the state's need to accommodate the surging market economy powerfully determined the timing, mode of implementation, and goals of these campaigns. For example, there is ethnographic evidence that many local campaigns were launched half-heartedly. In the mid-1990s, a cadre told me that the deputy governor of his province was not serious about "sweeping yellow" because he believed that economic development in the province heavily depended on attracting investors and tourists, and that the sex industry constituted a major part of that attraction (Hyde 2001; H. Zhang 2006). Indeed, this reasoning is sound: many business transactions were—and still are—carried out through *goudui*, which, as defined earlier, involves paid sex and sexual bribery (E. Zhang 2001; Zheng 2009). This provincial leader's reluctance to enforce sex work prohibitions in an effective manner is representative of many local cadres.

In addition, the rise of the entertainment industry, as well as the promulgation of regulations that officially set the entertainment industry apart from prostitution, created a rush of sex workers who packaged themselves as entertainers without changing their business. Both the taxes levied on the entertainment industry and the jobs the industry created became important ways for local governments to collect revenue and maintain social stability at a time when state-owned enterprises laid off a large number of employees and the flow of migrant workers from rural areas to urban areas intensified, making job competition ever more fierce. Also, many local governments found that starting an entertainment business was an easy way to deal with the consequences of their failed development projects (Pan et al. 2005a). For example, in my fieldwork in one big city, the government-owned site of a folded industrial supply depot had been transformed into a commercial complex hosting massage parlors, hair salons, karaoke bars, and so on, forming a complex of brothels under the guise of entertainment and service-sector businesses, and a needed source of revenue for the local government.

Local police also had their own "grievances," which created incentives for them to tolerate sex work (Liu 2007). All too often, authorities at higher levels of law enforcement judged the performance of local police in *saohuang* campaigns by the number of sex workers they rounded-up; the higher the number, the bigger the reward. Ironically, this motivated local police to refrain from regularly enforcing laws prohibiting sex work. It was of greater benefit to them to allow the sex industry to operate until a campaign was initiated, so that all arrests made in connection with sex work would count toward evaluations of their performance. At the same time, the context that had enabled the state to eradicate the sex industry in the 1950s had changed so dramatically in the post-Mao era that its reform strategy was no longer feasible (Hershatter 1997). For example, in the 1950s, the state either sent the prostitutes back to their homes, arranged for them to marry bachelors in the city or in remote areas (such as Xinjiang), or offered them jobs in the city. The market economy changed the capacity of the state to create jobs and the way that employment was arranged. It also diminished the ease with which the state could relocate sex workers, and made sex workers less willing to accept relocation. In the reform era, sex workers' new earning capacity, together with the changed attitudes regarding sexuality and consumption, on the part of the state as well as society, have enabled some sex workers to see increased worth in their work and selves, making them resistant to reform and relocation. In recent studies of the industry, sex workers tended to treat their work as a new kind of job, no different, qualitatively, from others available to them in commercial society. Depending on what kind of power relationship they were in with their employer—whether they were a free laborer or enslaved in some way—some sex workers were able to make a living as independent agents, courting interested clients while trying to keep themselves out of harm's way (Pan et al. 2005a, 2005b; Zheng 2009; Wang et al. 2009).

This is where the issue of how to regulate, rather than eradicate, commercial sex, becomes an important point of departure for rethinking the sex industry and the sexual revolution. Since the flourishing sex industry in China's economic transformation is not reducible to an issue of moral decadence, but is sustained by the economy of desire engendered by free-market reforms, the most effective way to control that industry is not to launch futile eradication campaigns, but to acknowledge its inevitability in the post-Mao state and to regulate it in ways that mitigate the most immediate public health and human rights risks it poses. This includes protecting sex workers to prevent the spread of HIV/AIDS and other sexually transmitted diseases. In traditional Chinese thought, such an approach may be described as *shudao* (dredging) rather than *du* (stopping up) the currents of wild desire. It would enable more humane treatment of sex workers as laborers and the provision of real protections to prevent sex workers from becoming victims of blackmail, enslavement, oppression, and infectious diseases. This is what is required from a public health perspective. Driving sex work further underground would contribute to the already substantial incidence of sexually transmitted diseases and make medical prevention and treatment less likely. In the end, having a successful sexual revolution in the general population is the best way to control the sex industry. One of the most vehement advocates for eradicating the sex industry argued that only if private ownership and the market economy are eradicated with the coming of a real communist society will the sex industry be eliminated (Liu 2007). And Chinese are all too well aware, based on decades of real experience, what abuses result from communist utopianism.

THE DISCONTENTS OF DESIRE: THE RESURGENCE
OF SEXUALLY TRANSMITTED DISEASES

Despite the lack of consensus about how the sex industry should be handled, there seems to be little disagreement that the spread of sexually transmitted diseases

(STDs) has become a serious issue, and that the flourishing of the sex industry is largely responsible for their spread. One afternoon in October 1999, when I was doing fieldwork in a sexual medicine clinic in a Beijing hospital, I met a young woman who looked no more than twenty years old. Accompanied by an older woman, she had come to the clinic seeking medication for genital warts. The doctor asked about her marriage status, to which she replied, "Single." Then, the doctor simply asked how many men she had had sex with. Hesitating a little, she answered, "about five." Then she said, "Let me put it this way: about 10." It seemed clear that this woman was a sex worker. She came from Zhejiang Province. What was alarming was that when asked whether she continued to have sex, she said, "Yes." She had sought medication in several places, but the irritation in her genital area had not been cured, and was causing acute pain and itching. The woman who accompanied her asked about the expense of the medication, because, according to her, the young woman was rather poor and hoped the medication was affordable.

After they left, this doctor filled out a standard STD report card, a mandatory procedure for a hospital assigned to the national STD surveillance network. This network was established in the 1980s and enhanced in the 1990s to counter the resurgence of sexually transmitted diseases. In the Republican period, sexually transmitted diseases such as syphilis were a serious public health threat. By the time the Communist Party took power in 1949, syphilis infection was reportedly present in as many as 84 percent of prostitutes and 5 percent of the general population in some large cities, as well as in 2 to 3 percent of rural residents (Z. Chen et al. 2007). Because prostitution played a major role in transmitting syphilis and other STDs, the policy of eradicating prostitution implemented in the 1950s facilitated the elimination of these diseases in the following ten-year period.

As the economic reform era began, the first cases of syphilis were reported in 1979. Not surprisingly, as the sex industry developed, STDs spread. According to data from the nationwide surveillance system, reported cases of syphilis increased from 184 in 1985 to 113,688 in 2005. The incidence of primary and secondary syphilis in 2005 was substantially higher than that in most developed countries. For example, there were 2.7 reported cases of syphilis per one hundred thousand individuals in the United States in 2004, compared to 5.67 cases per one hundred thousand individuals in China in 2005 (Z. Chen et al. 2007). A study conducted by Pan and Shi (2008) shows that these official numbers may not be accurate as a substantial number of hospitals did not report cases to the STD surveillance network; in addition, many who suffered from STDs might not have seen doctors at all. Pan and Shi concluded that the STD rate in China is alarmingly higher than the government's report estimated. For example, compared to the occurrence of syphilis reported by the state (about 16.54 per one hundred thousand persons in 2007), their finding in 2006 was twelve times higher; regarding the occurrence of gonorrhea, their finding in 2006 was seven hundred per one hundred thousand persons, a figure seventy times higher than the official figure in 2007 (Pan and Shi 2008). This difference may have to do with the fact that Pan and his colleagues focused on the prevalence of STDs over a number of years in order to gauge the rate at which the incidence was growing; in contrast, the government report examined the STD rate reported for each year separately, which may have created a less than accurate picture. Hence, the method of statistical analysis used in the government report contributed to inaccuracies, as did the underreported figures obtained from the imperfect monitoring system.

Winning the battle against STDs depends on dealing with the sex industry successfully. Among the high-incidence areas, Shanghai topped the list, followed by coastal provinces such as Zhejiang, Jiangsu, and Guangdong, and other economically advanced cities like Beijing, showing a high correlation between economic development and STD incidence. As I have noted, since it is impossible to eradicate the sex industry, the fight against STDs must focus on how high-risk groups of people are educated and their sexual contact regulated (e.g., by using condoms). There are different opinions as to which groups are at heightened risk for transmitting STDs, though observers agree that female sex workers constitute one such group. One view is that "surplus men"—predominately single, poor, and unmarried migrant male workers—are another major high-risk group (Tucker et al. 2005); the argument is that men who fall into this category have difficulty finding spouses as a result of the imbalanced sex ratio, and therefore are more likely to pay for sex—a readily available service in the urban areas to which they've migrated for work. China has 8.5 million more men than women among cohorts born between 1980 and 2000. If this trend continues, there will be a large number of "surplus men" in China in the years to come, another unintended social consequence of China's birth policy. Pan and his colleagues' findings call our attention to another high-risk group—men between the ages of thirty and thirty-four in the local, rather than the floating, male population. These men have had some education and generally earn higher incomes than those in the floating group. According to Pan and Shi's 2008 study, they also have higher STD rates. At present, it is unclear which research results are more accurate. Nonetheless, the increase in STD rates in post-Mao China represents one of the powerful and troubling discontents of the social body under the new regime of sexual revolution.

A SEXUAL REVOLUTION THE CHINESE WAY

In my view, China's sexual revolution has advanced through three stages. It started with the reemergence of "love" shortly after the Cultural Revolution in the late 1970s and early 1980s. At the same time, the implementation of the one-child policy opened the door, unintentionally, for the official justification of sexual pleasure in the 1980s. Then, the rapid rise of a consumer society that began after 1992 enhanced individual desire, to which sexual desire is integral, thereby integrating sexual behaviors into the emerging "consumer revolution" (Davis 2000). Finally, deepening social, economic, technological, and cultural developments, as well as the continued commercialization of China's economy in the new millennium have coalesced so as to decouple sexual desire from reproduction, and even sexual pleasure from love.

THE REEMERGENCE OF *AIQING* (ROMANTIC LOVE)

China's revolution shared with the earlier U.S. sexual revolution the same reality: both acknowledge, through delinking sexual desire from reproduction, that sexual pleasure is the most important and even the sole reason for having sex, and that sexual pleasure has its own ontological value of affirming life. This separation of desire and reproduction in sex has had enormous impact on everyday life in China. To understand this impact better, it is necessary to have an overview of the societal-wide change from the resurfacing of the discourse of *aiqing* (romantic love) at the beginning of the reform era in the late 1970s, to the rise of the discourse of *xing'ai* (sexual love) further into the economic reform era.

For most of the Maoist period, the word *ai* (love) did not refer to romantic love. From the 1950s to the 1960s—even before the Cultural Revolution—*aiqing* (romantic love) began to be modified by terms such as *revolutionary* in order to stress the proper link between passion and collectivism in the Communist ethos. As class struggle escalated in the 1960s, even the phrase "revolutionary *aiqing*" was purged. *Ai* (love) more often referred to one's dedication to the Party, socialism, and, ultimately, Chairman Mao. *Re'ai* (enthusiastic love) could only be directed toward the Great Leader, the Party, or the revolutionary classes and their cause. *Aiqing*, a phrase exclusively referring to romantic love since the Republican period, disappeared altogether from public discourse during the Cultural Revolution. Instead, during the first half of the Cultural Revolution, the general sentiment of hatred toward class enemies commingled with that of love toward Chairman Mao to energize frenetic rebellions and factional fights throughout China. A former Red Guard and rebel recalled how one evening during the days of factional fighting, a group of fellow rebels walked into an empty stadium in a provincial capital with guns in their hands. They spotted a man and a girl in the stands. Outraged by the scene of any possible sexual affection at the peak of asexual revolution, the rebels captured the man and, without evidence, denounced him as a rapist. Trembling, the man was unable to defend himself. The group of rebels then shot him in the groin, killing him.

"Desexualization," a term used by Pan Suiming (2006), refers to the same repressive phenomenon dubbed "sexual repression" (Zhang 2005). "Repression" does not refer to prohibiting sex within the boundary of marriage. It refers to strong vigilance and hostility toward sex outside marriage—premarital sex, extramarital sex, homoerotic relationships, and so on. It also refers to the discouragement of sex for pleasure and of the articulation of sexual desire, both through public discourse and through institutionalized practices that even affect the private lives of married couples. The birth rate rose at a great pace before it started to decline very gradually in the second half of the Cultural Revolution (Greenhalgh and Winckler 2005; Liang and Lee 2006). This is an unsurprising statistic, given that reproduction was the justification for married couples to have sex. The people born during this long period of robust reproduction rates, spanning from the end of the Great Leap Famine in 1962 to the latter half of the Cultural Revolution in the early 1970s, would become China's "baby boomer generation," which took the leading role in the sexual revolution (Pan 2006; Farrer 2002). During the period of their birth, however, the explicit articulation of sexual desire was greatly discouraged and even repressed, except for the empowered few. A middle-aged man who had been a sent-down youth in Heilongjiang Province in the late 1960s recalled, "Those who were in power were not sexually repressed." He explained,

At that time, youths wanted to return to the city, but needed to get the approval of the party branch for any opportunity of employment in the city, because, in addition to one's family class status, one's political performance in the countryside mattered a great deal. In order to get the approval, girls had to sleep first with the branch secretary, then the deputy secretary, and then the militia company commander, one after another. One girl was so pissed off that she swore that she would rather stay in the countryside. This was because when she had asked for the approval from the party secretary, she was told to talk to him. It was not a talk at all. The secretary simply caressed her body. The same secretary once boasted after getting drunk that he was satisfied with his whole life because he had slept with dozens of women. A militia platoon leader liked to take a young female militia member with him, pretending to train her in shooting. One day he thought most of the militia members were not good looking, so he picked up the daughter of a rich peasant and had sex with her in a big barrel.

It does not come as a surprise that authoritarian rule created a double standard whereby those few who were empowered by the state's legal and political apparatuses could act on sexual desire with impunity, while the majority of Chinese were compelled by the same mechanisms to repress such desire. While class struggle was on the rise in the 1960s, Mao himself reportedly loved to dally with young girls (Z. Li 1994). By the same token, the general ethos of class struggle launched and cultivated by Mao went against Mao's taste for more open sexual practice in some fields (Cai 1998). Mao ordered that the practice of sketching human nude models in art colleges be continued, but the ethos of *tanxing sebian* ("the talk of sex scares people") made it impossible to hire a nude model until the 1980s. Though the central government never explicitly ordered the repression of sexual desire, the ethos and structural constraints of collectivism, which were realized largely through the *danwei* (work unit) system around which all aspects of social life were organized, enforced the desexualization of social life for most Chinese (E. Zhang 2005).

When the Cultural Revolution ended in 1976, some authors lamented the loss of expressions of romantic love in the preceding decade, to the degree that a sent-down youth recalled that as soon as he heard the phrase *"aiqing"* (love) during the broadcast of Liu Xinwu's 1978 novella *The Place of Love* from the loudspeaker of a commune broadcasting station, what immediately came to mind was: "A coup is happening in China!" (Deng 1998). As one's political class status started to matter less and less in one's personal life, and the focus of the state and society shifted from class struggle to economic development, the phrase *"aiqing"* (love) regained currency. It was during this transitional moment that novels such as Liu Xinwu's *The Place of Romantic Love*, Zhang Jie's *Love Must Not be Forgotten* (1979), and Zhang Xian's *The Corner Left Behind by Romantic Love* (1979) were published, reintroducing and reanimating an age of romantic love.

However, the pursuit of sexual pleasure had not yet gained prominence or approbation in public discourse because it still sounded vulgar, and because "sexual revolution" was a much stigmatized phrase in the 1980s. It was at this time that the state made an intervention of unprecedented scope into the reproductive practices of the Chinese populace, which resulted in the decoupling of sexual desire and reproduction. This intervention, the one-child policy, was implemented forcefully across the country. Much has been said about the impact and consequences of this policy; my emphasis here will be on examining how China's one-child policy (or birth-control policy, to be more accurate) influenced the rise of desire in post-Mao China, as it has been charted thus far in this chapter.

THE ONE-CHILD POLICY:
WHERE SEXUAL PLEASURE WAS PROMOTED UNWITTINGLY

Before discussing the one-child policy, I will first examine the emerging movement among some citizens to justify sexual desire and pleasure through legal means, which proved to be a common method used to achieve sexual freedom and self-determination in the history of sexual revolutions in the West. Two cases illustrate how this approach has been enacted in China.

The first case has been dubbed by the Chinese news media and in popular discourse "The case of detention for watching pornography at home." In 2002, a couple in Yan'an, Shaanxi Province, was watching a pornographic DVD at home. The police stormed in and took the husband away. Later, the husband was officially detained. He was eventually released, but he had behavioral problems and was sleepy all the time, indicating that he had sustained a brain injury during his detention. Lawyers in Beijing who took his case alleged that his injury resulted from being beaten by police and reached an agreement with the Public Security Bureau responsible for overseeing the police station where he was detained. The husband received compensation of about thirty thousand yuan to cover medical expenses and wages lost when he was out of work during his convalescence. In addition, one police officer was fired and two others disciplined (Zhongxinwang 2003).

The second exemplary case occurred in Nanjing, Jiangsu Province, in 2002 and also involved compensation for an injury. A car ran over a man's leg, resulting in serious injury and sexual dysfunction. Together, the injured man and his wife took the driver to court. In its ruling, the court reasoned that sexual rights are citizens' rights; therefore, because the accident had damaged the plaintiffs' sexual lives, the defendant had infringed on their rights. Thus, the court ordered the defendant to make a financial compensation for the accident. It is notable that the court identified both the injured husband and his wife as victims and allowed the wife to stand in court as a plaintiff. The court ordered the driver's employer to pay the plaintiffs one hundred thousand yuan to compensate them for medical expenses and to provide disability support, along with ten thousand yuan as compensation for the damage to their mental health (Nanfangwang 2002).

These two cases expose the crucial, if slow, development of legal means by which to establish and protect sexual rights and one's entitlement to pursue sexual pleasure as one sees fit. The case concerning pornography reveals that the repressive practices and logic prevalent in the Maoist period persist in contemporary China. The encouraging outcome of this case, however, is that in the end, at least regarding the issue of sexuality, a highly publicized line was drawn between the legal and the ethical. People have started to learn to respect the legal rights of other people who were doing things they considered unethical.

Both cases represent a new trend in the production of desire in China: the desire for sexual freedom as it is articulated in the register of law. In this sense, sexual rights, to which citizens are legally entitled, have been produced as an object of desire. This development is more typical of sexual revolutions in the West. However, public debates surrounding these cases, and the issue of legalism and sexuality more generally, have not fully developed the concept of sexual citizenship, and therefore have not made inroads into legislation as in democratic societies. In China, powerful desire may be produced and made manifest in a twisted and surprising way, one that does not necessarily accompany the legitimization of sexual citizenship and the rights of citizens. China's one-child policy is a good example. The correlation between the increasing choice for sexual desire and the decreasing choice for reproduction, which resulted from delinking sexual desire from reproduction, cannot be understood adequately in terms of sexual rights. It is helpful to examine the crucial but sometimes hidden links between population and the body.

Despite there being well-developed studies of China's one-child policy, which focus on the regulation of the population (the species body), and also studies of sexuality, which tend to focus on the individual body, the link between population regulation and subjective sexuality has not been fully explored. Understandably, studies of the former tend not to see nonreproductive sexual practices, whereas studies of the latter tend to see sex but not in relation to social engineering policies designed to regulate the population.

It is Foucault, again, from whom we can draw inspiration for highlighting this link between the species body and individual bodies. He argues that "sex" emerges "at the juncture of the 'body' and the 'population' " (Foucault 1990: 147). The implication is that "sex" is at the heart of the economic and political problems of a population; for, as Foucault observes, "it [has been] necessary [for states] to analyze the birth rate, the age of marriage, the legitimate and illegitimate births, the precocity and frequency of sexual relations, the ways of making [persons] fertile or sterile, the effects of unmarried life or of the prohibitions, the impact of contraceptive practices" (25–26). This means that any change in the regulation of reproduction inevitably bears on individual sexual habits and experiences. Such was the case in China following the promulgation of the one-child policy, which transformed both the demographic profile of the vast Chinese population, and also the sexual desires, expectations, and practices of its constituents.

A notable exception to scholars of the Chinese history of sexuality, who have tended to pay less attention to the relationship between the change in reproductive pattern of the population and the change in individual experience of sexual desire, is Pan Suiming. In fact, Pan explored such a link as early as 1995 (Pan 1995). More recently, he claimed that China's one-child policy has been one of three directly important driving forces for the sexual revolution (the other two he identified are the new Marriage Law of 1980 and the demographic increase of youth in the population as a result of peaking birth rates from 1963 to 1968) (Pan 2006). Whether or not Pan has been influenced by Foucault, his longitudinal empirical studies of Chinese sexuality consistently explore the link between China's one-child policy and the justification and production of desire over the past several decades. Here is how I understand that link.

One major effect of the one-child policy is that it induced the use of contraceptives on an unprecedented scale. For a period of time, commencing with the policy's implementation, the state earmarked a portion of its funds for purchasing condoms, which were distributed in some areas without charge to married couples . By encouraging couples to use condoms in this way, the state sent out a clear signal that having sex to procreate was discouraged; at the same time, it implicitly acknowledged, and suggested it would tolerate, sex for nonprocreative ends, so long as it was protected. This signal was strengthened by the jural facet of the policy, under which having more than one child became a violation of the law. Doing otherwise— taking measures to prevent reproduction—was construed as a positive example of how responsible citizens should serve the interests of the nation in connection with the state-led effort to modernize. The state's show of approbation for the use of contraceptives arguably inflected the repressive moral sentiment surrounding nonprocreative sex, making it, and by extension, the pursuit of sexual pleasure, more permissible. Never before were sexual pleasure and reproduction so forcefully, openly, and officially separated, and the former so clearly justified. Even though population control was the surface script while the justification of sexual desire was the unintended hidden script, this hidden script could hardly go unheeded.

Subsequent changes in the way condoms were produced and distributed helped to promote sexual desire. When the one-child policy was first implemented, using condoms was far less popular than today, due to less availability, social resistance, and other factors. Many other prophylactic methods were practiced. Sterilization was practiced on men and women, and cottonseed oil was experimented with as a contraceptive. However, these methods may have been unpopular; for example, cottonseed oil was said to have unpleasant side effects for women. Some men I spoke to while doing fieldwork in Sichuan in the 1990s had been sterilized in the 1980s; they complained that the surgery later caused them to experience sexual dysfunction. The availability and use of prophylactic methods changed greatly in the 1990s. The production of contraceptives improved in quality and grew in quantity, and the consumption of condoms increased. After the turn of the millennium, both the consumption and production of condoms increased by 15 percent annually, outpacing the increase of national GDP (China News Net 2003). Also, different types of condoms, some of which were allegedly super thin to facilitate sexual pleasure, were introduced to the market and so advertised.

By this time, the acknowledged function of condoms had changed from preventing pregnancy to preventing pregnancy *and* sexually transmitted disease, which are two common sources of anxiety that diminish sexual enjoyment. One significant development was to place condom vending machines in public spaces, such as college campuses and neighborhoods. There was some resistance in the beginning to the attempt to place condom vending machines on campuses. Critics cited the danger of inciting sexual desire and indecent behavior. This reasoning is similar to that which motivated initial resistance to the importation of Viagra; in the latter case, critics cited the danger of openly encouraging the pursuit of sexual pleasure through the use of some kind of *yingyao* (lustful drug). Eventually, resistance to both evaporated.

By the same token, abortions have become much more common in contemporary China than they were in the Maoist period. Among women under forty years, 49.1 percent of urban women and 29.1 percent of rural women have had at least one abortion (Pan 2006: 105). This increase not only reflects a change in practice, but also in the moral sentiment surrounding abortion: it has become much less shameful for unmarried women than it was in the Maoist period, when a woman who underwent the procedure would surely be stigmatized if it became public knowledge, regardless of the circumstances surrounding her pregnancy. In contemporary China, easy access to and reduced stigmatization of abortion have reduced the fear of pregnancy and promoted sexual pleasure in relationships outside marriage. No doubt that the one-child policy also contributed to this reduction in the moral significance of abortion.

By discussing the important role the one-child policy played in separating sexual pleasure from reproduction, I mean to emphasize the uniqueness of China's sexual revolution, without downplaying other factors. One of the important characteristics of the sexual revolution in the United States was the role the existing civil society, under the protection of the Constitution, played in pushing to expand and protect sexual freedoms, including homosexuality, abortion, erotica, and so on. For example, in the famous sexual freedom forums on college campuses in the years of the Vietnam War, advocates couched their agenda in the language of national politics by using the now-iconic slogan, "Make love, not war!" Many organizations allied themselves in lawsuits to enshrine sexual freedom as a politico-legal right of citizenship (Allyn 2000; D'Emilio and Freedman 1998; Escoffier 2003; Li 2005). Thus, the U.S. sexual revolution was intertwined with contemporaneous social movements (the civil rights movement, the antiwar movement, the gay and lesbian movement, the feminist movement, etc.) and became a manifestation of the overall challenge to established values and practices. It was a way to call for open, diversified sexual practices, which translated into sexual rights through due process of civil liberty.

China's sexual revolution has occurred in a different social and political context. The contribution China's one-child policy made to the justification of sexual desire is an example of that difference. This policy was so swiftly enforced upon the whole population that the long-term outcome was largely unknown to the decision makers back in the late 1970s. This recalls Robert Merton's emphasis on the unintended consequences of purposeful social action. Not the least of the one-child policy's consequences is that sexual relationships became more salient than filial relationships—a fundamental shift in Chinese culture (see Yunxiang Yan's chapter in this volume). Just as the central government didn't intentionally condone sexual desire during the implementation of this policy, when the cadres in charge of family planning charted women's menstruation cycles on village blackboards, they were not aware that they were working toward the same result as sexologists like Dr. Ma on radio talk shows in the city in later years. Beyond the policy, ordinary people—sex educators, novelists, artists, photographers, bloggers, DVD vendors, entertainers, karaoke bar managers, travelers, fashion designers, filmmakers, condom sellers, rock-and-roll performers, advertisers, etc.—with divergent motives and intentions, did the on-the-ground work that led to the sexualization of China. If in the 1980s sexual practices such as premarital sex were still politically tinged in challenging state authority, then entering the 1990s, the rise of consumer society and the rise of individualism justified sexual desire directly, through straightforward appeals to that desire.

THE DISTINCTIVE FEATURES OF CHINA'S SEXUAL REVOLUTION

When the scholars of Chinese sexuality were debating the best translation of the English term *sexuality*, they were responding to the change in reality in which sex had expanded beyond the confines allotted to it in the Maoist period. They were also participating in the demand for a new set of terms through which to acknowledge and discuss this change openly. Many sexual behaviors popular now were either beyond people's imagination or simply hidden in the Maoist period. The change in sexuality is among the most significant changes in China's post-Mao transformation. No wonder calling it a "sexual revolution" is so telling.

As discussed previously, same-sex love is more and more tolerated in China, and in certain urban areas it is even flourishing. This tolerance derives partly from the cultural model of the androgynous body in Chinese cosmology and traditional medicine, and also from the fact that in Chinese history, intimate relationships between men or between women were not conceptually sexualized in the same way as they have been in Western thought. For this reason, they were less socially marked and did not pose a threat to the hierarchical gender/sex dichotomy that has, quite often in history, underwritten social orders. But the strategy of gays in China differs significantly from the gay-lesbian movement in the West, because many gay men believe that a radical stance on homosexual rights would prove ineffective and even counterproductive (Y. Li 2006). A large number of gay men manage to live in heterosexual families and feel indebted to family obligations, including producing a child, while still pursuing homosexual relations (Rofel 2007). This phenomenon may not result entirely from the political and legal limitations in China. Instead, it may have to do with the fact that sexual desire did not gain complete autonomy in social relationships because of social limitations on individual practices. This is where "homosexuality" or "same sex love" is not necessarily the same as *tongxinglian*, a term serving as the translation of "homosexual relationship" since the Republican period.

The practice of *bao ernai* may look like just a simple reintroduction of the practice of concubinage in pre-1949 China or a return to polygamy. However, "having a second pair of breasts" has become a way to satisfy the desire for an extramarital relationship, one that entails a longer commitment but less romance than a one-night stand, is more sustainable and intimate than seeing prostitutes, and is less "illegal" than polygamy. With regard to the naming of this phenomenon, it is the English language's turn to struggle with a suitable translation. "Second wife" is the term most often seen in English, but this is not accurate and could not be translated back into Chinese without looking awry, because the Chinese translation of "second wife" is *er laopo*, and means exactly that—a second wife. This linguistic uniqueness and its translational awkwardness reinforce the judgment that this phenomenon is neither complete innovation, nor is it a total return to old practice. Rather, it reveals a special character in China's mapping of desiring today. Again, we seem to have identified a space where practices in China's sexual revolution do not center around the autonomy of sexual desire. And in this instance, we see that China's sexual revolution includes counter-moves to the West's revolution in gender equality.

Today, *xiaojie* has become the most common name for sex workers or prostitutes. *Xiaojie* literally means "little elder sister" or young lady. The term used to be used for waitresses in restaurants, but can also refer to a woman who provides sexual services ranging from singing or dancing with some bodily contact, to erotic services of touching, grabbing, and stroking without having penile-vaginal intercourse, to having penile-vaginal intercourse. *Xiaojie*, which earlier on simply meant "Miss," has come to mean a person working as a bar hostess or massage girl, and for this reason many restaurant patrons try to avoid using it, substituting instead the more neutral term *fuwuyuan* (service worker). It is very interesting that more people prefer *xiaojie* to "prostitute," "sex worker," or any other names (mostly pejorative) such as *ji* (hen). *Xiaojie* not only reflects the range of services that may be provided, but also carries more social acceptance than "prostitute," while being more ambiguous than "sex worker." Because the sex industry figures more prominently in China than in the United States, the term *xiaojie* comes to represent that ambiguity between "legal" and "illegal," and provides the opportunity for somewhat greater social acceptance of sexual desire, but at the expense of stable protection of a basic human status for *xiaojie*.

In my research on sexuality and Chinese medicine, I discovered contrasting trends in dealing with sexual desire—the loss of *jing* (seminal essence, here meaning both sperm and vital energy), which means the rise of sexual desire at the expense of vitality and health; and the revival of *yangsheng* (the cultivation of life), which means having a cautious attitude toward sex not necessarily due to sexual repression but because of concern about health promotion. These two trends resonate with the contrast between the introduction of rock and roll and the rise of qigong in China (N. Chen 2003; Palmer 2007). The former is dynamic, while the latter is slow motion; the former is noisy, while the latter is quiet; the former features spontaneity and improvisation, while the latter features strict programming. Rock and roll originated in the West, whereas qigong originated in China. Some argue that the popularity of rock and roll in the United States in the 1960s is no accident, simply because it revels in all the characteristics of good sex (Pan 2006). Holding this view to the extreme would, however, dismiss one of the most important trends in post-Mao China—the rise of qigong as asexual. The reason for this dismissal is that from the perspective of rock and roll, which makes the body sexy, qigong simply desexualizes the body.

However, qigong could be viewed as sexy if we understand the function of sex differently. That is, in addition to reproduction and sexual pleasure, sex possesses a third dimension—the cultivation of life. One of the trends in post-Mao China is that the Daoist classics on sexual cultivation have been resurrected (e.g., in exhibitions on ancient sexual culture, festivals of sexual culture, and in a sex museum). If many traditional ideas and techniques, such as returning seminal essence to nourish the brain by practicing retrograde ejaculation, sound ludicrous today, then other techniques, such as paying attention to the flowing of *qi* in sex and stimulating the female partner into orgasm as a precondition for sexual cultivation, acknowledge a different type of sexual pleasure that resonates with current perspectives and partly accounts for the lower-than-expected reception of anti-impotence pills such as Viagra (E. Zhang 2007a). Self-discipline of the body through the exercise of qigong could counter the excesses of sexual desire.

To sum up, despite many similarities with the sexual revolution in the West, China's sexual revolution has unfolded in a greatly different social and cultural context. It has had different driving forces, taken different trajectories, and produced different effects. The examples above show that even if the separation of sexual desire and reproduction has been the leitmotif of the revolution, the pursuit of desire has not been the only motivational logic informing its experiential effects, as is seen in the emerging subjectivities of *xiaojie, tongxianlian, ernai,* and qigong practitioners and self-cultivators. They represent distinctive Chinese characteristics. This is where the difficulty of finding the exact Chinese translation of *sexuality* is a difference that represents a real difference.

It is also undeniable that sexual desire has become more prominent on its own terms. Just as the separation of sexual desire from reproduction has been developing strongly, another separation—that setting off sexual pleasure from romantic love—has become fashionable. *Xing'ai* (sexual love) has replaced *qing'ai* (sentimental, romantic love), as the former sounds a bit "sexier" than the latter, to become a more popular term for sexual relationships in the new millennium. While *aiqing* (romantic love) found its way back into the ordinary person's vocabulary shortly after the Maoist period ended, now *xing'ai* (sexual love) has taken hold, seemingly more appropriate for an age of consumption. Seeking sexual pleasure without falling in love has come to replace the idea of sexual desire embedded in romantic love as the center of many sexual encounters. This pleasure-centric practice indicates further detachment of sex from the relations and moral sentiments previously associated with it—reproductive, familial, romantic, and so on. It has become an independently valued means and end to the good life, no longer subordinate to other social values or experiential modes, as Pan's theory of "the primary life cycle" explains (Pan 2006). Pan argues that the ancient Chinese language did not include a term for the modern day notion of "sex." What was close to sex was *qing* (sentiment or affect) or *se* (lust). Moreover, the relationship between husband and wife was defined by *en 'ai* (reciprocal care and indebtedness) rather than love or sex. Building on his point, I argue that the word *ai,* which now means "love," is conceptually closer to "being close to" and "to care for" in ancient Chinese than any iteration of the root concept "sex." Yet, the fact that sexual practices undertaken for the sake of enjoyment per se appeared in erotica and many famous literary representations, even before the Qing Dynasty, shows that the distinctive connotation of sex did exist in the Chinese language, as well as social life, in the past. However, by and large, sex was presented via the pejorative words *se* (lust) or *yin* (lewd, lascivious). I make the bold proposition here that the legitimization of affection-based love was not accomplished until after the May Fourth movement (1919), which students and intellectuals launched for the modernization of China through democracy and science, whereas the legitimization of sex for the sake of sexual pleasure per se was not accomplished until the post-Mao sexual revolution. This may be unintended, but it is certainly a revolution.

Whether or not love is authentic depends on how profound it is, whereas whether or not sexual pleasure is authentic depends on how *shuang* (ecstatically pleasurable) it is. *Shuang* refers to sensual satisfaction. It is neither necessarily deep nor shallow, but it is undeniably pervasive, embodied, and exciting. This change in sensibility is profoundly altering ethical reasoning regarding what kind of person one may aspire to be, and also through what practices one may seek happiness. We can confidently say that, overall, sex has become more important in people's lives in China, compared to three decades ago. Having established that this is so, I must conclude this chapter by raising the crucial issue of the ethical implications of the sexual revolution, because the issue speaks so directly to *Deep China*'s emphasis on the implications of changing moral experience.

CONCLUSION: ARE PEOPLE HAPPIER?

Looking back, the need to find an adequate Chinese translation for the English term *sexuality* reveals the growth in scope of the space of sexuality. Many new phenomena have emerged to widen this space; their effects are reflected in experiential transformations, such as the novel sexual practices and values outlined earlier, and also in linguistic changes, such as the new terms and usages available for articulating a significantly expanded set of sexual relations and desires. That which had been confined to reproduction, which existed below the threshold of recognition, which was suppressed under the surface, or which perhaps did not exist at all, has been brought out into the light of day.

One ethical implication of China's sexual revolution is straightforward: Has it made people happier, freer, and more capable of realizing their human potential? There is no empirical answer as of yet. When Wilhem Reich, Herbert Marcuse, Norman Brown, and others called for sexual liberation, they were concerned about freedom and happiness, because they believed that the complete liberation of humans should and could be realized via sexual liberation (Reich 1963; Marcuse 1966; Brown 1966). Regardless of the feasibility of their ideas, their concerns persisted even in thinkers critical of their position. For example, Foucault commented, "this whole sexual 'revolution,' this whole 'anti-repressive' struggle, represented nothing more, but nothing less—and its importance is undeniable—than a tactical shift and reversal in the great deployment of sexuality" (1990: 131). That is, through the lens of sexuality, people who had been subject to one form of power—for example, repression—are now subject to a new form of power, biopower, which is the power exercised by the state and other institutions targeting biological life itself through affecting both the individual body and the population (species body) for the purpose of maximizing their productive potential and well-being. Foucault's argument that the shifts in Western history of sexuality, instead of freeing sexuality from power, only redeployed sexuality under different modes of power sheds light on China's sexual revolution. For example, when we know that desire was not recognized as an independent facet of sexual values, practices, and experience, but was subordinate to reproduction in the Maoist period, we understand how much the sexual revolution has accomplished in post-Mao China. However, this accomplishment has been accompanied by new forms of power, such as a regime of sexual health, that incorporate some mechanisms of older forms in unexpected ways. This is seen clearly in the history of the one-child policy, which led to an unintentional increase in sexual freedom for ordinary Chinese by tacitly acknowledging desire as a legitimate motive for intercourse, even as it provided a basis for the state to curb reproductive freedom through authoritarian means. In the final analysis, affirming the importance of the concerns of sexual liberation advocates, Foucault asked the following ethical questions: Have people gained more pleasure through the body (1990: 157)? And what kinds of subjects are shaped through this redeployment of power and pleasure (Foucault 2006: 190; Deleuze 1997)?

The question as to whether the sexual revolution in China has made people happier, freer, and more capable of realizing their human potential is worth exploring, regardless of however elusive, contradictory, and pluralistic the answer might be. I cannot help but recall some of my own experiences as I explore it. My grandmother on my father's side was born in Fujian Province before the fall of the Qing dynasty. She gave birth to ten children over her lifetime, but only five survived. Her ailing body, infirm posture, and bound feet are central to my memory. I doubt that she enjoyed much sexual pleasure. Her life leads me to conclude that we must not underestimate the significance of justifying sexual desire on its own terms, nor the freedom gained from delinking sexual desire from reproduction. I also recall a time during the late period of the Cultural Revolution when a female student's application for becoming a member of the Communist Youth League in a middle school was put on hold, because rumor had it that she liked to make friends with boys in her neighborhood. So much has changed since that time that it is hard now to imagine the history of repression or desexualization in the Maoist period. Here, in the roughest sense, we can conclude that China's sexual revolution, which is inseparable from the other changes addressed in *Deep China*, has had a number of positive effects for individuals, entire groups of people, and for the society. Because the sexual revolution has changed the experiences of ordinary Chinese so significantly, its future trajectory is a tantalizing question: Where will the rise in desire lead? Let me return to the ethnographic accounts for inspiration, rather than for firm answers.

One day in 2005, on a university campus in the United States, a Chinese gay activist and artist showed a documentary he had made about gay sex workers in China. The sex workers were young; some were called "money boys." Scenes he had shot in a gay bar in Beijing were very carnal and sensuous. One of the workers had sex with an older gay man in the basement of the bar, and then went upstairs where he had sex with a female. The flow of desire transgressed normative boundaries. Watching this documentary, I guessed about the possible effects it might have on different American viewers: a shock to somebody from a religious family in the Midwest, but a thrill to someone having a good time in a bar in San Francisco. The unevenness of sexual ideology in the United States recalls its unevenness in China. Just as the economic development in China is uneven, the mapping of sexuality and the distribution of access to sexual pleasure are uneven. We may witness bold transgressions of sexual identity and gender boundaries in one place, and the poverty of desire in another. When sexualization becomes a norm, we also hear complaints about sexual abuse at home and at work, violence against sex workers, and overwhelming pressure on sexual minorities. Even though more and more people know about orgasm, a large number of people remain unaware of the physical mechanisms of sexual pleasure. From 1991 to 2000, even though overall sexual activity had increased on college campuses, 30 percent of college students had still never spoken with their schoolmates of the opposite sex (Phoenix Television 2003). Women's confidence in expressing their desire may be rising, but more women than men still feel ashamed about sex (Parish et al. 2007).

Yet over the past decade, particularly in the past several years, one thing has become clear: fewer and fewer new developments in sexuality can produce as shocking an effect as events in the previous two decades. Anything sensational five years ago does not seem so today. A sex education radio talk show in Beijing, considered in the past to be "hot" or "racy," is much less so in contemporary China; a once busy clinic of sexual medicine now must relocate to a smaller consultation room because of a decline in patient visits. And entering a sex shop, one no longer sees curiosity and repressed excitement on the faces of shoppers, but yawning and sleepy employees acting like housekeepers in a summer home that has been shuttered for the off-season. Do these phenomena indicate that the sexualization of Chinese society has reached its saturation point? Or, as Pan Suiming has argued, do they signal that the revolution has reached its goal, so that sexual excitement, once concentrated in certain marked sites, has diffused into the settings of everyday life? Or has widespread sexualization, following the sexual revolution, just begun?

Three decades of change in sexuality might have carried China over a threshold beyond which sexualization may slow down on some fronts and gather momentum on others. Changes may be less dramatic in "hot" sites such as sex shops, red light districts, pornographic websites, or the *maopianr* vendors' stands, but become more pervasive in domestic spaces, as sexual pleasure becomes a routine part of lived experience in China. For most people, sex might finally become a private issue and one of individual choice. The majority of the population may want more sexual pleasure, while more and more people may prefer to have two or more children. Looking forward, we have reason to expect further changes—no doubt some will meet our expectations, while others may go well beyond them.

NOTE

1. These herbal tonics are believed to work by nourishing the kidney's *yang* or masculine element, in contrast to the *yin* or feminine element.

REFERENCES

Allyn, D. 2000. *Make Love, Not War: The Sexual Revolution: An Unfettered History.* New York: Little, Brown.

Brown, N. O. 1966. *Love's Body*. Berkeley: University of California Press.

Cai J. 1998. "Mao Zedong guanyu renti xiesheng moter wenti de pishi" [Mao Zedong's Directive on the Issue of Nude Models for Practicing Sketching Human Bodies]. *Zhongguo wenhua bao* [China Cultural News]. December 18.

China News Net. 2003. "Guojiajishengwei: Zhongguo meinian shengchan anquantao ershi yi zhi" [According to National Family Planning Commission: China Produces 200 Million Condoms a Year]. http://finance.sina.com.cn/b/20030129/0909307609 .shtml. Accessed August 2, 2008.

Chen, N. N. 2003. *Breathing Spaces: Qigong, Psychiatry, and Healing in China*. New York: Columbia University Press.

Chen, Z., et al. 2007. "Syphilis in China: Results of a National Surveillance Programme." *The Lancet* 369:132–138.

Chengshi Ribao [City Daily]. 2005. "Duihua Fudan jiaoshou Sun Zhongxin: Ta ba 'tongxinglian' tuidao qiantai" [A Dialogue with Professor Sun Zhongxin of Fudan: She Pushes Same-Sex Love to the Front]. November 5. http://news.enorth.com.cn/ system/2005/11/05/001157045.shtml. Accessed August 23, 2008.

D'Emilio, J., and E. B. Freedman. 1998. *Intimate Matters: A History of Sexuality in America*. 2nd ed. Chicago: University of Chicago Press.

Davis, D., ed. 2000. *The Consumer Revolution in Urban China*. Berkeley: University of California Press.

Deleuze, G. 1997. "Desire and Pleasure." In *Foucault and His Interlocutors*, edited by Arnold I. Davidson, 183–194. Chicago: University of Chicago Press.

Deng Y. 1998. "Cong zhongxin dao bianyuan" [From the Center to Margin]. *Chinese Market Economy Time*. March 6.

Engebretsen, E. L. 2009. "Intimate practices, conjugal ideals: Affective ties and relationship strategies among *lala* (lesbian) women in contemporary Beijing." *Sexuality Research & Social Policy* 6, no. 3:3–14.

Escoffier, J., ed. 2003. *Sexual Revolution*. New York: Thunder's Mouth Press.

Farquhar, J. 2002. *Appetites: Food and Sex in Post-Socialist China*. Durham, NC: Duke University Press.

Farrer, J. 2002. *Opening up: Sex and Market in Shanghai*. Chicago: University of Chicago Press.

———. 2007. "China's Women Sex Bloggers and the Dialogical Sexual Politics on the Chinese Internet." *China Aktuell—Journal of Current Chinese Affairs*, no. 4:1–36.

Foreman, W. 2009. "Gay Chinese Stand Up to Police Sweep of Hangout." *Associated Press*. September 14.

Foucault, M. 1990. *The History of Sexuality*. Volume 1. New York: Vintage Books.

————. 2006. "Omnes et Singulatim: Toward a Critique of Political Reason." In *The Chomsky-Foucault Debate on Human Nature*, 172–210. New York: New Press.

Greenhalgh, S., and E. A.Winckler. 2005. *Governing China's Population: From Leninist to Neoliberal Biopolitics*. Stanford, CA: Stanford University Press.

Hershatter, G. 1997. *Dangerous Pleasures: Prostitution and Modernity in Twentieth-Century Shanghai*. Berkeley: University of California Press.

Hyde, S. T. 2001. "Sex Tourism Practices on the Periphery: Eroticizing Ethnicity and Pathologizing Sex on the Lancang." In *China Urban*, edited by N. Chen, C. Clark, S. Gottschang, and L. Jeffrey, 143–164. Durham, NC: Duke University Press.

Kim. 1999. "Zhang Yue fangtanlu" [An Interview with Zhang Yue]. *Tiankong* [The Sky], no. 2. www.aizhi.org/jkwz/sky2.txt. Accessed August 5, 2008.

Li B. 2010. "Guanxi riji men juzhang bei shuangkai" [The Bureau Chief Caught Up in Diarygate is Double Demoted]. *Xinhua News Agency*. March 14.

Li C. and Sun L. 2008. "Jiemi wenge shouchaoben" [Shedding Light on Hand-Copied Books during the Cultural Revolution]. *Weekend*. August 22. http://news.sohu.com/20080222/n255305457_6.shtml. Accessed February 11, 2011.

Li Y. 2005. "Xifang xinggeming fenxi" [An Analysis of the Sexual Revolution in the West]. In *Zhongguo xingyanjiu de qidian he shiming* [The Point of Departure and the Mission of the Study of "Sexuality" in China], edited by Pan Suiming, 31–39. Gaoxiong: Wanyou chubanshe.

————.2006. "Regulating male same-sex relationships in the People's Republic of China." In *Sex and Sexuality in China*, edited by Elaine Jeffreys, 82–101. London: Routledge.

Li, Z. 1994. *The Private Life of Chairman Mao*. Translated by Tai Hung-Chao. New York: Random House.

Liang, Q., and C. Lee. 2006. "Fertility and population policy: An overview." In *Fertility, family planning, and population policy in China*, edited by D. Poston et al., 8–19. London: Routledge.

Liu W. 2007. *Zui yu fa: Zhongguo jinchang ershinian* [Crime and Punishment: Twenty Years of Striking against Prostitution]. Beijing: Zhongguo fulian chubanshe.

Marcuse, H. 1966. *Eros and Civilization*. Boston: Beacon Press.

McMillan, J. 2006. "Selling sexual health: China's emerging sex shop industry." In *Sex and Sexuality in China*, edited by Elaine Jeffreys, 124–138. London: Routledge.

Nanfangwang [Southern Net]. 2002. "Quanguo shouli xingguansi shengsu: Nanjing 'Qiuju' wei zhangfu chuqi" [The first lawsuit on sexual impairment: Nanjing's "Qiuju" seeks revenge for her husband]. www.southcn.com/news/community/fzzh/200211190369.htm. Accessed August 17, 2008.

Osburg, J. L. 2008. "Engendering Wealth: China's New Rich and the Rise of an Elite Masculinity." PhD dissertation, Department of Anthropology, University of Chicago.

Palmer, D. A. 2007. *Qigong fever.* New York: Columbia University Press

Pan S. 1995. *Zhongguo xing xianzhuang* [The Reality of Sexuality in China]. Beijing: Guangming ribao chubanshe.

————.2006. *Zhongguo xinggeming zhonglun* [An Overview of the Sexual Revolution in China]. Gaoxiong: Wanyou chubanshe.

Pan S. and Shi M. 2008. "Xingbing zibao fashenglu de shiduan gongxing jie yingxiang yinsu de huiguifenxi" [A Regressive Analysis of Shared Characteristics of Self Reports Concerning Sexually Transmitted Diseases within a Designated Period and the Relevant Factors]. *Hubei Daxue xuebao* 6:1–9.

Pan S. et al. 2005a. *Qingjing yu ganwu: Xinan sange hongdengqu tansuo* [Situation and Inspiration: A Study of Three Red Light Districts in Southwest China]. Gaoxiong: Wanyou chubanshe.

————. 2005b. *Chengxian yu biaoding: Zhongguo "xiaojie" shen yanjiu* [Performing and Labeling: An In-Depth Study of Female Sex Workers in China]. Gaoxiong: Wanyou chubanshe.

————. 2008. *Zhongguo xinggeming chenggong de shizheng* [The Empirical Evidence for the Accomplishment of the Chinese Sexual Revolution]. Gaoxiong: Wanyou chubanshe.

Parish, W. L., Ye, L., Stolzenberg, R., Laumann, E. O., Farrer, G., and Pan, S. 2007. "Sexual Practice and Sexual Satisfaction: A Population Based Study of Chinese Urban Adults." *Archives of Sexual Behavior* 36:5–20.

Peng X. 2005. "Dui 'sex' he 'sexuality' de taolun jiqi dingyi de Zhongwen fanyi" [A Discussion of the Terms "Sex" and "Sexuality," Their Definitions and Chinese Translations]. In *Zhongguo xingyanjiu de qidian he shiming* [The Point of Departure and the Mission of the Study of "Sexuality" in China], edited by Pan Suiming, 7–12. Gaoxiong: Wanyou chubanshe.

Phoenix Television. 2003. "An Interview with Sexologist Pan Suiming by Xu Gehui." http://v.ifeng.com/e/200808/e1f85092–6ebc-4900-a9a5–4a2e86598d84.shtml. Accessed September 26, 2009.

Reich, W. 1963. *The Sexual Revolution: Toward a Self-Governing Character Structure.* New York: Farrar, Straus and Giroux.

Rofel, L. 2007. *Desiring China: Experiments in Neoliberalism, Sexuality, and Public Culture.* Durham, NC: Duke University Press.

Ruan F. 2005. "Shi lun 'sexuality' de han yi" [On the Chinese Translation of "Sexuality"]. In *Zhongguo xingyanjiu de qidian he shiming* [The Point of Departure and the

Mission of the Study of "Sexuality" in China], edited by Pan Suiming, 13–30. Gaoxiong: Wanyou chubanshe.

Song Z. 2006. " 'Ziwo jieshi' yu 'jieceng rentong': Guanyu Beijing zhigao xuesheng
xingxingwei de ge'an yanjiu" ["Self explanations" and "status identification": A case
study of sexual behaviors of vocational school students in Beijing]. In *Zhongguo
xingyanjiu de qidian he shiming* [The Point of Departure and Mission of Chinese Sexuality Studies], ed. Pan Suiming. www.sexstudy.org/article.php?id=2711. Accessed
August 15, 2008.

Tucker, J. D., et al. 2005. "Surplus Men, Sex Work, and the Spread of HIV in China."
AIDS 19:539–547.

Uretsky, E. M. 2007. "Mixing Business with Pleasure: Masculinity and Male Sexual Culture in Urban China in the Era of HIV/AIDS." PhD dissertation, Department of
Sociomedical Sciences, Columbia University Mailman School of Public Health.

Wang, F., and Q. Yang. 1996. "Age at Marriage and the First Birth Interval: The Emerging Change in Sexual Behavior among Young Couples in China." *Population and Development Review* 22, no. 2:299–320.

Wang X., You Z., Liu J., and Jiang Q. 2009. *Zhuyi yu jiangou: Zhongguo xibei diqu xiaojie de shijie* [The Construction of Subjects: The World of xiaojie in China's North-
west]. Gaoxiong: Wanyou chubanshe.

Wen Y. 1979. "Zhi dazong dianying de zhubian he bianji tongzhi" [To Editor in Chief
and Editor Comrades of *Popular Films*]. June 10, 1979. http://i.mtime.com/liuhuang
su/blog/1484602/, accessed July 12 2010.

Woo, M. Y. K. 2006. "Contesting citizenship: Marriage and divorce in the People's Republic of China." In *Sex and Sexuality in China*, edited by Elaine Jeffreys, 62–81.
London: Routledge.

Xinmin zhoukan [Xinmin Weekly]. 2010. "Juzhang riji zhujiao hanfeng jiemi" [The
Hero in the Diaries of the Bureau Chief Han Feng Exposed]. www.cnd.org/my/
modules/wfsection/article.php%3Farticleid=25222. Accessed March 9, 2010.

Yan, Y. 2003. *Private Life under Socialism: Love, Intimacy, and Family Change in a Chinese Village, 1949–1999*. Stanford, CA: Stanford University Press.

Zhang B. 2004. "Zhang Beichuan dui Xinhua she 'guanzhu Zhongguo tongxinglian ren-
qun shengcun zhuangkuang' yiwen de jidian shuoming" [Zhang Beichuan on the
Article "Paying Attention to the Living Situation of Homosexuals in China" by Xinhua News Agency]. www.friendtongxin.com/2004xianzhuangshuoming.htm. Accessed August 12, 2005.

Zhang, E. Y. 2001. "Goudui and the State: Constructing Entrepreneurial Masculinity in
Two Cosmopolitan Areas in Southwest China." In *Gendered Modernities*, edited by
D. Hodgson, 235–266. New York: Palgrave.

―――. 2005. "Rethinking Sexual Repression in Maoist China: Ideology, Structure, and the Ownership of the Body." *Body and Society* 11, no. 3:1–25.

―――. 2007a. "Switching between Traditional Chinese Medicine and Viagra: Cosmopolitanism and Medical Pluralism Today." *Medical Anthropology* 26, no. 2:53–96.

―――. 2007b. "The Birth of nanke (Men's Medicine) in China: The Making of the Subject of Desire." *American Ethnologist* 34, no. 3:491–508.

―――. Forthcoming. "Flows between the Media and the Clinic: Desiring Production and Social Production in Urban Beijing." In *Trans/mediations: Erotics, Sociality, and "Asia,"* edited by Purnima Mankekar and Louisa Schein. Durham, NC: Duke University Press.

Zhang, H. 2006. "Female sex sellers and the public policy in the People's Republic." In *Sex and Sexuality in China,* edited by Elaine Jeffreys, 139–158. London: Routledge.

Zheng, T. 2009. *Red Lights: The Lives of Sex Workers in Postsocialist China.* Minneapolis: University of Minnesota.

Zhongxinwang [China News Service]. 2003. "Yan'an fuqi kan huangdie an 2002 nian zuihou yitian huashang juhao" [The Case of the Couple Watching Pornographic DVD Done Deal on the Last Day of 2000]. January 1. www.chinaelections.org/news info.asp?newsid=62759. Accessed August 12, 2008.

CHAPTER FOUR · Place Attachment, Communal
Memory, and the Moral Under-
pinnings of Gentrification in
Postreform Shanghai

Pan Tianshu

> Large scale changes in political economy and political
> power, as are taking place right now in our highly glo-
> balized world, change the cultural meanings we take for
> granted and the collective experience we are socialized
> into, and with them the self also changes, so that what
> we believe, how we act together, and who we are as indi-
> viduals also becomes something new. And that change
> extends to how we regard ourselves and others. The re-
> sult is that suffering, well-being, and the ethical practices
> that respond to human problems are constantly changing
> as local worlds change and as do we, the people in them,
> become something new and different.
>
> ARTHUR KLEINMAN, *What Really Matters*

Since the early 1990s, large-scale infrastructure projects have affected every corner
of Shanghai: ring roads, suspension bridges, tunnels, viaducts, subways, intercity
commuter trains, and a high-speed Maglev line were built simultaneously alongside
high rises, convention buildings, world trade centers, stadiums, and a host of shopping malls. Shortly after China's late paramount leader Deng Xiaoping completed
his carefully orchestrated and well-publicized "Inspection Tour of the South" (Nan
Xun) in 1992, Shanghai government officials launched a series of bold initiatives
that aimed to reclaim Shanghai's pre-1949 status as the most cosmopolitan city of
East Asia.[1] In March 2009, China's State Council gave the green light to speed up
the process of transforming Shanghai into a world-class international financial and
shipping center by the year 2020 against the backdrop of the current global financial crisis (R. Zhang 2009). As indicated clearly in the decision of the Central Government, Shanghai was expected to assume a key role in implementing the coun-

try's economic stimulus plan that would pour US$585 billion (RMB 4 trillion) into housing, water-and-energy projects, airport and railroad construction, and disaster relief.

"Development is the only hard truth," one of Deng Xiaoping's most quotable quotes, had already become an integral part of the hegemonic discourse exerting a profound impact on reform practices all over the country. As James Scott rightly points out, socialist leaders shared the same developmental logic as most believers in the transformative power of high modernism as more and more professionals, technicians, and engineers replaced amateurs after the revolutionary party achieved power (Scott 1998: 166–167). From an urban planning perspective, the insatiable desire to create an international metropolitan city arose from a significantly changed reconceptualization of megacities as globally oriented entities (Gaubatz 2005: 99). This reconceptualization was intensified during the late 1990s with the campaign for entry into the World Trade Organization (WTO) and the bids for hosting the 2008 Olympic Games in Beijing and the 2010 World Expo in Shanghai.

In the futuristic visions of the new generation of mayors and district officers, progress had to be measured in terms of the numbers and height of skyscrapers as if to demonstrate an unrivaled capability for transformation. Eager to become players and beneficiaries of China's unparalleled construction boom, the world's finest architects were drawn to various ambitious projects that would redefine the cities and the skylines (Jakes 2004). The official guideline dictated that the city of Shanghai should have "a new image every year, and every three years, a completely different image." The frequently updated city maps in the last decade best manifested the degree of spatial reconfiguration and urban sprawl.

Shanghai's landscape was altered not merely by the constant construction of roads and buildings, but more importantly by massive demographic shifts following the implementation of the economic reform in 1978. Owing to a rural-to-urban migration of unparalleled magnitude in Chinese history, the municipal authority could no longer retain the capacity to control and monitor the flow of the so-called floating population (migrant workers). The restructuring of the poorly managed and bankrupt state-owned enterprises (SOEs) significantly shrunk public-sector employment and created millions of *xiagang* ("those who stepped down from the sentry-post"), a euphemism for redundant and laid-off workers.

As casualties of the deepening economic reform, the *xiagang* proletariat witnessed in pain the collapse of a system of "organized dependency" (Walder 1986) along with the disappearance of the "iron rice bowl," a socialist metaphor for lifelong job security, affordable health care, subsidized housing, and retirement pensions. Millions of unemployed industrial workers in China found themselves in the anguishing process of adjusting to a new way of life centering on their community rather than their workplace. Unemployment drastically enlarged the marginal section of Chinese society that is officially labeled the "hardship population," traditionally including the elderly, the disabled, and the sick. Despite the fact that Shanghai had arguably the most sophisticated social welfare scheme in China, the fight against urban poverty was an uphill battle. For newly trained social workers, there seemed to be an endless supply of potential welfare recipients making all kinds of demands owing to Shanghai's socialist legacy. This legacy defined Shanghai as an industrial city, the locus of thousands of mills, plants, shipyards, and other industrial works that formed the nation's major rustbelt in the early 1990s. Meanwhile the steady, proportional increase of an aging population with a limited number of single children to assist them—an unintended consequence of the family planning policy—and the persistence of early retirement practices in SOEs also prompted experimentation with social-security schemes and community-based service programs, especially in the city's poor neighborhoods, where one could feel the devastating effects of the economic and social transition.

In the aftermath of the current world financial crisis, officials in Shanghai have had to confront an additional source of social instability: graduating college seniors and migrant workers searching desperately for jobs. Staff members from the various departments of the municipal government felt morally compelled to devote huge amounts of time and energy to accommodating the needs of the unemployed and underemployed, because they were acutely aware of the tradition of rebellion in the nation's "cradle of the proletarian class" and the birthplace of the Chinese Communist Party. If no concrete actions were carried out to alleviate the agony of those who had yet to partake in the economic bonanza, the lofty goal that the party-state set for itself to "build a harmonious society" would remain a cruelly distant dream.

Shanghai's ongoing transformation of geographical and social spaces—unprecedented in magnitude—has changed the nature of moral experiences and reshaped power relationships among individuals, institutions, and localities. One of the most popular sayings that one encountered during conversations with friends and colleagues in recent years best summarized the impact of such rapid socioeconomic restratification on the way the city's space was reimagined. According to the bitter truth this quip conveyed: the English speakers had taken over the inner ring of the city, the Mandarin speakers had moved into the middle ring, and the Shanghainese speakers could only find their niche in the outer ring. While far from being an accurate depiction of empirical reality, the saying did indicate noticeable changes occurring in China's most cosmopolitan city: the gradual expansion of an international community (subsumed under the broad category of "English speakers"), the increase of "new Shanghainese," the specially talented people from other regions who possessed the credentials to qualify for household registration status,[2] and the marginalization of those "Shanghainese speakers," unemployed workers, impoverished and displaced residents or evictees who could no longer afford to live in gentrified neighborhoods in the city.

To a certain extent, the three rings corresponded to differing degrees of cultural and moral worth among those who inhabited the core, semiperiphery, and periphery of the everyday social world of postsocialist Shanghai. More importantly, the aphorism suggests that the profound social and economic transformations had hardly blurred the age-old dichotomy between the lower quarter (low end) and upper quarter (high end). In the Shanghainese dialect, the "upper quarters" *(shang zhi jiao)* indicates "uptown" or "the right side of the tracks." The "lower quarters" *(xia zhi jiao)* is a synonym for shantytown housing or shacks *(penghu)* located on the "wrong side of the tracks." In everyday discourse, the lower/upper quarter dichotomy remains a linguistic device strategically appropriated by the Shanghainese to delineate the cultural and moral boundaries of their neighborhoods and their perception of the social and economic reality of where they belonged. If the upper quarters continue to stand for modernity and civilization in the popular imagination, the lower quarters beyond the neon lights remain a symbol of backwardness and moral inferiority.[3]

Based on ethnographic research and field observations that I conducted intermittently in different urban communities from 1999 to 2009, this chapter examines the impact of the spatial memory of the city's neighborhoods, dichotomized as the "upper and lower quarters," on the ways in which notions of locality-based citizenship are essentialized and reified. As the Shanghainese equivalent of English terms such as *uptown/downtown* or *upscale/ghetto* that encode the race and class relations in many North American cities, the dichotomy between the lower quarter and the upper quarter is a "disparity index" that can be used to measure the social and moral distance between the powerful and the marginal. Such a binary opposition between the high and low, as I will argue in this chapter, has furthered a preexisting discourse on how cultural and moral personhoods can be identified, differentiated, and judged on the basis of spatial hierarchy in a diverse and internationalized society. Mapping neighborhood Shanghai in time and space thus helps me to locate the cultural symbols in actual sites, so that upper quarters and lower quarters can be observed and analyzed as segregated moral worlds. Using the intimate perspectives provided by ethnographic fieldwork, I explore how the lower/upper quarter dichotomy embeds what I will call locality power, place attachment, and meanings of moral self-worth. I show how this prevailing dichotomy is exploited, and I also emphasize the individuated memories to which it is linked, and more importantly, the justifying legitimacy it provides for present-day reconfiguration of the physical and moral landscape. This chapter treats the spatial dichotomy as a lens for the examination of the ways in which city-dwellers go about meeting the exigencies of their everyday lives as they try to make sense of the ongoing gentrification processes in neighborhood Shanghai.

In the context of urban renewal in the postindustrial world, "gentrification" has often been interpreted as middle-class settlement or resettlement in older inner-city neighborhoods formerly occupied mostly by working-class and underclass residents (e.g., Anderson 1990; Butler 2003; Caulifield 1994). In this chapter, gentrification refers to a cultural and moral process of urban change brought forth by socialist engineering and community development during the reform era (1978–present). As far as spatial reconfiguration in neighborhood Shanghai is concerned, we are able to discern two parallel forms of gentrification in the upper and lower quarters. Within the former French Concession and the International Settlement, the ongoing gentrification process can be explained in its conventional sense, except that inner-city neighborhoods in post-1949 Shanghai were never a "downtown," despite the signs of urban decay in certain parts. Many such neighborhoods retained the status and self-image of being coupled with a sense of the cultural and moral superiority of the upper quarter. As a subtle but vivid expression of the spatial dichotomy, the current urban design ideology intersects with gentrification practices that have shaped Shanghai's neighborhoods in the past as well as recent appropriations and transformations of those spaces.

The 1990s witnessed the emergence and growth of "Shanghai nostalgia," a multifaceted process of manipulating collective memories for the rediscovery, reevaluation, and reinvention of Shanghai's pre-Communist colonial past (e.g., X. Zhang 2000). As a cultural industry, Shanghai nostalgia was actively promoted by the city's social and economic elites as well as by government officials. The officially sanctioned nostalgia for a selectively remembered and reimagined colonial Shanghai served the long-term goal of turning an increasingly global city into a commercial hub of East Asia. As a simultaneous development, Shanghai nostalgia has given rise to aggressive gentrification schemes in the former colonial concessions and international settlements exemplified by the restoration and renovation of old-style villas and mansions along with the construction of skyscrapers and modern apartment buildings. Despite the fears of a real-estate bubble, the housing market has remained robust for Shanghai's inner ring, especially the upper quarters.

This chapter begins with a discussion of the everyday discourse on lower quarters and upper quarters, which corresponds to different and unequal kinds of morality and citizenship. From the colonial past to the late socialist present, these notions were among the most meaningful categories for articulating one's socioeconomic position and moral status in society. The persistence of the dichotomy points to the limits of the social engineering attempts (1949–78) and postreform community building efforts (1978–present) aimed at eliminating inequality and promoting brotherhood within and between Shanghai's residential quarters.

In the second section, I examine the local management of the remnants of a failed socialist system, a system that not long ago was the key provider for the hundreds of thousands of industrial workers in Shanghai. In this chapter I use the term *debris* to describe the material realities of East China's main rustbelts, a plain social fact in a Durkheimian sense. The term *debris* also refers to the moral and psychosocial consequences that resulted from the loss of a major Maoist legacy for laid-off workers in gentrified neighborhoods such as Bay Bridge, which I will introduce later.

The last section on showcasing citizenship examines the impact of the global flow of knowledge and ideas in the late 1990s on community-building practices. The younger generation of street officers adopted a selective strategy that aimed at turning a gentrifying neighborhood into a showcase "civilized community." Their efforts to help the lower quarters attain the prestigious kind of cultural citizenship previously reserved for the upper quarters, as indicated by my field observation, achieved limited success owing to the discrepancy between the modernist and futuristic visions of municipal officials and the harsh local conditions in a depressed and demoralized lower quarter.

WHY PLACE MATTERS: THE MORAL
UNDERPINNINGS OF THE SPATIAL IMAGINATION

Over the past 150 years, the twin process of urbanization and industrialization have transformed Shanghai from a rural county seat into a cosmopolitan city, and in the process produced strata that represent radically different lifestyles, local histories, native place identities, and living environments. Like nearly every Chinese metropolis, Shanghai proclaimed itself, and even felt itself to be, a city of quarters divided and marked by different strands of communal memory and cultural identities. As a reflection of both historical imagination and economic reality, the notion of "quarters" was employed self-consciously by local residents, municipal officials, and real-estate agents as a strategic device to position themselves in everyday social life and gauge the moral and cultural quality *(suzhi)* of the inhabitants of particular locales.

Historically, the upper quarters were the neighborhoods with enclaves of foreign populations—the French, the British, the Americans, and the Jews who had fled Russia and Eastern Europe. Under socialism most of the Western-style buildings located on the Bund continued for over fifty years to perform their former functions as commercial (banks and trading companies) and government (a customs office and municipal court) institutions. Within the upper quarters, a beautiful house with a garden and backyard, well protected by an iron gate and thick walls, would often be the residence of a top government official. Yet in the same neighborhood, a colonial-style apartment building might house more than a dozen families who had moved in after the original owner fled Shanghai on the eve of the Communist takeover in 1949. It is important to note that for most of the ordinary residents living in the former International Settlement and the French Concession, their sense of moral and cultural superiority derived from the very location of their home and not necessarily their actual housing conditions.

Owing to the historical legacy of the Maoist urban planning scheme, which aimed at both limiting population and controlling residence, inner-city neighborhoods in Shanghai have retained their upper-quarter status despite the profound changes of Shanghai's city landscape brought forth by the construction boom of the 1990s. The old Chinese city, officially referred to as Nanshi ("the Southern District"), which occupies the middle ground between the upper and lower quarters, is a good case in point. Now part of Huangpu District (previously the International Settlement) as a result of recent redistricting, Nanshi has been turned into a tourist attraction, exhibiting a reinvented local culture with an origin that could be traced back more than seven hundred years. While feeling proud of the Temple of City Gods, the Yu Garden and nearby teahouse, and the restored Confucian Temple, the local residents are rather embarrassed by their living environment. Until very recently, the Nanshi District had been the most densely populated residential area in the city. Old wooden houses and alleyway buildings were the major forms of housing. Despite the inconvenience of having to put up with communal kitchens and public toilets, many would choose to remain in the district for both nostalgic and practical reasons. On the one hand, their sense of belonging originated from being the residents of a unique place rich in history and traditions. Each accidental archeological discovery (e.g., remnants of a chamber dating back to the Song dynasty) during the current wave of infrastructural development further affirmed their belief in the cultural and moral worth of a dilapidated neighborhood. Living within walking distance of the upper quarters, on the other hand, makes them feel protected from the bad influences from the lower quarters, only minutes away to the west of Nanshi.

In local terms, the lower quarters had always been associated with stereotypical images of narrow lanes inhabited by the Subei people, the descendents of migrants and refugees from northern Jiangsu who spoke a dialect distinctively different from Shanghainese. The derogatory term *Subei* might be just a designation that was conceived by residents elsewhere in the city and not necessarily an objective description of their place of origin, as Honig rightly argues (1992: 28–35). Yet the lower quarters, the very source of cultural prejudice against the Subei people in Shanghai, has remained a material reality and a mental category for decades. Shanghai's lower quarters were seen as the armpit of the city, and were stereotyped as undesirable places where one would expect to see the vicious cycle of urban poverty, illegal housing, family breakdown, moral degradation, and social disorganization.

The dichotomy between lower and upper quarters has been a key reference point for the city administrators as they proceeded to identify the social and economic characteristics of a particular neighborhood and mark out the boundaries of residential enclaves. After 1949, the districts within the entire Shanghai municipality were reorganized in such a way that a district became an administrative region of several subdivisions referred to as "streets and avenues," or *jiedao* in Chinese. Each subdistrict formed a constituency governed by the street office appointed by the district government. Because of the desire of Communist city planners to eliminate or at least minimize the inequalities in income and housing conditions between districts, the goal of redistricting was to combine administrative spheres that fell into the pre-1949 categories of the lower quarters *and* upper quarters. The geographical boundaries that separated poor districts from the rich ones disappeared on the city map of the new Shanghai after 1949. Yet, within each newly configured district, the cultural and moral boundaries that used to separate the lower quarters from upper quarters continued to exist.

While demarcation lines between the quarters, such as walls, fences, and paths, became less visible, the establishment of subdistrict street offices served to reify the difference between the socioeconomic statuses of those inhabiting neighborhoods that represented two totally different social worlds. In everyday bureaucratic practice, the leaders of the street office actually acknowledged existing differences by establishing residents' committees based on the types of neighborhood, the living conditions, and even the native-place origins of the inhabitants. The alleyways and lanes within the jurisdiction of the street office as well as the allocation of space to particular uses and sizes of buildings, therefore, became an overt expression of the total gamut of social and moral behavior characteristic of a certain residential quarter.

As if to rid the city of its colonial past and to reflect the changes brought by the founding of New China in 1949, the English and French names of the streets within the upper quarters were changed into Chinese ones. Ford Lane became Fujian Road while Route Lafayette became Fuxing Road (which literally means "the street of revitalization"). The street names within the lower quarters, for the most part, were purposefully kept. Socialist citizenship was not only defined by class affiliation but also reflected in the official spatializing strategies in neighborhood Shanghai. According to my observation, it was a common practice for the local officials to keep the names of the lanes within the lower quarters (e.g., those indicative of the residents' native place such as "Subei Lane" and "Nantong Lane") until the 1970s.

Redrawing administrative boundaries between the urban districts and renaming streets and lanes after the Communist takeover in 1949 failed to dissolve the upper/lower quarter dichotomy. The fundamental divide among segregated residential quarters was not only reflected on the social and political maps but also materialized on the ground. Luwan District, where the primary field site for my inquiry is located, is one such example in which one can actually see the reclaiming of gentility in its upper quarter and the sweeping of the debris of socialism down to its lower quarter. After 1950, Luwan had within its jurisdiction four subdistricts under the control of four street offices. Three of the four subdistricts were located in the former French Concession (1842–1945). Within these subdistricts, Avenue Joffre was renamed Huaihai Road, commemorating a military campaign that led to the revolutionary victory in China's civil war (1947–49). The upper quarter remained the upscale section of the residential areas of Luwan where the district leaders lived and worked. In contrast, Bay Bridge, the fourth subdistrict added to Luwan after 1949, like its counterparts elsewhere in Shanghai, had retained its lower quarter status, and was inhabited by the descendants of migrants, refugees, and farmers who were not able to properly speak the Shanghai dialect. As described in the following pages, Bay Bridge seemed to share all the defining characteristics of a lower quarter in terms of geographical location, native place of origin, and the social and moral standing of the local population.

MANAGING THE SOCIAL
AND MORAL DEBRIS IN BAY BRIDGE

Having grown up in a mixed neighborhood in Huangpu District (a borderland between the pre-1945 International Settlement and the French Concession) that was separated from the northern section of Luwan District by one street, I myself had never heard of Bay Bridge as a teenager, even though I had visited a dental hospital on its east end (belonging to another district). When I appeared embarrassed at such an oversight of the actual existence of a real community, my cadre friends and even residents of the community assured me that there was no reason why one should know about Bay Bridge in the first place; "it was a lower quarter after all."

Aunt Lu, a veteran staff member of the residents' committee located in Pingming, the most crowded housing community of Bay Bridge, told me that her youngest son, who held a PhD in electrical engineering from the University of Texas, would choose to stay at a hotel nearby during his homecoming visits. With mixed feelings Aunt Lu remarked that her boy had worked hard to change his fate and would surely earn a place in the upper quarter. As an improved moral and cultural being, he would never come back because he didn't belong to Bay Bridge any more. Later Aunt Lu told me that her son had been a role model for the children in the neighborhood who dreamed to "get out of the place." Inspired by the success stories of Aunt Lu's son, one of "the boys next door" became a top athlete on the National Basketball Team. Hailed as "Yao Ming's best teammate" from Shanghai, the hometown hero never cared to acknowledge that he was born and bred in Bay Bridge.

The lower quarter status of Bay Bridge was reified, as I gradually learned over the course of my field research, because of the additional sources of moral and social stigma attached to the entire locality. First, a well-established funeral site prior to 1949 was believed to have disrupted the system of geomancy *(fengshui)* that augured well for good fortune. The locality was further "polluted" in the aftermath of the notorious Japanese bombing of Shanghai in 1937 that had effectively turned Bay Bridge into one of the city's biggest graveyards, where thousands of dead bodies were discarded without proper burial. During the civil war, the "ghost land" of Bay Bridge became a haven for both the bandits evolved from the defeated soldiers of the Nationalist Army and the landlords who had fled their home villages in the aftermath of the Communist Land Reform (1945–50). Even during the present construction boom, the inauspicious indications of an unspoken and unspeakable past often disturbed those living in the present as human bones and skeletons were unearthed in virtually all the sites upon which high-rise office and apartment buildings were being built.

The pre-1949 Bay Bridge had more than enough attributes to qualify as the lowest of the city's lower quarters—graves and garbage, dirty ponds and stagnant creeks, squatter settlements, beggars and tramps, mosquitoes and flies. The historical connection with death, funerals, filth, and starving beggars became a major source of stigma that reinforced the marginalization of the area even after 1949. The lack of decent schools, hospitals, movie theaters, and other cultural institutions confirmed its social and economic status. The people of Bay Bridge could never expect to be treated equally by the "legitimate" Shanghainese in the upper quarters, even though they were legally registered as permanent residents of Shanghai under the *hukou* system. Small wonder that the local cadres dispatched from the Luwan District Government (which was, ironically, located in the upper quarter, the former French Concession) referred to Bay Bridge as "Luwan's Siberia," a "heartbroken island." In the eyes of these civilizing agents (colonial administrators and communist cadres alike), Bay Bridge was a special reserve for the disenfranchised people who had no culture, no traditions, no history, and, ultimately, no morality.

What set Bay Bridge apart from other comparable underclass neighborhoods in the city's periphery was, however, its proximity to the northern section of Luwan District, which claimed upper-quarter status because it had been part of the French Concession. To the best knowledge of the urban planners I interviewed, Bay Bridge was among the very few lower quarters in the city that were in the vicinity of historical landmarks. To its north was the restored holy site of the "Birthplace of the Chinese Communist Party," where the First Congress of the CCP was held in July 1921. To its south was Jiangnan Shipyard (an arsenal during the later Imperial era), which was called the "Cradle of China's Proletarian Class" in the official history. To its east and in the center of Nanshi, the "City of Temple Gods," a walled city for the Chinese residents in the colonial days, had become a showcase exhibiting local cultures and customs. Located to its far west was a Catholic cathedral known for its pivotal role in promoting the Chinese understanding of the West three centuries ago.

In Luwan's northern section (i.e., the upper quarters), colonial style villas, hotels, and clubs were well preserved and restored, while the red-brick terrace buildings that once housed the pre-1949 middle class were meticulously renovated and refurbished. On the once hallowed ground of socialist Shanghai, the pre-1945 "borderland" between the French Concession and the International Settlement, where the first CCP congress convened in 1921, a cluster of restored nineteenth-century colonial row houses emerged. This US$150 million project was the brain child of

Hong Kong's Victor Lo, the chairman of the Shui On Group, who had long dreamed of turning this old part of the French Concession into a picturesque tourist attraction that showcased Shanghai's colonial era with designer boutiques, hip cafes, and a shopping mall. With the collaboration of Luwan District officials, the architectural face-lift involved the razing of five square blocks and displaced hundreds of families, some of whom had lived in the neighborhood for decades. The project also led to the demolition of a century-old French manor house that belonged to I. M. Pei's family, despite the official aim to set a precedent for the preservation of Shanghai's cultural heritage.

As if to make an overt statement, this project was named "Xin Tian Di," meaning the "New Heaven and Earth" where "yesterday meets tomorrow in Shanghai today," as indicated in its promotional brochure. Since the founding of the CCP was said to represent a new era with the promise of creating a new heaven and earth for the Chinese people, the establishment of Xin Tian Di seemed to proclaim the postsocialist triumph of capitalism over communism right at the heart of the CCP's birthplace. It is important to note that the completion of the Xin Tian Di project in 2001 coincided with President Jiang's "theory of three representations." That theory had been incorporated into the revised Constitution of the Chinese Communist Party on the eve of its eightieth anniversary. According to Jiang's three representations, the CCP in the future should represent the most advanced forces of production, elite culture, and the interests of the majority of Chinese people. In light of this theory, the high modernist principles and futuristic visions embedded in gentrification practices started to make sense. Yet one could not help wondering what such a grand scheme of cultural differentiation and moral orientation would mean to those living in the city's lower quarters.

Although within walking distance of historical landmarks that monumentalized the city's past, Bay Bridge has remained a marginalized lower quarter that was never a part of the pre-1945 French Concession. Xujiahui Road (now a four-lane expressway) has always served as the demarcation line separating the upper quarter of Luwan District from the unfashionable south, where Bay Bridge is located. The continuing presence of both upper quarters and lower quarters in Luwan is evidenced by the coexistence of built forms within the district. As I walked from northern Luwan to Bay Bridge, I could detect a gradual change in housing patterns, from the fancy if small European-style villas sandwiched between the postmodern highrises, to the more traditional terraced houses that blended into rows of matchbox-shaped six-story walk-ups. Within Bay Bridge, the match box-shaped buildings and the century-old dilapidated wooden houses were the typical forms of dwelling and settlements for the local residents. Even in the twenty-first century, it is not difficult to spot traces of squatter settlements in Bay Bridge's oldest and poorest community, "the commoners' village" (a homonym with "the paupers' village," both pronounced *pinmin* in the Shanghai dialect).

Until it became an officially designated "Model Community" in 1995, Bay Bridge had rarely been considered a place worth writing about. As the biggest territorial subdivision of Luwan, occupying an area of 3.07 square kilometers inhabited by 81,634 registered residents, Bay Bridge is given hardly any attention in the District Gazette's 244 pages—merely two pages of introduction to its population and neighborhood organization structure. For the district officials who set their visions high, Bay Bridge could not possibly match the standard of the prosperous Luwan District, whose public image recalled colonial gentility while also symbolizing postsocialist prosperity. The conspicuous absence of an official account of everyday life in the city's underclass neighborhood can be explained by the social and political context of post-Deng Shanghai's relentless bid for an internationally oriented millennium. So how could a lower quarter like Bay Bridge represent itself in an increasingly global city? In the summer of 2000, I presented a street office with a report on the undocumented history of the pre-1949 past of Bay Bridge with the hope that they could use some of my findings for an upcoming exhibition on the past and present of the neighborhood. To my surprise and dismay, the street officer and his colleagues acknowledged the time and effort I took in "writing so much about so small a community," but showed very little interest in what I wrote about. They implicitly criticized me for being too obsessed with the past of Bay Bridge. The past had practically nothing to do with their present, let alone the future they envisioned for themselves.

My cadre friends' lack of interest in my work could be conveniently explained by the fact that the newly acquired knowledge of Bay Bridge's past had allowed me to intrude not just into the private lives within the community, but also the privacy of their collective space. However, after several follow-up visits to Bay Bridge, I realized that aside from the potential damage that such intimate knowledge of a previously "contaminated" locality could do to the image of Bay Bridge, there is a serious economic interest at stake. In 2001, the difference in the sales value of a housing unit located in the lower quarter and that of a unit in the upper quarter could be as significant as one thousand yuan (approximately US$150) per square meter. There was very little the local cadres could do to stop the *fengshui* (geomancy) masters of Hong Kong, Macao, and Taiwan from collecting and disseminating such "dangerous" information about the fact that Bay Bridge was once a highly polluted locality haunted by "hungry ghosts."

Like their counterparts in charge of other lower quarters in neighborhood Shanghai, the cadres of Bay Bridge seized every possible opportunity to elevate the social and moral status of their neighborhood and developed various strategies of competing for community resources, media coverage, and attention from the municipal officials. The community construction movement, beginning in the early 1950s, became their best chance to change the image of the lower quarter by erasing its unspeakable past and monumentalizing its present for the purpose of creating a model community of a civilized and scientific way of living in a modernist city. Each generation of street officers shared the idea that, as a typically marginalized place, Bay Bridge was no more than a blank sheet of paper on which they could paint beautiful pictures and implement their well-conceived plans to improve the cultural and moral quality of the inhabitants of this lower quarter. Some of the pictures, as I show in the following sections, faded as time went by while others turned into hollow showcases or even figments of the imagination.

Since the early 1990s, the global flow of knowledge and ideas has had a profound impact on local bureaucratic practices in both the upper and lower quarters. Along with the introduction of Western concepts of efficient business management, city administrators replaced outmoded socialist jargon with such terms as "social work," "sustainable development," and "community service." These modernizing terms were appropriated to authorize the gentrification and revitalization process. As post-Deng Shanghai engaged in a relentless bid to regain its pre-1945 status through establishing new central business districts on both sides of the Huangpu River, state factories located in the city's periphery, where most of the lower quarters were, marched toward an inevitable end of their productive life.

Determined to bid farewell to the city's recent past as the nation's industrial hub, the Shanghai political elite chose to terminate the operation of many SOEs, which included run-down steel plants, mechanical works, and textile factories. At a highly publicized event known as *yading* ("smashing the spindles") in 1999, hundreds of thousands of spindles were smashed as cameramen from all the major media networks faithfully recorded this historical moment on the eve of China's ascension to the WTO. What the official cameramen failed to capture was the sense of disorientation and demoralization of the unfortunate victims of Shanghai's accelerating industrial restructuring and urban revitalization processes.

The gradual emergence of transnational and private firms and the death of SOEs in post-Deng Shanghai made the city a place where different modes of living were on display under the same neon lights reminiscent of Shanghai's colonial era. On the one hand, gated communities managed by local or transnational real estate developers made their appearance on the land acquired from the owners of bankrupt or poorly managed SOEs. In a sense, the built forms of high-rise apartments in a typical "lower quarter" such as Bay Bridge were literally the sprouts of capitalism grown out of the debris of socialism. On the other hand, the advent of gated communities did not immediately result in the forceful relocation of the local residents. In fact, the process of gentrification was relatively slow, especially in comparison with what went on in the upper quarter. The upper quarter (the pre-1945 French Concession), which used to be part of a famous shopping street named after Joseph Joffre, a French general, came to relive its glorious past as overseas investors assumed an active role in transforming its cultural and political landscape. More and more shopping malls (one of which is Sincere, whose owner fled to Hong Kong on the eve of the 1949 liberation) were put up, often with Hong Kong money. The historical building of the colonial French Municipal Council was completed revamped and became home to cafes, restaurants, and designer clothing and accessory stores.

As recipients of a culture of conspicuous consumption and avid consumers of "Shanghai nostalgia," the new generation of yuppies in Luwan's upper quarter tended to be employees of joint ventures and foreign companies working in the office highrises concentrated in the district's Pacific Hong Kong Plaza, which appeared to be a recast of its original in Hong Kong. As college postgraduates born in the 1970s, the yuppies were well educated, with good computer and English-language skills. The beneficiaries of the economic reform that favors the young, the beautiful, and the affluent, many of the yuppies became local representatives of transnational corporations and earned an annual income equivalent to what their parents might have made as factory workers over a span of ten or more years. A decade ago the upper quarter of Luwan District allegedly had the highest concentration of head-hunting companies serving the needs of "job hoppers" working in the adjacent buildings.

The images of affluent yuppies that dominated the covers of fashion magazines, unabashedly showcasing economic prosperity in the upper quarter, stood in stark contrast to what went on in the lower quarter of Bay Bridge, which witnessed the emergence of a new generation of *xiagang*. For the ordinary residents in the neighborhood, "Shanghai nostalgia," experienced by those living in the upper quarter, represented nothing more than a lifestyle and mode of consumption they could not afford. As more and more state-owned factories (mostly in the textile and steel industries) declared bankruptcy, hundreds of thousands of laid-off workers became members of the "urban poor," eligible for welfare assistance. A sad truth for the Luwan District bureaucrats to confront at the ground level was that the increase of *xiagang* clearly outpaced the growth of yuppies in Luwan and elsewhere in Shanghai. While a yuppie was enjoying a cup of cappuccino in Park '97 (a cafe modeled after its Hong Kong prototype) or a recently opened Starbucks and planning to buy a second or third apartment in the old French Concession, the *xiagang* in Bay Bridge were worrying about how to pay their monthly bills. Widely publicized annual events such as the "Rose Wedding" in October (organized by the District Tourist Bureau), starring one hundred yuppie couples in shiny limos parading in the upper quarter, only heightened the sense of distance and despair on the part of the gradually marginalized *xiagang* in the lower quarter.

In Bay Bridge, the small- and medium-sized state-owned factories reached such a deteriorated condition that they were either on the verge of bankruptcy or sold to corporate real-estate developers. Recall that in the 1950s, most of these factories and processing plants were constructed to replace the temples, shrines, and guild halls as the landmarks representing the new socialist social and moral order. Prior to the reform era, industrialization had characterized the Maoist approach to urbanization in China. Smokestacks were auspicious signs of triumphant socialism practiced in and outside the city's neighborhoods. Four decades later, the smoke had stopped and the rusty iron gates could barely survive amid the debris of torn-down buildings and workshops.

Psychologically unprepared for the sudden loss of the "iron rice bowl" of secure lifelong employment, the *xiagang* of Bay Bridge, like their comrades elsewhere in China, found themselves in the midst of a mid-life crisis, struggling to restructure their everyday life. And this occurred while they became increasingly dependent on their neighborhood rather than the work unit that once gave them institutional and collective identity. They were afraid of reentering the labor market because they thought that they had long lost the ability to compete. Whenever they became nostalgic for the "good old days," they felt they were being shortchanged.

Identifying *xiagang* as a key source of social instability, if not a potential cause for labor insurgencies, the Shanghai Municipal Government decided to tackle the pressing issues of unemployment and welfare reform with the aim of assuaging the disgruntled workers. Huang Ju (1938–2007), then the party secretary of Shanghai, made the point repeatedly at meetings with district officials that "we must resolve any social conflicts at the grassroots level" for the sake of social stability. Since the mid-1990s, the party secretariat has made numerous visits to residential communities in the city's lower quarters where *xiagang* are concentrated. During an informal interview in 2001, the general manager of the Shanghai Textile Group (formerly

the State Textile Bureau) told me with much relief that his effort in cutting the total number of textile workers from 550,000 to 250,000 did not lead to any collective
action such as public protest. One of the community beat cops confided to me that
confronting the desperate *xiagang* ("who had nothing to lose and nothing to fear")
in Bay Bridge was actually more challenging than handling the student protesters
back in 1989 or hunting down the adherents of the Falun Gong cult in 1999.

In preparation for the large-scale downsizing of state-owned factories, government officials in Shanghai in recent years devised various reemployment schemes
and piloted welfare assistance and reemployment programs that have been cham-
pioned as a model to replicate nationwide. During an interview conducted in 1999,
an official working in the local branch of the Ministry of Civil Affairs boasted to
me that he and his colleagues were pioneers in setting the first poverty level in China;
they also developed schemes such as food coupon books and poverty relief funds
as early as 1993. Yet, he acknowledged with candor that despite the systematic
changes in social welfare reform, the municipal government still lacked the capacity to deal effectively with the greatest crisis in urban management since 1949.

From the perspective of the municipal officials, official neighborhood organizations, represented by the street office and the affiliated residents' committees, should
enhance their dual role as grassroots institutions of social control and also welfare
service providers. In routine practice, my cadre friends on the residents' committee
found the *xiagang* to be the most difficult to deal with among all welfare applicants.
This was because their unemployment status did not automatically make a *xiagang*
an eligible welfare recipient.[4] The committee cadres in charge often had a hard time
figuring out the "real income" of the applicant. For most *xiagang*, the sudden loss
of the "iron rice bowl" of secure lifelong employment was totally out of the blue.
While some *xiagang* were fortunate enough to receive a portion of their original
salary as compensation, many of their comrades had to "return home empty-
handed." If they became sick, they would rather stay at home than go to see a doctor because there was no guarantee that the medical expenses would be reimbursed
under the new circumstances.

For well over four decades, China's industrial workers had worn the badge of
honor as members of the vanguard class. As legitimate city-dwellers, their sense of
cultural and moral worth was affirmed by the affiliation with a state-owned enterprise or government institution. Yet as *xiagang*, the unemployed workers found
themselves in an irreversible process of making a transition from "work-unit persons" *(danwei ren)* to "society persons" *(shehui ren)*. Such a transition was both demoralizing and undignified. In order to get back what they believed the state owed

them, the desperate *xiagang* in Bay Bridge would try to do whatever they could to fight for what they deserved (even if they were deemed "not eligible"). The small office of the resident's committee became an outlet for them to vent their anger and despair. The residents' committee cadres, unfortunately, were misidentified by some frustrated *xiagang* as bureaucrats who lacked "human feelings and sympathy." In one case, a frustrated applicant who was told that he failed to qualify as a welfare recipient because of the recent change of policy, shouted at the committee cadre, "If you do not let me eat, I won't let you shit!" What he meant was he would go on strike in the office until the cadres gave in. In another case, a *xiagang* unabashedly said, "Listen, I am a member of the Communist Party . . . the party-state has an obligation to take care of me! And *I* am entitled to all the welfare benefits." The committee cadres were shocked and speechless. Such words of anger not only pointed to the obvious failure of the Party's ideological effort in educating its members to be "selfless and patriotic," but also indicated a sadly ironic sense of moral confusion among the working class members of the "Party for the Workers."

No doubt the current urban crisis had reemphasized the role of the neighborhood organization as the buffer between the state and the people. In practice, residents' committee cadres were constantly confronted with the dilemmas of social and moral transformation: without a well-developed social safety net, who would be willing to care for those who are not "making it" in the new, globalizing economy? Within the local community, who would possibly be able to manage the debris of the system created under Maoism?

In Bay Bridge, the "granny cadres" from the residents' committees were once champions of social rights and welcomed by the majority of the residents, especially among the poor and needy. The power of these seemingly weak elderly women derived from the moral legitimacy built up slowly over the several decades they had worked for the community. Most of them started working as volunteers or activists for the neighborhood organization in the 1950s or the early 1960s. Even in the 1990s, these granny cadres still remained an indispensable and formidable force in maintaining the order and stability of the local community. In the absence of a well-structured judiciary court system, the residents' committees often played an important role in mediating and settling disputes among feuding neighbors and even between relatives. In Bay Bridge, the elderly, the sick, the disabled, the widowed, and the relatives of "revolutionary martyrs" (parents and widows of deceased military personnel) had long been the beneficiaries of state welfare policies. As the neighborhood became increasingly gentrified, some granny cadres expressed acute concern over the possible loss of a moral tradition of caring that they had prided themselves on upholding as the government attempted to professionalize the social services and its local agencies.

Although seldom treating these granny cadres as their social equals, the current generation of forward-looking street officers and district leaders confided to me that these old ladies had been crucial in helping implement state welfare policies over the decades at the "base level" (i.e., grassroots). Unfortunately, the street officers also believed that the historical mission of the granny cadres had been fulfilled and that these elderly women could no longer function effectively to deal with new challenges. Since the mid-1990s, the granny cadres in Bay Bridge were gradually replaced by the "textile sisters" *(fangsao)*, the laid-off workers from bankrupt state-owned factories. After these textile-sisters went through a program of reemployment sponsored by the district government, they were recruited by the street office as social workers as part of the ongoing scheme to professionalize the neighborhood organizations.

Unlike the granny cadres, these textile sisters were not embedded in the local communities. Most granny cadres believed that ideally, the workers of the neighborhood organizations should not only implement but also "humanize" (rather than professionalize) the state welfare policies. For the younger generation of social workers, getting too personal with the welfare recipients was not a preferred style. The young and relatively well-educated professional social workers lacked (and did not care to gain) the intimate local knowledge, interpersonal skills, ability to strategize in an increasingly diverse urban environment, and attention to "caregiving." In the short run, the textile sisters were not likely to become moral authority figures like the snoopy and seemingly "unprofessional," but really quite remarkable, granny cadres.

UPSCALING BAY BRIDGE: SHOWCASING CITIZENSHIP IN A GENTRIFYING NEIGHBORHOOD

In the futuristic visions of Shanghai's ambitious leaders, community building serves the long-term goal of turning a late socialist city into the financial center of East Asia. They needed to beautify both the upper quarters and the lower quarters so that Shanghai residents could claim the prestigious kinds of cultural citizenship associated with a considerably higher moral standard. The need to compete with other global cities became even more urgent after the party secretary's visit to Rio de Janeiro and other Latin American cities in June 1995. During an interview with district officials, I learned that the leaders of the Shanghai delegation were said to be dismayed at the degree to which most of the Brazilian cities they saw were divided. The graphic coexistence of scenic spots for the rich and rundown houses for the poor in the inner-city neighborhoods or *favelas* bore too much resemblance to the remaining ramshackle constructions in Shanghai's lower quarters and the emerging squatter settlements on the city's outskirts, where illegal housing construction went on everyday. Delegation members reportedly feared that Latin America's present could be Shanghai's future. This was the lesson that the party secretary insisted that his colleagues must learn while looking for the gentrification strategy most suitable for China. The focus of the citywide model community building program would be on both the lower and upper quarters. As base-level organizations, the street office and its residents' committees were once again on the front lines of campaigns for promoting both citizenship and morality.

In everyday practice, such revitalization schemes were translated into a series of civilizing projects that captured the attention of the party-state, the mass media, and academics across the nation. Participation in model community contests was a top priority of Shanghai neighborhood organizations. Street officers in the lower quarters seized every possible opportunity to improve the social and economic status of their neighborhood and developed various strategies to compete for media coverage and attention from the municipal government. The street officers invested a considerable amount of their time, energy, and resources in preparation for the monthly inspections and unexpected visits of the officials from the various departments of the municipal and central governments. These official visits would often determine the final outcome of the neighborhood's annual bid for the model community award.

As of 1998, eleven street offices in Shanghai had been officially recognized for their achievement in community building as a reward for their effort in putting on a show that pleased the inspecting authorities. Among those who had successfully garnered the official awards was the street office of Bay Bridge, which had emerged as a dark horse in the competition for fame and honor. Many local cadres insisted that the current elevated status of Bay Bridge was indeed hard earned considering its competitive disadvantages in location (as a lower quarter- area) and the low educational levels of its residents.

Bay Bridge's achieved status, in the form of brass plaques on permanent display as a badge of honor at the entrance of the residential compounds, was proudly flaunted as a symbol of cultural citizenship. Varying in size depending on at what level of model community the residential unit was accredited (district or municipal), the plaques were all engraved with the same red characters, *wenming shequ,* which literally means "civilized community." But did it really make sense for cadres in Bay Bridge, an underdeveloped urban community iconic of Shanghai's lower quarters, to become so preoccupied with such an impractical game of fame? How could they balance the overwhelming problems created by the debris of socialism with the need to showcase citizenship in a less than average community where the economic reforms were eroding residents' social and cultural citizenship?

In order to deal with these questions, we must first look at the connections between ongoing community-building processes and neighborhood gentrification during the 1990s urban reforms, as well as institutional restructuring and individual strategizing at the local level. The overnight disappearance of state factories in the city's depressed industrial areas coincided with the neighborhood gentrification of lower quarters like Bay Bridge. Gated communities managed by local or transnational real-estate developers started to appear on the land acquired from the owners of bankrupt or poorly managed state-owned factories. In a sense, the built forms of high-rise apartments in a lower quarter were literally the sprouts of capitalism grown out of the debris of socialism. But the advent of gated communities did not immediately result in the relocation of poorer residents. A gated community in Bay Bridge was often located in the mist of several "workers' new villages" *(gongren xincun)* made up of dozens of six-story walk-ups in the typical form of government housing projects built during the 1970s.

Between 1997 and 1998, two brand-new housing complexes (named "Volkswagen Town" and "Redbud Pavilion") were completed in north and southwest Bay Bridge. Accordingly, two residents' committees were established in order to manage the life of the newly arrived 3,552 residents (as of September 1998). Volkswagen Town, for example, was the fourth residential housing project in Shanghai funded by the famous German automobile company in order to improve the living conditions of its employees (mostly scientists and engineers recruited from throughout China). Redbud Pavilion was a residential community of 426 residents who were mostly mid-level government officials. With financial support from their own work units, they managed to buy homes in these modern apartment buildings.

The most active gentrifying agents in Bay Bridge were the young, well-educated street officers who formed an alliance with property and real-estate developers, local entrepreneurs, and urban planners with the same vision of high modernity and scientizing principles divorced from the social and economic realities of the locality. The new technocrats who had taken control of the neighborhood were pleased with the presence of Volkswagen Town and Redbud Pavilion, because these gated residential communities were essential to the rapid process of gentrification that would "improve" the cultural and moral quality of the neighborhood by attracting potential homebuyers. The granny cadres of the residents' committees, however, became increasingly suspicious of whether these new residents in the gated communities would identify themselves with the rest of the locality, because it was once part of the lower quarters. Such concerns on the part of the granny cadres proved to be legitimate, because the community building schemes implemented in the late 1990s served to justify the existence of a variety of communities representing very different interests in a gentrified Bay Bridge.

For the technocrats of the district government and subdistrict street officers, the gated community, whose residents were total strangers in the neighborhood, represented the ideal form of a "model community"—a perfect showcase for cultural and moral citizenship that was promoted and rewarded by the state. In the eyes of the young and forward-looking street officers, it would make perfect sense to showcase a garden-like model community (otherwise known as a "civilized community") supervised by an elected neighborhood council or homeowners' association. In so doing, they believed they would help the local residents forget their dark past, restore their confidence in the present, and envision the future of Bay Bridge as a transformed "modern" locality. However, balancing the needs of managing the debris of socialism and showcasing modern citizenship was a daunting task. With a mountain of unresolved problems from unemployment to housing shortages, Bay Bridge hardly stood a chance in the model community contest and other beautification campaigns. As a result, the street officers resorted to a selective strategy by showcasing one or two newly established gated communities, such as Volkswagen Town, in order to attract media attention and official recognition.

By choosing only a few new housing communities to represent a significantly improved lower quarter, however, the technocrats also reminded the remaining majority of those living in Bay Bridge of "what we used to be," *not* "what we are supposed to be." It was as if the "urban villages" and other elements deemed to be morally undesirable were now airbrushed from the social and political map. Underneath the false façade of a harmonious, hygienic, and crime-free environment, however, Bay Bridge continues to be treated (by its inhabitants and the rest of Shanghai) as if it were atypical, yet still a lower quarter.

CONCLUDING REMARKS

The earth-sháttering developments in Shanghai that left indelible imprints on its cityscape within the past decade made it easy for us to assume that the old hierarchy of center and periphery, of downtown and outskirts, ought to be replaced by something diffuse and amorphous, and held together through interconnected grids (i.e., telephone wires, electricity, television and Internet cables). The futuristic images of technological innovation and economic sustainability presented at the 2010 World Expo seem to reaffirm jingoistic assumptions about the rise of a formidable powerhouse on the world stage. Located at an edge, distant from the Expo site, the rapidly gentrifying Bay Bridge provides perhaps a better point of departure for analyzing the role of lived geography in contemporary Shanghai's social and moral transformations.

After the municipal government launched a six-hundred-day citywide beautification campaign in preparation for the 2010 World Expo, state-led initiatives and community-based volunteer mobilizations became highly sensationalized and politicized media events. The carefully stage-managed and well-publicized model community contests turned out to be eye-catching promotional showcases of cultural citizenship and helped the young street officers earn credentials and rewards as they climbed up the career ladder. But the modernist visions of the technocrats who have become key actors in local governance are still in great tension with the harsh conditions of lower-quarter neighborhoods. Moreover, the fundamental structure of inequality exemplified by the spatially dichotomized upper quarters and lower quarters remains. The strong degree of place attachment among generations of residents of China's most cosmopolitan city has maintained an abiding smell of the local beneath the revolutionary rhetoric of socialism, the commercial practice of capitalism, and the inhuman engineering quest for a sanitized modernity free of dirt, danger, offending smells, and local people.

Echoing Arjun Appadurai's call to "put hierarchy in its place" (1988), I have described in this chapter the reappropriation and redeployment of familiar terms and recognizable spaces in new contexts, practices, and situations in postreform Shanghai. As empirical social categories, "lower quarters" and "upper quarters" are highly inaccurate, even though they have been used polemically to represent two distinct polarities. Yet as cultural categories, which formed owing to a complex interplay of environmental and socioeconomic influences, the seemingly obsolete notions of lower quarters and upper quarters continue to inform our understandings of the material and moral processes that have shaped Shanghai's neighborhoods in the past and are at the core of transformations that are remaking Shanghai's current designs. It is this change in the built and lived environment that has created the deep moral context for the new Chinese subjectivity.

NOTES

1. See Deng Xiaoping's comment on his regret about not having included Shanghai as one of the first four special economic zones in the initial stages of the economic reform in *Selected Works of Deng Xiaoping*, vol. 3 (Beijing: Foreign Languages Press, 1994), 376.

2. In theory "new Shanghainese" should include all the people working and living in Shanghai. In actual practice, however, it's an achieved status that would almost certainly exclude migrant workers.

3. In "Questioning the Modernity of the Model Settlement," Jeffery N. Wasserstrom questions the prevalent views of prior writers that Shanghai's colonial settlement was a thoroughly modern place in which one would expect to see strong evidence of the development of modern citizenship (2002). While acknowledging his historical insights and sharing his doubts about the uniqueness of the foreign concessions in Shanghai, in this chapter I place my emphasis on the impacts of the essentializing differences between the two quarters in terms of their symbolic meanings and the strategies of utilizing such a dichotomy to mark the high and the low.

4. As of July 1, 1999, the qualified coupon applicants were those who received a monthly income of less than 280 yuan (approximately US$35).

REFERENCES

Anderson, E. 1990. *Streetwise: Race, Class, and Change in an Urban Community.* Chicago: University of Chicago Press.

Appadurai, A. 1988. "Putting Hierarchy in Its Place." *Cultural Anthropology* 3:36–49.

Butler, T. 2003. *London Calling: The Middle Class and the Remaking of Inner London.* Oxford: Berg Publishers.

Caulfield, J. 1994. *City Form and Everyday Life: Toronto's Gentrification and Critical Practice.* Toronto: University of Toronto Press.

Gaubatz, P. 2005. "Globalization and the Development of New Central Business Districts in Beijing, Shanghai and Guangzhou." In *Restructuring the Chinese City: Changing Society, Economy and Space,* edited by L. J. C. Ma and F. Wu, 98–121. London: Routledge.

Honig, E. 1992. *Creating Chinese Ethnicity: Subei People in Shanghai, 1850–1980.* New Haven, CT: Yale University.

Jakes, S. 2004. "Soaring Ambitions: The World's Most Visionary Architects are Rebuilding China." *Time* (Asia Edition). May 24.

Kleinman, A. 2006. *What Really Matters: Living a Moral Life Amidst Uncertainty and Danger.* Oxford: Oxford University Press. 227.

Scott, J. 1998. *Seeing Like a State: How Certain Schemes to Improve the Human Condition Have Failed*. New Haven, CT: Yale University Press.

Walder, A. 1986. *Communist Neo-Traditionalism: Work and Authority in Chinese Industry*. Berkeley: University of California Press.

Wasserstrom, J. N. 2002. "Questioning the Modernity of the Model Settlement: Citizenship and Exclusion in Old Shanghai." In *Changing Meanings of Citizenship in Modern China*, edited by M. Goldman and E. J. Perry, 110–132. Cambridge, MA: Harvard University Press.

Zhang R. 2009. "Shanghai Aims at International Financial and Shipping Center." *China Daily*. March 26. www.chinadaily.com.cn/china/2009–03/26/content_7617756.htm. Accessed February 21, 2011.

Zhang, X. D. 2000. "Shanghai Nostalgia: Postrevolutionary Allegories in Wang Anyi's Literary Production in the 1990s." *positions: east asia cultures critique* 8, no. 2:348–387.

CHAPTER FIVE · Depression

Coming of Age in China

Sing Lee

A U.S.-CHINA PARADOX OF DEPRESSION

Depression today has been found to be a highly prevalent illness in the United States and other Western countries. Epidemiological surveys indicate that one-third of the general population in the United States suffer from lifetime depression based on diagnostic criteria of the illness drawn up by the American Psychiatric Association. Depression has been equated with the common flu, in that it can be easily detected by general practitioners or laypeople using a variety of self-screening tests. Individuals who screen positive on the tests may simply request antidepressants from their doctors. By 2005, unsurprisingly, antidepressants surpassed antihypertensives to become the most widely prescribed class of drugs in the United States. Apart from being the signature diagnosis of contemporary psychiatry, depression has become such an encompassing lay category for unhappiness that normal sadness is said to be lost in the United States (Horwitz and Wakefield 2007).

By contrast, depression was almost an unknown category in China until the early 1990s. Among the general public, the term "depression" (*youyuzheng* or *yiyuzheng*) or "depressed" (*yiyu* or *youyu*) was rarely used. Likewise, Chinese psychiatrists uncommonly made a diagnosis of depression as it is recently understood in the West. Two national epidemiological surveys conducted in 1982 and 1993 respectively showed that depression occurred in less than 0.5 percent of people in China (Lee et al. 2009). They suggested that depression is thirty-five times less common in China than in the United States.

The discrepancy is intriguing when we compare the prosperity and political stability of the United States to the massive amount of sociopolitical turmoil that has occurred in China. Suffering has been a hallmark of Chinese society. This is because disasters continued to plague the country beginning with the fall of the Qing dynasty, followed by disruptive warlordism, partial and chaotic reunification under the Nationalist Party, a vast dislocation caused by the war with Japan, and the civil war. Times after the establishment of the People's Republic of China (PRC) were marked by poverty, famine, high death rates, devastating upheavals during the Great Leap Forward and Cultural Revolution, the June 4 incident, large-scale natural disasters including floods and earthquakes and, more recently, rampant capitalism and uneven growth. It is true that the Chinese Communist Party (CCP) has suppressed sociopolitical turbulence with a measure of success. But it is hard to believe that collective fear, sorrow, and other heartbreaking emotions have been rare among Chinese people.

This chapter discusses how emotional expression, mental disorder, and sociopolitical context interrelate in Maoist and postcollective China. It traces how repression of emotions during the Maoist period promoted neurasthenia as a popular physical idiom of distress and a ubiquitous medical diagnosis. It also describes how a partial retreat of the state and economic reform that liberalize both everyday life and psychiatric practice have unleashed emotional disclosure in Chinese people and encouraged the clinical substitution of neurasthenia by the "Western" disease of depression. While arguing that the proliferation of the diagnosis of depression follows a complex cultural and historical contingency, this chapter arrives at the perspective that social change in China has real social consequences in the mental health arena. The latter include the growth of moral challenges to psychiatry, rising prevalence of depression, a huge psychiatric treatment gap, and an upsurge of talk therapy.

NEURASTHENIA AS A SOMATIC IDIOM OF DISTRESS

Inner feelings and their outward expressions can be cautiously controlled and distinct in Chinese people. Consequently, emotions are often expressed in an indirect manner. For example, Chinese parents, instead of hugging their children and telling them that they love them, will commonly communicate affection by cooking their children's favorite food, asking them to dress warmly, or giving them pocket money. By holding their inner feelings back, Chinese people may even appear to deny their emotions. A woman who is fond of a man may reply "I don't know" or "Of course,

I don't love you!" when he asks if she loves him. When a girl becomes unhappy with her boyfriend and he asks her what is wrong with her, she may say "nothing" while avoiding any eye contact with him. These indirect expressions of emotions are admittedly changing among younger generations of Chinese people. In the area of psychopathology, anthropological and psychiatric research indicates that Chinese people often hold in their inner depression and are inclined to express interpersonal distress by way of physical symptoms such as headaches, insomnia, chest discomfort, and dizziness. There is a widely used cultural category for expressing these physical symptoms. It is known as neurasthenia or, in standard Chinese, *shenjing shuairuo* (Lee 1998).

The English term *neurasthenia* was coined well over a century ago by the American neurologist George Beard to denote "exhaustion of the nervous system." Beard believed that the condition was composed of a varying mixture of many symptoms. The latter included, among others, weakness, fatigue, poor concentration, memory loss, severe headache, and poor appetite. Neurasthenia steadily acquired popularity with both physicians and the general public in North America up to the early years of the twentieth century. The term subsequently fell into disuse and has apparently been supplanted by *depression*.

Neurasthenia has run a different social course in China. The term *shenjing shuairuo* was probably introduced to China from Japan in the early 1900s. *Shen* is emblematic of vitality, the capacity of the mind to form ideas, and the desire of the person to live life. *Jing* originally refers to the meridians or channels that carry *qi* (vital energy) and *xue* (blood) through the body. Conceptually, *shen* and *jing* are treated by Chinese people as one term *(shenjing)* that means "nerve" or "nervous system." When *shenjing* becomes *shuai* (degenerate) and *ruo* (weak) following undue nervous excitement, a variety of somatic symptoms may ensue. Although traditional Chinese medicine does not originally contain the term *shenjing shuairuo*, the neurasthenic notion of weakness closely resembles the popular and nonstigmatizing illness category of *xu* (weakness). Unsurprisingly, *shenjing shuairuo* readily found acceptance among laypeople and health practitioners alike.

Previous community surveys showed that neurasthenia was by far the most common mental disorder in China. For example, a 1959 survey in Chengdu, Sichuan, demonstrated a current prevalence of 5.9 percent (X. H. Liu 1982). This is comparable to the current prevalence of depression in contemporary Western communities. From the 1950s to 1970s, 80 to 90 percent of psychiatric outpatients and a high number of medical outpatients in China received a diagnosis of neurasthenia.

A COMMUNIST DISEASE

I had not been aware of such a high incidence
of neurasthenia under the Guomindang
government. . . . In time, I came to regard
neurasthenia as a peculiarly communist
disease, the result of being trapped in a
system with no escape.

Z. S. Li, The Private Life of Chairman Mao, 1994

During Maoist China, the focus of public health was on sanitation and infectious diseases. The notion of "emotional disease" or "mood disorder" was unimaginable. Psychiatry was brought to a standstill and viewed with suspicion by the Chinese state as an imperialist import. Social sciences that formed the scientific basis of psychiatry, such as psychology, anthropology, and sociology, were highly restricted or banned. "Mental health" was about developing moral character via a continuous struggle between the proletariat and the bourgeoisie. Mental disorder was attributed to the failure of the old political system and the injustices brought about by moribund capitalism. It was thus to be rectified with thought reform, especially readings of Mao's writings and imposed work therapy. Given such an antipsychiatric ethos, it would seem surprising that a "mental disorder" such as neurasthenia could flourish. Most notably, Mao himself was said to suffer from it (Li 1994).

In 1980, American psychiatrist-anthropologist Arthur Kleinman carried out a psychiatric-ethnographic study of neurasthenia at the psychiatric department of Hunan Medical University in south central China (Kleinman 1982). By carefully interviewing in Mandarin one hundred Chinese outpatients with a clinical diagnosis of neurasthenia, he examined not only their medical symptoms but also how their illness retold the pains of sociopolitical change. Kleinman found that the patients were conversant with the diagnostic label of neurasthenia. Even after they improved with "antidepressant" drugs, they still believed they suffered from neurasthenia. Unlike depressive American patients who readily volunteered the symptom of low mood, their presenting complaints consisted predominantly of physical symptoms such as headache, insomnia, dizziness, and other pains. Specifically, 30 percent of the patients presented entirely with physical complaints while 70 percent viewed physical complaints as most important. None of the one hundred patients made an entirely or mostly psychological presentation.

Kleinman found that the patients' physical symptoms were not the direct manifestation of diseases of physical organs. When they revealed their illness experience in a confiding interview, it became apparent their physical symptoms were embedded in a matrix of social and emotional difficulties that would otherwise have been concealed in socially prohibitive settings. Most of them perceived their illness to be due to work (61 percent), political (25 percent), and separation (25 percent) problems. The most common meaning (93 percent of cases) of the patients' illness was to communicate personal or interpersonal distress.

Several case vignettes described by Kleinman illustrated how physical symptoms served as idioms of distress in a sociopolitical period that inhibited emotional disclosure. One of them was about a thirty-five-year-old female physician who presented with a decade of chronic headache and other neurasthenic symptoms. Her illness followed the realization that she had made a mistake in leaving her boyfriend in order to join the Cultural Revolution and, in the quixotic ideology of the day, serve the people selflessly. The headache worsened whenever she was criticized by coworkers and unit leaders for not having worked hard enough. Another patient was a fifty-two-year-old cadre who presented with chronic abdominal pains, headache, insomnia, and poor appetite. Her illness was connected with her husband having been labeled a rightist and severely criticized during the Cultural Revolution. The latter led to substantial work difficulty and social pressures on the family as well as school problems for their children.

Although neurasthenic patients presented with physical symptoms, Kleinman was able to actively elicit the psychological symptom of persistent low mood from most of them. Using the same American diagnostic criteria that he would have used to diagnose depressive patients in the United States, he made a diagnosis of depression in eighty-seven of the one hundred neurasthenic patients. Kleinman concluded that the physical symptoms of neurasthenia represented "somatic idioms of distress." By that, he meant socially and politically acceptable ways of experiencing and expressing interpersonal distress. In situations of trust and safety, these physical symptoms could become patients' mnemonic device for recapturing their past emotional difficulties. This finding indicated that emotions might be concealed or even lost among people who lived through the turmoil of Maoist China.

CONCEALMENT AND LOSS OF EMOTIONS

Notwithstanding Kleinman's finding on somatisation and substantial evidence that the Chinese party-state has powerfully shaped people's social spaces and expression of their individuality, there is a dearth of research on using the emotional dimension of the person to understand the Chinese social and political world. There is, nonetheless, a rich Chinese lexicon for expressing a variety of emotional states. For example, somewhat different versions of the so-called seven emotions *(qiqing)* have been described in traditional Chinese medicine and in Confucian and Buddhist writings. Depicting a miscellany of emotions and complex psychological states in Chinese people, they include happiness, anger, sadness, anxiety, disgust, panic, grief, lust, hatred, yearning, and fear. The manifestation of these emotional states is, however, context dependent.

During the Maoist era, the boundaries between individual and political bodies were blurred. Compulsory allegiance to the Communist Party, continuous class struggle, and heeding the state's call to forsake individual and familial interests to serve the people and their revolution were given primacy. Private ownership was confined to items of personal use, such as clothing, which were rationed by the state. Everyday life consisted of an endless cycle of work and "study sessions" aimed at thought reform. There was little social space for recreation. Entertainment (e.g., model operas and movies about the class struggle of the old society, followed by routinized discussion) was primarily a means of indoctrination. Although weary workers and peasants were allowed to sleep, this had the specific purpose of restoring energy for doing more work. Since resting was considered "unproletarian," leisure was sacrificed to boost production or spent on "voluntary" labor. Failure to comply with state-mandated directives might be followed by public criticism, lengthy interrogations, ideological brainstorming, and daily writing of "confessions" on mistakes allegedly made. As people strived to survive in such dangerous times, there were perhaps valid reasons for concealing individuality and, with it, personal sadness as well. The cardinal symptoms of depression (such as low mood, loss of drive, psychomotor retardation, and social withdrawal) could easily be criticized as the manifestation of magnified individualism that alienated people from the masses. These complaints could also be denounced as evidence of laziness, malingering, and an inability to advance personally to a more proletarian mindset.

Although there is little published work on how people expressed their emotions during Maoist China, there are both semifictional and biographical accounts of the concealment of emotions. Jung Chang wrote in *Wild Swans* about the moral dilemma over expressing sadness when her mother evidently experienced the symptoms of depression: "At the end of all this, my mother's two comrades voted against full Party membership for her. She fell into a deep depression. . . . She dreaded seeing people and spent as much time as possible alone, crying to herself. Even this she had to conceal, as it would have been considered as showing lack of faith in the revolution" (1991: 165). Importantly, Chang's semifictional account echoed Kleinman's ethnographic research. Yan Zhongshu, a male physician who lived a morally taxing life through the Cultural Revolution and its aftermath, is one example. He explained emotional concealment and the need to maintain a politically correct and low-key public self as follows: "To survive in China you must reveal nothing to others. Or it could be used against you. Use only indirection and . . . ambiguous language. . . . Sometimes you even should block your own thoughts, because you know at those terrible times you can't trust yourself. . . . Let your public self be like rice in a dinner: bland and inconspicuous, taking on the flavours of its surroundings while giving off no flavour of its own" (Kleinman 2006: 80).

In *Enemies of the People* too, Anne Thurston (1987) interviewed in depth various kinds of participants of the Cultural Revolution. She found that they "lost a sense of trust and predictability in human relations as colleagues, friends, and sometimes even relatives and immediate family turned against them." Some of them, like Qiu Yehuang, Li Meirong, and Bai Meihua respectively, reckoned that the Communist Party taught people "not to say the truth" and to lie, and thus they "never say what they really think" (Thurston 1987: 207–208, 256). Thurston was often able to elicit the symptoms of depression and post-traumatic stress disorder in her interviews, but the manifestations of these symptoms were context dependent. For example, Jiang Xinren described in his father the symptoms of forgetfulness, insomnia, withdrawal, retardation, and bouts of anger toward family members at night even though he would not say anything all day while he was at work. Jiang noted that in the workplace his father "was afraid that if he said anything, he would be attacked," so the anger "would gradually build up during the day, and at night he would take anger out on us. It was *shenjing shuairuo*—neurasthenia" (Thurston 1987: 261).

People's nondisclosure of true thoughts and feelings was perpetuated by a constant fear of these being distorted and indelibly documented in their dossiers. In *Ten Years of Madness—Oral Histories of China's Cultural Revolution*, a forty-one-year-old editor at a publishing house explained why this was so:

My experience has proven that when people speak favourably of you, it isn't worth anything, because no one puts this in your dossier. If you are accused of, or simply suspected of, having done something wrong, however, it is most likely written in your dossier. Once something gets into your dossier, it is never taken out and follows you throughout your life. Can you guarantee you are a good guy in your dossier? You know you are honest and loyal to your country and your work. You think that you have nothing to hide, and that you are guileless. But in your dossier, you may appear to be a completely different person, one with smirches all over. When it comes to others making a judgment about you, you will be viewed and treated according to what your dossier says. (Feng 1996: 211)

These accounts suggest that sadness (whether labeled as depression or not) did occur in connection with the many forms of profound brutality and loss that were inflicted on people during the Maoist era. It could, however, be socially unutterable and thereby concealed as people would not say how they felt or what they thought for the sake of self-preservation. If concealment was routinely carried out, nonetheless, it might become automatized and indistinguishable from emotional flattening. Since love for family members could be publicly condemned as bourgeois sentimentalism, some people, be they victims, perpetrators, or often both, could lose their ability to feel basic human emotions. Writing about life in a labor camp in *Grass Soup*, Zhang Xianliang recounted how emotions could be lost: "I never met a man in the camps at this time who talked about his parents, wife, lover or children in warm, earnest, loving terms—not even the shortest sentence. . . . A mention of one's home, that is one's real home, was bound to be related to receiving a package of things to eat in the mail. . . . Other than that, home had no place in a man's emotions, because he had lost his emotions" (Chang and Zhang 1994: 227–228).

Based on twenty years of field research that involved four hundred in-depth interviews with villagers in Da Fo in north China, Ralph Thaxton demonstrated how disastrous policies and brutal cadres inflicted forced labor, mass starvation, and suffering on peasants during the Great Leap Forward from 1958 to 1960 (Thaxton 2008). The latter was Mao's economic plan to rapidly transform China from a predominantly agrarian economy into an industrialized society. But it turned out to be a deadly famine and humanitarian disaster that claimed twenty to forty-three million lives. Based on the villagers' recalled experience, Thaxton showed that the calamity of the Great Leap was not merely about serious food shortage. He wrote that when people articulated their anger over the Great Leap Forward, this was often indirect by focusing on forced labor, citing one of them as follows:

The problem with the Great Leap Forward was not only food shortage, but also the demand for everybody to come to work in the fields or to work on a project. Some leaders became simply crazy. The Dongle County leaders declared that we had to mobilize everybody to work to build socialism. On the surface, there was nothing wrong with a slogan like this. However, the Liangman People's Commune and Da Fo village leaders would then push this policy to the extreme, taking it to mean that literally everybody, including the blind, had to do something. As long as you could move your body, you had to work in the collective fields or appear to be working in the fields. (Thaxton 2008: 132–133)

Apart from forced labor, Thaxton described other kinds of dehumanizing experiences inflicted on noncompliant peasants. They included public criticism, humiliation, and physical torture. Regarding how peasants reacted to these catastrophic circumstances, Thaxton described their modes of suffering as "utter exhaustion," "sick from overwork," "ruined health," "walking skeletons," "sleep disorder," "great pain," "fear," "humiliation," "indignation," and "disgust." He did not record any narratives that included the word *depression* or its cognates. Nor did he use it to describe the emotional condition of the villagers. It is worthy of note, however, that Thaxton found the practice of *ganqing* (emotions of human concern) to be so completely demolished by the Great Leap Forward that it was very difficult for villagers to recover from illnesses caused by forced labor and other brutalizing experiences (2008: 142).

Whether people denied, concealed, or simply lost their emotions, the principal conclusion of Kleinman's study of somatisation and depression in Hunan was that neurasthenic experience might function as a somatic camouflage for many individuals to communicate interpersonal distress with less risk of political denunciation during the always dangerous Maoist times. As political victimhood was transmuted into personal patienthood, criticisms, oppression, and alienation were clothed and reexperienced in the neurasthenic body as pain, insomnia, dizziness, and exhaustion.

DEPOLITICIZATION AND UNLEASHING OF EMOTIONS

Since 1978, Chinese society has continued to change profoundly and at high speed. The 1980s was a period for many local communities to recover from collective trauma and to resurrect their heritage. Most people were relieved that they did not have to continue to live under the constant threat of surveillance and could begin to disclose their own thoughts and feelings more freely. For others, it was a time to unleash previously silenced emotions such as anger, corrosive cynicism, and memories of injustice and deep loss. As economic reforms have continued today to progress, a robust private sector that is less directly fettered by the Party has flourished. Albeit selective, the retreat of the party-state has facilitated a dramatic reconfiguration of the material and psychological life of people in China. This is shown by the state endorsement of relaxation, entertainment, and private ownership as valid ingredients of social life. In May 1996, Saturday was recognized as a nonworking day throughout China.

Along with the expansion of personal freedoms, self-expression—including that of emotions—has become more open. This is especially noticeable for younger people among whom values of autonomy, privacy, emotional communication, and entitlement to consumption grow rapidly. This is true of both urban and rural youth. In a remarkable longitudinal study of rural youths in northeast China, anthropologist Yunxiang Yan, a contributor to this volume, wrote that "contemporary youths have become more vocal and open in expressing their most intimate feelings" (2003: 83). Yan believes that changes in the local world of living following loosening of political control in the era of economic reform have played a vital role in expanding the imaginative world and emotionality of rural youth.

New market forces that operate within the ideological and social space of Chinese people have also shaped their moral and emotional experience. As thought reform of the collective era quickly lost its salience, a single-minded devotion to business values and profiteering has permeated much of the population from 1990 onward. This is evidenced by a counterfeiting epidemic, often conflated with entrepreneurship, that has swept across China. Despite an oft-mentioned intention to "beat forging" *(dajia)* by both the public and the government, an extensive variety of fake goods have become commonplace. These include, among others, rice wine, shark's fins, medicines, infant formula, bank notes, dinosaur fossils, brand-name products, electronic products, and graduate theses. As making money and enjoying oneself become the new order of social life, there has been concern over the fall of public morality. N. Xie, an eighteen-year-old vocational school student, had this to say about the Cultural Revolution and moral quandaries in post-Mao China: "The problem with the Cultural Revolution was that political relations became more important than any other kind of relations. The problem these days is that money relations are more important than any other kind of relations. . . . In the Cultural Revolution, one man spoke for millions; these days, nobody listens to anything anyone says" (Feng 1996: 256).

The downside of economic reforms notwithstanding, there is little doubt that both urban and rural people can now express their emotions more freely. As Feng observed, the twentieth anniversary of the collapse of the Cultural Revolution was marked by Chinese people tending "more towards the emotional," and "a mixture of a hundred emotions" (1996: 247). Indeed, in everyday interactions, popular writings and the media, the terms "psychological" *(xinli)*, "stress" *(yali)*, "mood" *(xin-*

qing), "feeling" (*qingxu* or *ganjue*), "unhappiness" (*bukaixin* or *buyukuai*), "feeling bad" *(nanguo)*, and "depressed" *(youyu)* have become increasingly popular. Moreover, people's daily hassles consist of problems that are decidedly less political in nature than during the Maoist era. In the cities, this may be reflected by the emergence of numerous telephone counseling services that appear to be the equivalent of mind therapy in the West. By assuring the callers' anonymity, these services have become popular especially among young people. Several studies of telephone counseling services in Beijing, Shanghai, and Nanjing in the 1990s revealed that the most common problems for consultations were about emotional upset, broken love, marriage, teenage education, parental intrusiveness, financial loss, and self-labeled depression. Whereas declaring stress and low spirits would appear to risk political incorrectness in the past, reporting being stressed out and depressed evokes common problems of living nowadays.

There has also been an explosive growth in cyberspace. This is reflected by the fact that the number of Internet users in China exceeded those in the United States in June 2009. Online messaging tools such as QQ have enabled a fast-growing number of rural people to access the Internet simply via their cell phones. This is bringing about a profound shift of the primarily urban base of the Internet in China. It is true that the Internet is still monitored by an online police force who may detain netizens for posting information deemed challenging to local authorities. Nonetheless, it is clearly too vast to monitor fully, especially as posts can be written in subtly subversive ways. The Internet is by any measure the most democratized social space in China today. Increasingly, netizens' activism to resist new threats of censorship has become more open and may be successful, such as in delaying the implementation of the Green Dam filtering software (supposedly for blocking violence and pornography on the Internet) on all personal computers. They can even become online heroes by challenging the judiciary that privileges officials against common people. Generally, the Internet has brought about unprecedented levels of communication between geographically dispersed people both within China and around the globe. By weakening the CCP's mechanisms of social control, it is turning out to be a powerful tool for interpersonal expression and profound social change in the country.

In contradiction to the Maoist notion of "working to boost production for the country," multistory fitness clubs, and the accompanying idea of "working out" the individual body, have become increasingly popular among China's new middle class. Once considered Western "culture-bound syndromes," clinical eating disorders in the form of anorexia and bulimia nervosa are increasingly seen among young Chinese women. There is also, as Zhang's chapter in this volume illustrates in great detail, an exponential growth of the sex trade and karaoke clubs that generate enormous financial gains as well as challenges to public health and morality. China was officially atheist for more than half a century and religious practice is still highly regulated by the Bureau of Religious Affairs. But an increasing population of people resort to religious activities in apparent violation of a law that they should worship under a state-sponsored religious body. This may speak to the rising spiritual need of Chinese people amidst the collapse of communism and unchecked capitalism. In an ethnographic study of a thriving high-tech company in the southern coastal city of Beihai, anthropologist Xin Liu described the feelings of boredom and meaninglessness of a successful business woman as follows:

> *There is nothing worth living for.* . . . The woman who said this was a great business woman, able to send her child to a private suburban boarding school that was costing more money than most people can afford. A few minutes earlier, the same woman was so decisive while playing cards and was discussing investing millions. . . . She had fun. She went to the beauty parlour, she had lunch with her husband's friends, she played *cuodadi*, she was happy, she was busy . . . she was indicating a loss of direction in her life. . . . Or, more precisely, where are we going? . . . People can conceive of what to do next, but they cannot conceive of the significance of what should be done. Life goes on, but the perspective and orientation of life have begun to disappear. (X. Liu 2002: 168–169)

To varying degrees, these feelings of existential uncertainty are arguably present among Chinese people in the current time of both prosperity and social adversity. They can provide a fertile ground for the interpersonal experience as well as social construction of depression in postreform China.

SOCIAL CONTEXT OF DEPRESSION

The medical apparatus for recognizing pathological sadness, no less than the experience of sadness, occurs in a social context. Although a recognizable syndrome of morbid dejection could be traced to ancient Greece and Rome, the descriptive content of such a syndrome and its causal explanations have varied considerably over the centuries. Historical accounts of melancholia emphasize prolonged periods of marked mental and behavioral derangement that could reach a delusional degree. Consequently, melancholic depression was often equated with madness or "partial insanity" (Jackson 1986). But the contemporary version of depression, as described in recent versions of the Diagnostic and Statistical Manual of Mental Disorders (DSM) globally circulated by the American Psychiatric Association, has focused on a noticeably milder and shorter period of negative emotional change. A depressive episode is defined by an individual having frequent low mood for two or more weeks, gloomy thinking, and a number of other mostly psychological symptoms that health practitioners judge to be "of clinical significance." In *The Loss of Sadness*, Allan Horwitz and Jerome Wakefield (2007) argue that the DSM definition of depression fails to draw an adequate boundary between normal sadness and mental disorder. By artificially disconnecting symptoms and context, it has turned much of normal sorrow into a medical disease.

As Paul Starr persuasively argued in *The Social Transformation of American Medicine*, "The history of medicine has been written as an epic of progress, but it is a tale of social and economic conflict over the emergence of new hierarchies of power and authority, new markets, and new conditions of belief and experience" (1982: 4). In the specific case of psychiatry, Horwitz and Wakefield believe that powerful social forces reinforce the resilience and social impact of the contemporary psychiatric portrayal of depression. They call them the constituencies for depressive disorder. Thus, the profession of medicine and in particular psychiatry can expand its sphere of control by transforming previously nonmedical problems into a disease. Mental health clinicians, equipped with the unique power of determining whether sadness constitutes clinically significant depression, can rationalize reimbursement from third-party insurers for treating a wide range of problems in living. Psychiatric researchers have successfully argued for more funding for a rampant disease that may camouflage controversial social problems and existential despair. Advocacy organizations have used a broadened definition of depression to drive anti-stigma programs and achieve insurance reimbursement parity for mental disorder with medical conditions like diabetes and heart disease. Pharmaceutical companies are motivated to increase revenues by sponsoring educational activities that emphasize the high prevalence of nonsevere depression and the benefits of early-intervention pharmacotherapy. Distressed individuals may welcome a professional diagnosis as a useful label for personal problems. By making debatable projections to the year 2020, the World Health Organization has disseminated an authoritative message that there is a massive disease burden of depression. It says the burden is global and should be treated as a public health priority.

The popularization of depression and its drug treatment has led to a belief that America has been overdosed because of a massive increase in the prescription of antidepressants. The latter's use in the United States nearly doubled from 1996 to 2005.

According to 2005 figures from the U.S. Centers for Disease Control and Prevention, they accounted for some 5 percent of all prescription medications recorded in outpatient files. This would mean doctors writing some 150 million prescriptions for antidepressants a year. A *Time* magazine article even posed the question of whether antidepressants should be available as over-the-counter drugs (Blue 2008).

Do similar contextual factors described by Horwitz and Wakefield operate in China? Is the DSM also becoming psychiatry's bible there? If so, what are the local uses and consequences of medicalization?

CHINESE POLITICS OF DEPRESSION

> Politics plays as big a role as science in current descriptions of depression. . . . The vocabulary of depression, which can be enormously empowering to marginal people who have no way to describe or understand their experiences, is endlessly manipulable. Those more advantaged members of a society experience their illness through that vocabulary, which is nonconspiratorially spun by Congress, by the American Medical Association, and by the pharmaceutical industry.
>
> A. Solomon, The Noonday Demon, 2001

Unlike many physical diseases, there is at present not a single laboratory test to confirm the authenticity of mental disorders. The clinical diagnosis of a mental disorder (be it depression or neurasthenia) involves three interconnected steps over which physicians possess considerable cultural authority whereas patients experience a special vulnerability to professional belief (Jackson 1986; Starr 1982). The first step involves a physician's taking a comprehensive history of the symptoms of a patient and observing the latter's clinical behavior. During the second step, the physician organizes the symptoms into a familiar cluster called a syndrome. In the final step, he or she applies a set of diagnostic criteria to find out the best match between the symptom cluster and a professionally defined mental disorder and determines if those symptoms are "of clinical significance." Through these steps, physicians offer patients what Starr called "a kind of individualized objectivity, a personal relationship as well as authoritative counsel" in "the very circumstances of sickness"

that "promote acceptance of their judgment" (1982: 5). The clinical process of transforming symptoms lived in daily lives into diagnosed depression depends critically
on how a physician asks about and makes sense of the patient's illness experience
according to the professional definition of depression and his or her motivation to
make the diagnosis in a particular context. As Horwitz and Wakefield argue, this
process is socially constructed and has a politics of its own.

Chinese psychiatrists' concept of the depressive syndrome was previously confined to melancholia, that is, severe forms of psychotic mood disturbances (Jackson 1986). Clinical depression as it is currently understood in the United States, which
often creates dilemmas of differentiation from ordinary sadness, was a little-used
diagnostic category. Consequently, when Kleinman's study revealed that 87 percent
of neurasthenic patients in Hunan could be rediagnosed with depression, the finding stunned Chinese psychiatrists. Published by an American researcher when
China was adjusting to the drastic change from Mao's anti-imperialist harangue to
Deng's utilitarian imperatives, the study seemed to get at the "to-copy-or-to-resist"
complex of Chinese psychiatrists toward American culture (of which the system of
psychiatric classification is a part). To endorse the findings of the Hunan study was
therefore to risk incurring further national shame. The latter dated much further
back to the ruthless force of foreign imperialism, the Opium War, and the disintegration of first the Qing court and later the Republic. Reacting with a blend of awe
and xenophobia, Chinese psychiatrists initiated a series of psychiatric studies in order to prove that neurasthenia was a real disease.

Although the diagnostic results of the Chinese studies mostly confirmed the Hunan study, Chinese psychiatrists maintained that the overlap between neurasthenia
and depression was only partial. In a thematic issue of *Culture, Medicine, and Psychiatry*, Zhang Mingyuan, then president of the Chinese Society of Psychiatry, submitted that "the diagnosis of neurasthenia helps to establish a desirable physician/
patient relationship," and that switching neurasthenia to depression would be "accompanied by the risk of jeopardizing the doctor/patient rapport which is essential for successful treatment" (Zhang 1986).

Yet, the fate of neurasthenia has turned out to be vastly different from what Chinese psychiatrists had anticipated. By 2000, the use of this once ubiquitous disease
label has practically disappeared among Chinese psychiatrists. Few, if any, studies
can be found in medical journals in China that address the clinical or epidemiological dimensions of neurasthenia. By contrast, the diagnosis of depression has come
to symbolize modernity, scientific advancement, and universality. In July 1998, a senior psychiatrist at a psychiatric conference in Shanghai had the following to tell me

about the Hunan study: "The work of Dr. Arthur Kleinman in Hunan was like an alarm clock that woke up psychiatrists in China. It made them realize that antidepressants could make neurasthenic patients recover, and suggested that neurasthenia was mostly a kind of misdiagnosed depression."

Neurasthenia used to occupy a cardinal nosological status in earlier versions of the Chinese Classification of Mental Disorders (CCMD, first edition 1979). But the third and latest classification, called the CCMD-3 (2001), has marginalized it dramatically. Now neurasthenia can only be considered after depression, anxiety disorders, and somatoform disorders (a heterogeneous group of chronic pain and other somatic syndromes with no obvious physical causes) are excluded. As such, it exists merely as a ghostly apparition in the new diagnostic system (Zhonghua Yixue Jingshenke Fenhui 2001). Unsurprisingly, a recent epidemiological survey using such a marginalized definition of neurasthenia found the once common illness to hardly exist in China anymore (Phillips et al. 2009). GW was a thirty-five-year-old psychiatrist who worked in a university-affiliated psychiatric department in Sichuan. When asked his experience with neurasthenic patients in China, he replied in July 2008: "I have worked as a psychiatrist since 2000 and have never diagnosed any patient as having neurasthenia. I think most of the so-called neurasthenic patients could match the diagnostic criteria of depression, though depression may include a series of heterogeneous problems."

COMMERCIALIZATION OF DEPRESSION

I don't understand why. The kind of neurasthenic patients that I routinely encountered in the 1960s and '70s, who presented with insomnia, pains, difficulty in thinking and weakness, are rarely seen nowadays. By contrast, depression is a common illness.

A Chinese professor of psychiatry, 1995

The Chinese government did not previously allow foreign pharmaceutical companies to operate in the country. It manufactured its own drugs at a very low cost and had a fairly equitable system of distribution. As a result of new laws on the patenting of drugs that China created to follow the dictates of the World Trade Organization, drugs patented after 1986 in the United States are currently protected in China. The Chinese drug market is now quite sophisticated. It consists of a large number of competing international, joint-venture, and domestic pharmaceutical companies, as well as distributors from whom hospitals purchase drug products. The great majority of new psychotropic drugs known in developed countries are now available in China. By hook or by crook, drug companies are keen to push their products into each local government's list of reimbursable drugs.

Following China's trade liberalization, practically all global pharmaceutical firms had opened offices in China by the mid-1990s. Their influence on the different medical specialties, including psychiatry, has grown rapidly. Psychiatric conferences have witnessed an escalating number of marketing activities. Apart from sponsoring the meetings, drug companies make themselves highly visible in ways unimaginable in the past. There is plenty of razzmatazz, such as strategically located banners and booths with all varieties of product-driven freebies, from pens and T-shirts to multicolored pamphlets. Sumptuously sponsored dinners are attended by the most distinguished Chinese professors of psychiatry and senior hospital administrators. The latter often include powerful Communist Party secretaries. Via generous sponsorships, drug companies have been able to insert promotional discourse into academic meetings that otherwise have little to do with their pharmaceutical products. At one national conference on schizophrenia and psychopharmacology that I attended in Hangzhou in 1996, the first keynote lecture was, curiously, about Prozac (i.e., fluoxetine). The latter is a drug for depression, not schizophrenia. The lecture was given by a senior sales manager from Eli Lilly that sponsored "Prozac prizes" for the three best papers presented at the conference. Chinese psychiatrists did not start the dinner until such hard-sell activities were over.

In the United States, it has been shown that commercial sources of information provided by drug companies typically overstate efficacy and minimize negative reports. This can overshadow scientifically based material and powerfully sway doctors. Bias is especially likely when the information is delivered during extravagantly sponsored educational activities. There is little doubt that drug companies exercise considerable influence over the American Psychiatric Association and the FDA. A recent study in the *New England Journal of Medicine* found that FDA-registered clinical trials on antidepressants with negative results are either not published or published in such a way as to convey a positive outcome (Turner et al. 2008). It warns that such biased reporting leads to unrealistic estimates of drug effectiveness and risks. Adverse consequences for researchers, study participants, health care professionals, and patients may follow.

For several reasons, pharmaceutical advertising makes a particularly poignant impact on doctors in China. First, many Chinese psychiatrists do not have direct access to the English-language scientific literature on new psychotropic drugs. Others may be barred from understanding it because of language barrier. As a result, they have to rely on Chinese-language educational information that is usually provided by drug firms. Second, there is little consumer organization that lobbies for psychiatric patients' rights, and access to legal help is very limited. Drug-related complications are therefore less likely to be documented than in the West. Finally, the economic power differential between salespersons and doctors in China is different from that of most Western countries, Hong Kong, or Taiwan.

These "detail persons" in China consist of friendly, pleasant looking, and gracefully dressed young women and men who confidently market their products. Unlike their counterparts in developed countries, they are carefully selected medical graduates who receive training from Western-style marketing managers. Typically, they earn a salary several times higher than that of medical doctors. In many other countries it may be considered "working down" for doctors to become salespeople. But this career change in China was frequently legitimized in the market ethos of the 1990s.

Among Chinese psychiatrists there is a popular saying that depicts the poor financial prospect of working in the mental-health field. It is *jiaoshou yuejiao yueshou* ("the longer a professor teaches, the poorer he becomes"). Nonetheless, a senior academic psychiatrist in Shanghai did not think that young doctors who become salespeople are merely lured away by high salaries. In October 1997, he observed:

> I do not blame young psychiatrists for choosing to work as salespersons. It's not merely about everybody going into business in China these days *[quanmin jingshang]*. If somebody has to be blamed, blame the government! Our doctors' salaries are despicably low compared to those overseas, even lower than waitresses. Their job also offers little satisfaction and opportunity for personal development. Their supervisors, the so-called associate professors who were poorly trained during the Cultural Revolution, are hardly qualified to teach them and provide no academic stimulation at all. In China, we have a common problem of finding competent middle-aged doctors to succeed the retiring senior professors *[jiebanren wenti]*. These professors have worked hard and are learned despite the difficult times they went through. They are like old yellow cows *[laohuangniu]*—they eat grass themselves but they produce milk for their students to drink. If I were a young doctor, I would work for drug firms too.

His view was echoed by a fourth-year female resident: "The associate professors frequently teach me wrong things during ward rounds, but I keep quiet in order not to offend them. After all, if something bad happens to patients, it will be their responsibility, not mine. At other times, they solicit other junior doctors' views and simply re-present the information as their own!" Partly because of improved income for doctors in the new millennium, the trend for medical graduates to work for drug companies has decreased. As in other parts of the world, a number of successful academic psychiatrists have quit their work units to take up leadership positions in these companies. Such developments suggest that the medical profession is steadily gaining sovereignty in postreform China where prestige is measured by market power and in monetary terms.

At least two reasons have made it timely for pharmaceutical companies to expand the Chinese world of clinical depression since the 1990s. First, new classes of antidepressants, especially the "Selective Serotonin Reuptake Inhibitors" (SSRIs), have become available. These drugs, such as Prozac, have swept across the United States. They seem to work as efficiently as old-style antidepressants. Unlike older antidepressants, however, they cause fewer side effects and are not lethal during overdose. These characteristics make them safer drugs for patients and have become the focus of considerable pharmaceutical marketing. Nonetheless, SSRIs are as expensive for patients as they are lucrative for drug companies. For example, one tablet of imported Prozac (20mg, E Lilly), Seroxat (20mg, GlaxoSmithKline) and Efexor (75 mg, Wyeth) cost in 2008 about eleven RMB (about US$1.60), twelve RMB (about US$1.70) and fourteen RMB (about US$2) respectively. On a daily dose basis, this is about thirty-five times the cost (0.35 RMB) of one hundred milligrams of locally made imipramine, an equally effective old-generation antidepressant. The cost of domestically manufactured SSRIs is lower (e.g., *Youke* or fluoxetine is four RMB per 20mg tablet) than the imported ones. But it is still over ten times the cost of imipramine therapy. Since the recommended period of acute and preventive treatment for depression is at least one year, the total yearly cost of new antidepressant therapy for a patient will be several thousand RMB. This is beyond the means of most working-class and unemployed people in China. Nonetheless, China has a 1.3 billion population. Even if only the insured and more affluent classes can afford new drugs, the Chinese antidepressant drug market is still lucrative.

The second factor that benefits the pharmaceutical industry is the government pricing policy. Because of radical health care privatization, hospital expenditure in China is no longer largely subsidized by government budgets. Decentralization of the fiscal system and the need for the government to make up for the huge losses incurred by SOEs have dramatically limited the government budget for health care. Since hospitals have to generate their own income to cover the escalating cost of operations, they no longer provide free medical services as in the collective era. Apart from over-ordering high-tech services, the other main method of maximizing profit is to prescribe new or imported drugs rather than domestically produced basic drugs. New and invariably more expensive drugs, unlike basic drugs kept within the reach of ordinary wage earners by the Central Pricing Commission, have an allowed mark-up of 15 percent or more. It is noteworthy that the bonus payments that doctors receive in addition to their regular salaries are tied to the revenue they generate for their hospitals. Additionally, doctors may get kickback *(huikou)* from drug companies (Blumenthal and Hsiao 2005). From the 1990s onward, some 40 percent of the income for hospitals in China has come from pharmaceutical sales (Chinese Center for Disease Control and Prevention 2007). Unlike other medical specialties such as surgery, there are few investigatory and surgical procedures for charging patients in psychiatric practice. Surely, provider-induced demand has encouraged the use of new antidepressants.

In their effort to launch the new generation of antidepressants, drug companies have meticulously embellished neurasthenia as a pharmacoresponsive form of biological depression. Aware of most Chinese psychiatrists' then greater familiarity with neurasthenia than depression, they strategically advertised Kleinman's finding, without his rich anthropological interpretations, that 87 percent of neurasthenic patients suffered from major depression. A colorful pamphlet on fluoxetine issued in 1996 by Watson Pharmaceuticals says:

It's been estimated that over ten million people in China suffer from depression, which causes prolonged suffering to patients and their family members. According to the CCMD-2-Revised, the diagnosis of depression is based on the presence of persistently depressed mood and 4 of the following symptoms. . . . In one study in China, 50–87% of patients diagnosed as neurasthenia (the common symptoms of which are headache, insomnia, dizziness, forgetfulness, anxiety, and loss of energy) fulfilled the criteria for depression. Fluoxetine is indicated for mild depression, severe depression, psychogenic depression and depressive neurosis.

For better or worse, pharmaceutical companies are ahead of Chinese academic psychiatrists in broadening the concept of depression. Substituting depression for neurasthenia also facilitates their seeking approval for marketing new generations of antidepressant drugs. In fact, new antidepressants nearly always make their way into the reimbursable drug lists in China's cities. It is worth noting that Prozac was aggressively translated as *baiyoujie*, meaning "undoer of all kinds of worries or sorrow." This connotes a broad-spectrum therapeutic effect and encourages prescription across multiple disease categories. The translation was later required by the State Food and Drug Administration to be changed. The subsequent alteration, involving the middle character, from "worry" to "excellence," was creative. This is because these two characters are phonetically identical *(you)* and ideographically near-identical, thereby preserving the drug's connotation as a panacea.

BIG PHARMA AND EXCHANGE OF FAVOR

In Western countries, the medical-industrial complex has aroused considerable public concern over conflicts of interest and prompted serious attempts to reform physician-industry relations in regard to medical research, education, and practice. Professional bodies have issued increasingly stringent regulations on competing interest disclosures that doctors must comply with when they work with drug companies, including online disclosure of physician-industry relationships. Exceptionally, the British Royal College of Psychiatrists has conducted its annual meeting at Imperial College, London, without any industrial sponsorship since 2008. By contrast, there is as yet no official policy in China for doctors to disclose conflicts of interest. Unsurprisingly, some Chinese professors are more ready than others to speak for the virtues of new antidepressants. At a national conference on biological psychiatry held in November 1995, for example, a well-known professor was asked to give a short lecture on fluoxetine. Although empirical evidence was lacking, he listed neurasthenia as an indication for treatment because it was a form of "atypical depression." At a dinner symposium sponsored by Eli Lilly during the 1997 Regional Meeting of the World Psychiatric Association, a senior Chinese professor who used to defend the disease validity of neurasthenia, reported on an open (i.e., non-blind) clinical trial of twenty-nine patients with neurasthenia. He concluded that "treatment of neurasthenia with fluoxetine appears to produce clinically more significant effects on some aspects of the symptoms of neurasthenia and to have fewer side effects than does doxepin [an old generation antidepressant]." This statement contrasted with his clinical impression in May 1979 that the response of neurasthenic patients to antidepressant medications was "not as good as had been hoped" (Kleinman and Mechanic 1980). This is despite the fact that Chinese patients with a diagnosis of neurasthenia in the 1970s were much more likely to suffer from depression than they were in the 1990s.

Depression has also been appropriated for medicalizing other social problems.

At a psychiatric conference I attended in 1996, a female pediatrician concluded in her paper that two to three weeks of treatment with Prozac achieved "pleasing results" in ninety-six children who refused to go to school. Several participants questioned the ethical basis of the study. But she defended that Prozac helped these children because they all suffered from "underlying mild depression." She also cautioned that the age at onset of depression had decreased, and that depression could present in all sorts of ways in young children.

Besides funding clinical trials, drug companies have supported leading Chinese psychiatrists to attend international conferences that few of them could afford by themselves. There is, of course, no such thing as a free lunch. By tactfully manipulating the exchange of favor *(renqing)*, drug firms have subsequently "invited" these psychiatrists to give promotional lectures. Although such transactions are a routine element of the medical-industrial complex in the West, they represented a novel and sometimes morally taxing experience for Chinese academics in the 1990s. As one senior professor told me right after he talked about the effectiveness of Seroxat in 1996: "I was quite uneasy *[nanweiqing]* with the talk as it made me feel I was working for the drug company *[tiyaochang dagong]*. But I could not turn down the request because I owed the company a favor. Do overseas academics do this too?" After lecturing on Zoloft (an SSRI, Pfizer) at the same conference, another well-known professor of psychiatry asked me: "What do you think of my talk? Maybe I shouldn't have mentioned that Prozac is not as good as Zoloft. That may have offended some people. Anyway, I don't want to give such a drug-selling *[maiyao]* talk in the future." By 1997, this professor had become more comfortable with such lecturing: "I have already become the academic consultant for three major drug companies, which have kept me really busy lecturing. It's so hard to turn them down. . . . I used to have a lot of interesting conversations with my academic friends during conferences. But I am now so occupied with the pharmaceuticals that I can hardly talk with them any more. . . . I believe this is just a transitional period for Chinese psychiatrists. Things will become better in the future."

Since the late 1990s, drug companies have also targeted unrecognized depressive patients in medical departments. A professor of psychiatry from Shanghai was critical of this form of "general hospital psychiatry." In December 1997, he commented:

> The drug firms give a lot of money to general doctors with no psychiatric training. They ask them to give SSRIs to medically ill patients who simply don't feel happy. A television program in Beijing has recently revealed that a general hospital doctor can get "grey" income of as much as 5,000 RMB

per month, which is three times his salary. I do think the SSRIs are good drugs that can reduce the misuse of benzodiazepines. But the drug companies manipulate our non-psychiatric doctors, who often prescribe blindly *[xiayongyao]*. And there are so many drug salesgirls speaking out for them nowadays.

A chief resident in the southern city of Shenzhen was similarly concerned: "Doctors in general hospitals are now quite heroic in using the SSRIs. Some of them simply administer the Hamilton Depression Rating Scale. Once a score of 20 or more is obtained and provided patients can afford it, they will prescribe without making a clinical assessment of depression." Shen Qijie, a well-known professor and researcher on depression in China, has this to say about the increase in diagnosis of depression:

> Both drug companies and psychiatrists are obliged to educate general doctors and the public on the recognition and treatment of psychiatric disorders, including depression. . . . But we must beware that unwholesome reward systems can cajole doctors into over-extending the ambit of depression, and consequently misusing antidepressants as "happiness pills." The neurasthenia label is widely used in general hospitals. So drug firms have recently pushed the use of new antidepressants among these so-called neurasthenic patients. Despite the absence of empirical evidence that such treatment is effective, the use of these drugs is increasing. However, this attempt to resurrect neurasthenia for the sake of encouraging prescription may run counter to psychiatrists' efforts to teach general doctors how to recognize depressive disorders among patients indiscriminately labeled with neurasthenia. I therefore urge that drug companies should carry out such commercial activity cautiously!

Nonetheless, the new millennium has witnessed a continued increase in the clinical diagnosis of depression in China. This is true of both psychiatrists and general hospital doctors. Moreover, the notion of mild depression *(qingxing yiyuzheng)*, previously unknown among Chinese psychiatrists, has become increasingly fashionable. The Chinese professional definition of clinical depression has slackened. There was a three-month duration requirement for depressive neurosis in the previous Chinese diagnostic system. By contrast, the current diagnosis of depression only requires a patient to report two or more weeks of frequent low mood or low energy as in the American diagnostic system (Chinese Society of Psychiatry 2001). Articles on how depression is caused by inadequate brain serotonin function, early recognition of mild depression, and randomized controlled trials of SSRIs are readily found in Chinese medical journals. By 2008, the new antidepressants have become much more commonly prescribed than earlier generation antidepressants in China. The influence of drug companies on professional practice becomes rampant as global companies expand their sales forces and distribution channels to tap into the country's enormous drug market. For example, sponsorships from five drug companies can be found on the third page of the authoritative CCMD-3 manual. A "Wyeth Pharmaceuticals" logo likewise appears on a widely used webpage on mental health hosted by the Chinese Society of Psychiatry and Beijing Huilongguan Hospital.[1]

SUICIDE AS DEPRESSION

Suicide has an ancient provenance in Chinese society. It is often considered a moral act in trying circumstances. This is illustrated by the quintessential example of Qu Yuan, a Chinese poet and official during the Warring States period, who committed suicide by jumping into the Miluo River. His suicide expressed his moral repugnance for the government of his time. By conveying his uprightness, the suicide had a wide social impact. Even today, Chinese people still commemorate Qu Yuan's sacrifice at the Dragon Boat Festival by eating glutinous-rice dumplings and participating in dragon boat races. Although reliable statistics are wanting, popular literature and anecdotal accounts suggested that suicide was alarmingly common during the Maoist era. It affected particularly the "four bad types," namely, landlords, wealthy peasants, intellectuals, and dissidents. In those chaotic circumstances, suicide might represent a way out of humiliation and moral resistance against oppressors.

Some of the most recent examples of suicide in China are of a morally reverse kind. These have come from Chinese government officials suspected of corruption as they resort to suicide as a way out of shame and punishment. One of them was Song Pingshun, the sixty-two-year-old chairman of the Tianjin municipal People's Political Consultative Conference and director of the municipal party politics and law committee. Amid the central government's investigation of corruption, Song asphyxiated himself in an office building of the Chinese People's Political Consultative Conference on June 3, 2007. He did so by sealing his mouth with tape, wearing a mask, and covering his head with a plastic bag. Song had worked in the city's public service for more than forty years. He was the first ministerial-level official to kill himself since former Beijing mayor Wang Baosen did so in 1995.

Suicide thus reveals societal ills and makes a moral impact on people. This explains why it had been a taboo subject for research, health intervention, and media coverage in China. The Chinese government did not begin to report suicide data to the World Health Organization until 1989 (see chapter 6 by Wu Fei in this volume).

This was long after suicide had become a well-established field of academic and policy research in other countries. The statistics indicate an alarming picture that counterbalances the optimistic accounts of prosperity and its much acclaimed effect on everyday life as a result of economic reform. There were 343,000 suicides in China in 1990. When converted into suicides per one hundred thousand people, the rate is three times the global average. Over nine hundred people kill themselves in China each day. Recent estimates of suicide in China are somewhat lower (about 230,000 deaths per year) but the number remains high by international standards.

Suicide has complex social antecedents (e.g., impulsivity in the setting of serious family, financial, and work problems) and consequences. This complexity is well illustrated by an alarming chain of ten suicidal deaths and several suicide attempts among young migrant workers at the Foxconn Technology Group between January and May, 2010. The giant Taiwanese contract manufacturer in Shenzhen makes some of the most well-known global products, such as the iPhone, and has responded to the suicide crisis by sharply increasing workers' wages, asking them to sign no-suicide pledges, and calling in mental-health experts to examine the risk factors for workers' suicides in order to prevent them. Whether or not such measures help to diminish suicide rates, this approach may oversimplify the complexity of suicide because social discrimination against migrant workers, exploitative employment practices, and other nonmedical causes may play a role.

The complexity of suicide notwithstanding, the contemporary psychiatric perspective considers that people who kill themselves are victims of untreated clinical depression. In this biological model, depression is ultimately a disease of chemical imbalance in the brain. Therefore, psychiatric treatment (typically pharmacological) is justified for preventing suicide. The medical method of research for establishing the causal link between suicide and depression is known as "psychological autopsy." This is carried out by researchers asking one or more persons who know the dead person whether the latter exhibited the diagnostic symptoms of depression prior to suicide. Psychological autopsy research worldwide has shown that 80 to 90 percent of people who died by suicide suffered from depression. The findings from studies carried out in China, though lower in number, are not very dissimilar. About 70 percent of suicide in China is said to be caused by depression.

Most symptoms psychiatrists use for diagnosing depression are subjective and people with depression may conceal their feelings for one reason or another. Nonetheless, psychological autopsy research assumes that the subjective experience of a dead person can be accurately retrieved from people around him or her. Because the researchers are nearly always psychiatrists who subscribe to the medical model of suicide and the research findings cannot be disproved by interviewing a dead person, considerable doubt exists as to whether this research method prematurely excludes alternative ways of understanding the complex origins of suicide. Anthropological research in rural China by Wu Fei (see chapter 6 in this volume) suggests that the contribution of depression to suicide may be much less than currently claimed.

There is little doubt that psychological autopsy is a tool of medicalization. By "scientifically" transforming social problems into a medical disease, it can muffle the moral voice of the suicidal individual, render the study and prevention of suicide acceptable to governments, as well as secure funds for researchers. Indeed, the suicide-as-disease discourse may help explain the Chinese government's somewhat softened stand after decades of embargo on suicide research and prevention. Regular national and international conferences on suicide and depression have been held in China since the late 1990s, though the government continues to impose restrictions on the content of academic presentations. Constraints on media reporting on suicide have generally been relaxed. Resources have been allocated to the development of crisis intervention centers for preventing suicide in many regions of the country. The Beijing Suicide Research and Prevention Center was established in 2002 as a model for the country. Its website says that "one of the best methods of preventing suicide is to promote public knowledge of depression and suicide. Many sufferers of depression (the most common cause of suicide) do not recognize that it is a mental disorder . . . current treatment for depression is very effective, so that not seeking treatment will bring about a vast number of 'unnecessary suicide[s].' "[2] The center has pledged to reduce the annual suicide rate of China by 20 percent within the next eight years, thereby saving fifty to sixty thousand lives per year. In 2009, its researchers published in *The Lancet* a multiprovince community epidemiological study based on an innovative and yet controversial methodology. They argued that Chinese individuals with depression might not present with depressed mood or low energy, which are the two core diagnostic symptoms of depression in the current DSM system. Accordingly, they broadened the DSM definition of depression to include people feeling "emotionally constricted, gloomy/dejected, negative, pessimistic, and tough to get through the day." They also believed that depression that was subthreshold in degree (i.e., not reaching the internationally standardized number of depressive symptoms required for diagnosis) but judged by psychiatrist-interviewers to be "clinically significant" was a genuine psychiatric disease. Based on these controversially slackened criteria, a person who reported tough days or feeling pessimistic for two weeks and a few other symptoms of depression could be considered as having clinical depression. Although the methodological strategies of the study are of interest to cross-cultural research, they are medicalizing in their consequences. Unsurprisingly, the study reported a high current (one-month) prevalence of depressive illness of 6.1 percent (Phillips et al. 2009). In stark contrast to the findings of previous national psychiatric surveys, this elevates China to one of the most depressed countries in the world today![3]

MEDICALIZATION OF TRAUMA

The concept of "post-traumatic stress" has become increasingly popular in Western society. Research has shown that more than half of people in the United States reported during their lifetime at least one traumatic or disastrous event that may be natural, political, or psychological in origin. Besides, 7 percent of Americans suffer from a mental disorder known as post-traumatic stress disorder (PTSD). This is characterized by the development of distressing or impairing anxiety and hyperarousal symptoms for one month or more following exposure to an extreme traumatic stressor. PTSD is usually accompanied by depression. Its treatment is pharmacological and/or psychological.

Large-scale traumas and disasters have been common in modern Chinese history, but the concept of post-traumatic stress or PTSD is alien to China. Political traumas, such as those brought about by the Great Leap Forward, Cultural Revolution, or the June 4 event, were managed by political means. The usual response of the CCP was repression in the service of societal stability and economic growth. Survivors of trauma suffered silently and/or were made to collectively forget the bad experience. There was not a tradition of addressing psychological trauma and offering medical treatment. When traumas took the form of natural disasters, very little of their details and consequences was typically released. For example, the great Tangshan earthquake that occurred on July 28, 1976, is considered to be the biggest earthquake of the twentieth century. Official figures indicated that 242,419 people were killed; some sources suggest a death toll three times higher. Despite the alarming mortality and morbidity, the Chinese government declined international aid. Even today, very little is known about the suffering of the victims of the disaster. The tendency to suppress information is still true of recent disasters such as floods, landslides, and coal mine accidents. China has probably the most deadly mining industry in the world as owners push production beyond safe limits in response to rapidly growing demand and soaring profits. Mine accidents may be man-made rather than natural. The exact number of victims and the postdisaster status of survivors and their relatives remain largely a mystery.

By contrast, the Chinese government demonstrated a distinctly different response to the Sichuan earthquake that occurred on May 12, 2008. This "5.12 earthquake" had the same magnitude (nearly 8.0 on the Richter scale) as the Tangshan earthquake and killed some ninety thousand people. It occurred in a mountainous region that greatly obstructed relief efforts as well as media access. But the government swiftly appealed to the international community for aid and initially allowed the media unprecedented access to the disaster zone. There was moment-to-moment coverage on state-run television of scenes of rescues, shocked survivors, weeping relatives, and other tribulations. These projected powerful public images of traumatic grief and psychological distress. It is noteworthy that there was a state-mandated call for psychological counseling services for victims even though the usefulness of these services remained uncertain. By May 20, 2008, the Ministry of Health dispatched a total of 171 mental health professionals to work with medical personnel, teachers, and volunteers at the earthquake sites to carry out what was the largest mental health crisis intervention in the history of China. The Department of Health, Beijing Military Area, appointed three mental health professionals to quickly publish a manual known as *A Brief and Easy Guide to Helping People with Psychological Trauma after a Major Earthquake*. On June 2, 2008, three thousand copies of this manual were distributed to the army, health staff, and voluntary workers at the disaster sites. At the same time, there has been a noticeable growth of mental health information including websites, training courses, and conferences on post-traumatic psychology (*zaihouxinli* or *chuangshanghouxinli*).[4]

The consequences of "natural" disasters such as the Sichuan earthquake are not necessarily all natural because questions of political accountability are often involved. Victims whose trauma is rooted in social injustice may resist psychiatrists' attempt to pathologize them as patients with PTSD. Even if they do receive medical treatment that partially relieves grief symptoms, traumatic memory can outlive any "successful" treatment. Its moral essence may oblige sufferers to seek out justice and reparation even if this means trespassing state-mandated limits on collective action. It is not surprising that the Chinese government's tolerance of the public demonstration of post-traumatic emotions is often short-lived. In the case of the Sichuan earthquake, many grieving parents had openly expressed their anger and pressed their demands for an investigation into government officials and construction contractors who might have contributed to the death of their children. They believed that corruption was responsible for poorly built schools that readily collapsed and brought about the death of some ten thousand schoolchildren. This aroused extensive public concern and media attention. In response to this, the government detained parents who staged protests outside government offices and tightened control over media reporting. It was only half a year after the earthquake that government officials acknowledged substandard school construction could be a problem in China. Regarding the school buildings that collapsed in the Sichuan earthquake, nonetheless, the Chinese government maintained that they were properly built. What caused the massive collapse of schools remains a delicate issue. On August 12, 2009, police officers in Chengdu detained Hong Kong reporters in their hotel rooms by alleging that they possessed illegal drugs. Although no drugs were found after a seven-hour search, these officers successfully blocked the reporters from covering the trial of human rights activist Tan Zuoren. The latter had been imprisoned for probing into the deaths of schoolchildren in Sichuan.

Traumatic emotions may thus be politically sensitive because of the moral resistance they produce. Although PTSD, like depression, can be treated with SSRI therapy, it has not yet become a target for pharmaceutical marketing in China. The Chinese diagnostic system does contain the diagnosis of PTSD. As the history of the study of suicide shows, however, what the psychiatric profession can legitimately embrace is still under considerable influence from the Chinese state. It remains to be seen whether PTSD may become a popular category of illness in China.

IMPLICATIONS

Much of this chapter has focused on depression. But the big picture of emotional liberalization in China must be one of Chinese people becoming not only sadder but also happier and more self-confident, especially in the post-Olympic and post-Expo era of triumphant glory and national pride. The rich and yet divided subjectivity they experience is embedded in a complex pathway of development clearly different from those of Chinese people in Hong Kong, Taiwan, or Western countries. Although the Chinese Communist regime remains a dictatorship, it has expanded individual liberty in multiple recognizable ways that have brought about a profound transformation of everyday life. For one thing, interpersonal communication can be expected to become increasingly expressive of feelings. These feelings will become ever more discriminating, especially among younger and middle-class individuals. This new mode of articulation needs to be considered in understanding the multiple realities of change in China today. In the mental health arena, there are a number of consequences.

One of these is the finding of rapidly increasing rates of depression in community epidemiological surveys. Indeed, a survey conducted in 2001 and 2002 in Beijing and Shanghai found that depression occurred in 3.5 percent of Chinese adults in their lifetime. This rate, though still lower than that found in the latest Chinese studies, is considerably higher than those rates estimated in the previous national surveys. The same survey indicates that depression along with alcohol and drug problems are going to rise significantly among younger generations of Chinese people. Specifically, the relative risk of depression among people born in 1967 or later was 22.4 times that of those born earlier than 1936. The study also projected that by the time the participants in the survey reach seventy-five years of age, 7.2 percent of them will have developed depression (Lee et al. 2007). This suggests that depression exhibits intergenerational differences in prevalence and is becoming as common in China as in Western countries.

What is bringing about more depression in China? Is the increase real or merely a product of people's greater openness in expressing complaints and of clinicians and researchers' effort to medicalize? The answer is probably both. Increased emotional self-expression and the growing power of psychiatric diagnosis certainly contribute. But the replacement of egalitarian values by meritocratic norms and a hastily widening income gap that follow the uneven transition from a collective economy to a market economy may also play a role. By overwhelming people's mental capacities, these volatile changes may bring about frustration, cynicism, and demoralization in a background of an accelerating rise of individualism. There is no doubt that many entrepreneurs do get rich first in accordance with the call of Deng Xiaoping *(rang yibufen ren xian fuqilai)*. However, many more people have been frustrated by not being able to fulfill the higher expectations that come with economic progress. A study based on the World Values Survey provided empirical evidence that people in China are getting objectively richer but subjectively are not happier. In 1990, 28 percent of Chinese people considered themselves very happy, but by 2000 only 12 percent did so. This drop was found across rural and urban China and in nearly every income bracket (Brockman et al. 2009). Although financial dissatisfaction played a minor role in predicting happiness in 1990, it had by 2000 become a leading predictor of people's happiness. The authors suggested that it was how people perceived their financial position relative to "winners" in China's economic reform, not their absolute income, that explained the loss of happiness.

The people who fare worst are laid-off workers from bankrupt SOEs, exploited migrant workers, impoverished farmers, and the poor elderly with little filial support. In postcollective China generally, everyday life with regard to education, employment, health service, and social and retirement benefits is experienced with a heightened sense of uncertainty. This is partly because the party-state has substantially reduced its protective net of state welfare services. Rapidly growing in numbers, elderly people may be especially likely to feel insecure. They are confronted with barriers to health service access and dwindling filial support, the time-honored Confucian foundation of old-age security in Chinese society, and often continued demands for financial and domestic help from their grown children.

A scary sense of danger is also created by the mass media, which can report on the down side of social change more freely than before. It is now routine to read sensational media accounts of murder, misfortune, traffic accidents, suicide, stock market frenzy, pollution, fraud, food poisoning, communicable diseases, unethical medical practice, counterfeit drugs and food products, carcinogens, corrupt officials, labor disputes, ethnic riots, and the like. After years of double-digit growth, the sense of uncertainty has recently escalated as China eventually found itself drawn into the global financial crisis of 2008 and experienced (albeit briefly) an economic downturn and a fall in export trade. This has led to a surge of social unrest as shrinking jobs and incomes affect growing legions of frustrated university graduates and migrant workers who have become emboldened to express their unhappiness.

Thus, although this chapter has demonstrated the complex cultural-historical contingency of the rise of depression and other psychiatrically defined health problems, it also considers that social change has real consequences for people in their subjective lives. Rampant capitalism is globally known to have real adverse consequences on health. It breeds depression and a cluster of other health problems such as alcoholism, drug addiction, sexually transmitted diseases, HIV/AIDS, domestic and ethnic violence, pathological gambling, deadly traffic injuries, industrial accidents, and the multiple injurious effects of pollution. All these problems are known to be rising in China, a nominally socialist nation. A government-funded seven-thousand-person psychiatric survey conducted in the southern city of Shenzhen in 2006 revealed that over 20 percent of people aged eighteen or over reported a lifetime DSM-defined mental disorder (Hu et al. 2009). This suggested that, using a comparable method of epidemiological research to define mental disorders, the level of psychiatric morbidity in China is catching up with that of high-income countries.

In clinical settings, there has been an obvious increase in the diagnosis and treatment of depression. This is partly because both patients and doctors are now more open in communicating depressive emotions. But this does not mean that most people with depression in the community can go through the barriers to health service access and receive clinical care. Thus, the same survey in Beijing and Shanghai indicated that only 5.6 percent of people who developed depression received treatment during the year of onset of illness. This was despite the relatively high concentration of health care resources in Beijing and Shanghai compared to other regions of China (Lee et al. 2009). The level of treatment is about six times below that of the United States, though comparable with that of other large developing countries with marked disparities in wealth among urban and rural populations. Among the small proportion of people who did receive help, they did so primarily from general medical practitioners who did not confer psychiatric stigma. This indicates that stigma cannot be the main reason for the low rate of help seeking among people with depression in China today. The low rate of treatment is more likely to be due to structural barriers to care, especially among those with more severe mental disorders. Increasingly limited access to health care in China can be traced back to economic reforms that cut back on government support and progressively eroded the collective health care system. Government and work unit-funded health insurance is now available to less than half of the urban population and almost no one in rural China. A major illness may wipe out the savings of an entire family. Consequently, financial barriers have prevented many people from perceiving the need for clinical care as well as access to care. Since even very poor people enjoyed basic health service access prior to the reform era, the treatment gap for depression is cogent testimony to the paradoxical nature of China's socialist modernity as it has been guided by the invisible hand of the market.

As a further sign of unmet mental health needs and the growth of the private health care sector in China today, demand for Western-style talk therapy that focuses on emotional release and psychological growth is increasing among the new middle class. Nowadays, it is not unusual to see on television a Chinese "psychologist" analyzing and healing people's disturbed psyches. Although most people cannot afford the relatively high costs of psychotherapy, variously labeled counseling clinics have sprung up in the cities. Among health workers, teachers, and self-labeled psychologists, seminars and courses on psychological treatment have become quite popular. These activities are often jointly run by local institutions and Western professionals from a variety of psychotherapeutic traditions. Many university departments of psychology, previously shut down during the Cultural Revolution, now offer longer courses in order to churn out more qualified psychologists. Though not affordable for poorer people, the rapidly growing market for talk therapy heralds a new era in the management of emotions and other problems of the Chinese psyche. It suggests that many Chinese people no longer deny or conceal emotional problems as in the Maoist period. Nor are they obliged to keep their problems within the family in accordance with traditional cultural values. Instead, it is becoming socially acceptable to pay to talk to an outsider for venting private emotions and solving the problems of living created by the malaise of modernizing China.

But it is worth remembering that the familiar professional disciplines of clinical psychology, psychiatric social work, and occupational therapy have barely been established in China. Not unlike other developing countries, professional and ethical issues such as ensuring the standard of training, supervision, board examination, licensing, mandatory continuing education, confidentiality, and protection of patients' rights are matters that mental health professionals in China have only begun to tackle recently. In fact, there are fewer than twenty thousand doctors working in psychiatric settings in China, and they are unevenly distributed across the country. This gives a psychiatrist/population ratio that is about fifteen times lower than in the United States when China's population of 1.3 billion is considered. Most of these doctors have not received official psychiatric training of a kind available in developed countries. Expectedly, a national specialist board examination of an internationally acceptable standard has yet to be set up.

A low standard of psychiatry can make doctors vulnerable to exploitation, collusion, and even corruption, especially if they were poorly trained and worked in *Ankang* ("Peace and Health") hospitals run by the Ministry of Public Security (i.e., the police). To the author's knowledge, there is no evidence of systematic abuse of psychiatry in China as in the former Soviet Union where dissidents were politically diagnosed and mistreated for "sluggish schizophrenia." I have personally assessed patients with psychoses induced by the inappropriate practice of Falun Gong and other forms of qigong during China's qigong boom (Lee and Kleinman 2002). The latter was a period in the late '80s and early '90s when qigong, a therapeutic practice based on controlling and channeling one's vital energy (Chen 2003), was widely practiced by Chinese people as an inexpensive and beneficial antidote to the social chaos brought about by the Cultural Revolution. It was long before 1999 when the silent vigil of over ten thousand Falun Gong practitioners outside the CCP leaders' compound in Zhongnanhai prompted an official crackdown on the practice. Nonetheless, even if the Falun Gong could genuinely induce psychotic breakdown in susceptible individuals, and some of them might even turn out to suffer from bona fide schizophrenia, inadequate ethical and clinical training could put psychiatrists at risk of being used by police officers entrusted to suppress the practitioners. If, for example, Chinese psychiatrists who carried out forensic assessment did not distinguish between delusion (defined psychopathologically as an unshakable and usu-ally false belief that is out of keeping with a person's cultural and personal back-ground) and legitimate cultural beliefs (such as shared religious beliefs), they could have colluded with local police in detaining and even maltreating otherwise men-tally normal dissidents and petitioners who were confined for psychiatric assessment (Mirsky 2003). One important way to prevent the abuse of psychiatry is therefore to improve the ethical standard and professional autonomy of psychiatrists in China. And this is something China's leading psychiatrists seek as their field slowly professionalizes.

Likewise, of the large number of self-labeled counselors and psychotherapists in China today, it has been estimated that only about two thousand are professionally qualified. Their standard therefore varies considerably. At present there are few for-mal mechanisms to ensure the quality of psychological treatment even though psy-chotherapy is known to be capable of causing harm. It is not even clear what the quality of services is like in the new private sector where consumers may conceiv-ably exercise more rights over the treatment services they receive. This is not even to speak of the vast and under-staffed public psychiatric system. As with many other social phenomena that emerge during China's unique and uncertain engagement with global modernity, it is hard to predict how professional psychiatry and psy-chotherapy will evolve. Suffice it to say that there are no quick fixes and what we know about professionalization in developed countries may not apply. It remains to be seen whether mental health services will improve following the recent economic challenges as Chinese leaders consider increasing health care investments to boost domestic consumption and maintain economic growth. Here, the same uncertainty that emerges from changes in subjectivity is emerging in the professions (psychia-try and psychology) legitimized to manage those changes.

NOTES

1. Chinese Psychiatry Online, www.21jk.com/p/index.asp.

2. Beijing Suicide Research and Prevention Center, www.crisis.org.cn/.

3. In 2010, Phillips, a Canadian, stepped down as leader of the Beijing Municipal Sui-cide Prevention Center and transferred to become director of the Shanghai Suicide Re-search and Prevention Center. It may be that this change reflects a continuing sensitiv-ity in China's capital about the way its suicide problem is perceived both within China and abroad.

4. E.g., www.21jk.com/zhxlrx/zhxlrx.asp.

REFERENCES

Blue, L. 2008. "Prozac over the Counter?" *Time*. May 26. www.time.com/time/health/article/0,8599,1809504,00.html. Accessed February 21, 2011.

Blumenthal, D., and W. Hsiao. 2005. "Privatization and its Discontents: The Evolving Chinese Health Care System." *New England Journal of Medicine* 353, no. 11:1165–1170.

Brockmann, H., J. Delhey, C. Welzel, and H. Yuan. 2009. "The China Puzzle: Falling Happiness in a Rising Economy." *Journal of Happiness Studies* 10:387–405.

Chang, H. L., and X. L. Zhang. 1994. *Grass Soup*. Boston: David R. Godine.

Chang, J. 1991. *Wild Swans: Three Daughters of China*. New York: Simon and Schuster

Chen, N. 2003. *Breathing Spaces*. New York: Columbia University Press.

Chinese Center for Disease Control and Prevention. 2007. *Chinese Health Statistical Digest*.

Feng, J. C. 1996. *Ten Years of Madness: Oral Histories of China's Cultural Revolution*. San Francisco: China Books.

Horwitz, A. V., and J. C. Wakefield. 2007. *The Loss of Sadness: How Psychiatry Transformed Normal Sorrow into Depressive Disorder*. New York: Oxford University Press.

Hu J., Hu C. Y., Duan W., Gao H., Zhang X., and Tang Z. 2009. "Shenzhenshi huji ji feihuji jumin jingshenjibing xiankuang diaocha" [Survey on mental disorders among registered residents and non-registered residents in Shenzhen]. *Zhonghua Liuxingbingxue Zazhi* [Chinese Journal of Epidemiology] 30, no. 6:543–548.

Jackson, S. W. 1986. *Melancholia and Depression: From Hippocratic Times to Modern Times*. New Haven, CT: Yale University Press.

Kleinman, A. 1982. "Neurasthenia and Depression: A Study of Somatization and Culture in China." *Culture, Medicine and Psychiatry* 6, no. 2:117–190.

———. 2006. *What Really Matters: Living a Moral: Life Amidst Uncertainty and Danger*. New York: Oxford University Press.

Kleinman, A., and D. Mechanic. 1980. "Mental Illness and Psychosocial Aspects of Medical Problems in China." In *Normal and Abnormal Behaviour in Chinese Culture*, edited by A. Kleinman and T. Y. Lin, 331–356. Dordrecht: D. Reidel Publishing Company.

Lee, S. 1998. "Estranged Bodies, Simulated Harmony, and Misplaced Cultures: Neurasthenia in Contemporary Chinese Society." *Psychosomatic Medicine* 60, no. 4:448–457.

Lee, S., and A. Kleinman. 2002. "Psychiatry in Its Political and Professional Context: A Response to Robin Munro." *Journal of the American Academy of Psychiatry and the Law* 30, no. 1:120–125.

Lee, S., A. Tsang, M. Y. Zhang, Y. Q. Huang, Y. L. He, Z. R. Liu, Y. C. Shen, and R. C.

Kessler. 2007. "Lifetime Prevalence and Inter-Cohort Variation in DSM-IV Disorders in Metropolitan China." *Psychological Medicine* 37, no. 1:61–71.

Lee, S., A. Tsang, Y. Q. Huang, Y. L. He, Z. R. Liu, M. Y. Zhang, Y. C. Shen, and R. C. Kessler. 2009. "The Epidemiology of Depression in Metropolitan China." *Psychological Medicine* 39, no. 5:735–747.

Li, Z. S. 1994. *The Private Life of Chairman Mao: The Memoirs of Mao's Personal Physician.* London: Chatto and Windus.

Liu, X. 2002. *The Otherness of Self: A Genealogy of the Self in Contemporary China.* Ann Arbor: University of Michigan Press.

Liu X. H. 1982. "Shenjing shuairuo 1982" [1982 Neurasthenia]. In *Zhongguo yixue baike quanshu–Jingshen bingxue* [Chinese Medical Encyclopedia—Psychiatry], 75–76. Shanghai: Shanghai Publishing House of Science and Technology.

Mirsky, J. 2003. "China's Psychiatric Terror." *New York Review of Books* 50, no. 3:38–42.

Phillips, M. R., J. Zhang, Q. Shi, Z. Song, Z. Ding, S. Pang, X. Li, Y. Zhang, and Z. Wang. 2009. "Prevalence, Treatment, and Associated Disability of Mental Disorders in Four Provinces in China during 2001–05: An Epidemiological Survey." *The Lancet* 373, no. 9680:2041–2053.

Solomon, A. 2001. *The Noonday Demon: An Atlas of Depression.* New York: Scribner.

Starr, P. 1982. *The Social Transformation of American Medicine: The Rise of a Sovereign Profession and the Making of a Vast Industry.* New York: Basic Books.

Thaxton, R. A., Jr. 2008. *Catastrophe and Contention in Rural China: Mao's Great Leap Forward Famine and the Origins of Righteous Resistance in Da Fo Village.* New York: Cambridge University Press.

Thurston, A. 1987. *Enemies of the People.* New York: Alfred A. Knopf.

Turner, E. H., A. M. Matthews, E. Linardatos, R. A. Tell, and R. Rosenthal. 2008. "Selective Publication of Antidepressant Trials and Its Influence on Apparent Efficacy." *New England Journal of Medicine* 358, no. 3:252–260.

Yan, Y. X. 2003. *Private Life Under Socialism: Love, Intimacy, and Family Change in a Chinese Village.* Stanford, CA: Stanford University Press.

Zhang M. Y. 1986. "Shenjing shuairuo de zhenduan wenti" [The Diagnostic Problem of Neurasthenia]. *Zhonghua shenjing jingshenke zazhi* [Chinese Journal of Neurology and Psychiatry] 19:261–263.

Zhonghua Yixue Jingshenke Fenhui [Chinese Society of Psychiatry]. 2001. *Zhongguo jingshen zhang'ai fenlei yu zhenduan biaozhun, di san ban* [The Chinese Classification of Mental Disorders, 3rd ed. (CCMD-3)]. Shandong: Shandong Publishing House of Science and Technology.

CHAPTER SIX · Suicide, a Modern
Problem in China

Wu Fei

On December 5, 2007, Yu Hong, a well-known literature professor at Renmin University in Beijing, committed suicide by jumping from the tenth floor of a high-rise building.[1] Given that Yu Hong was a prominent intellectual figure in China, his death provoked numerous discussions about suicide and reminded people of other famous suicides over the past three decades. On March 26, 1989, Haizi, indisputably the best Chinese poet of his time, threw himself in front of a train in Shanhaiguan; on January 4, 1991, Sanmao, a writer celebrated on both sides of the Taiwan Strait, hanged herself in a hospital; on September 24, 1991, Gemai, another poet, drowned himself in a river near Peking University. This is far from a complete list.

After each suicide, people were thrown into anxious debates about the meaning of life and death; but such heated concern would not have lasted long if it weren't for the finding that the suicide rate in China is one of the highest in the world. In 2002, in a paper published in *The Lancet,* Michael Phillips (who has devoted his research career to the study of this condition in China) and his colleagues found that the suicide rate in China is twenty-three to thirty cases for every one hundred thousand people (Phillips, Li, and Zhang 2002). This rate is more than two times greater than that in the United States. Phillips's study attracted great attention from practitioners in many fields, and suicide thereafter became a hot topic in China studies. Key findings in several studies are that women, young people, and the elderly (in contrast to middle-aged people), particularly among the rural population, are most inclined to commit suicide. These findings—save for the high suicide rate among the elderly—are different from what is observed in most other countries. Also notable is the finding that the rate of mental illnesses seems significantly lower among Chinese suicides than in most Western countries.

These differences are not arbitrary. While some scholars try to explain them using a global public health perspective, clinical psychiatric principles, and large-scale social factors, it seems to me that the best way to understand the particularities of suicide in China is to dig deep into its cultural roots. By understanding suicide, we end up also inquiring into profoundly important aspects of Chinese culture today.

An important factor related to suicide is family politics. There are multiple causes for different suicides, but among the two hundred cases I examined in Mengzou County (a pseudonym) in northern China, where I conducted seventeen months of anthropological fieldwork, more than 90 percent appear to be due to family politics. In another survey, conducted recently in six counties in Hebei Province by the NGO Rural Women, 83.3 percent of respondents said they regard family problems as the most important cause of suicide (Rural Women 2008: 10).

The family has long been held to be the central institution in Chinese society (Fei 1975; Freedman 1971). For a Chinese person, the most crucial indicator of happiness is whether she or he has led what the Chinese refer to as a harmonious family life. The fact that family life is essential to a Chinese person's happiness, however, does not mean that it is easy to handle or cope with. In a family, it is necessary to deal with people whose personalities, needs, and experiences are different from one's own. This leads to all manner of conflict between family members as they confront and negotiate divergent stakes and obligations in the process of articulating collective interests and undertaking decisions and actions that will serve those interests. In other words, there is always politics in any given family. Family politics is different from public politics in that deep emotional engagement is always involved, as is moral commitment to what is most at stake. When family members are at odds with each other, they not only seek to get an upper hand in family politics, but also want to earn each others' love and respect. Family members are not usually enemies. The principle behind family politics is not hatred—though that emotion may be stimulated by events—but rather deep emotional attachment and moral responsibility (what is meant by the word *love*, in common-sense terms).

It is these principles—of love, emotional attachment, and moral responsibility—that make family politics much more complex than public politics between strangers. The following anecdotal example illustrates why this is so. A young woman named Qiongzhi had established a very good relationship with her husband. However, this status was challenged when a thief was able to steal Qiongzhi's tape recorder because she was not watching it carefully. When she told her husband of the theft, he said some extremely rude things and blamed her for it. Qiongzhi could not bear his reaction. She later said, "He was never so rude to me. How could my husband blame me like that?" Then, on impulse, she attempted suicide. She did so in order to express a grievance, to protest, and to resist, because a family member's behavior violated her moral expectation for respectful and just treatment (Wu 2009: 10–11).

I term the sense of injustice in family politics "domestic injustice." Domestic injustice occurs when a family member fails to meet another's expectation—for instance, when one is not treated as well as expected, or when one's words are not listened to by another. Family politics in China is also about respect, and hence it is a moral politics. In family politics, a family member wants to get the upper hand, but it is not good to do so by plunging the family into conflict. Hence there are many games of power, as I shall call them, in the family. And an unusual aspect of family politics in rural China is that suicide becomes a strategy in playing these family games of power. These moral and emotional struggles are changing as China changes, yet they also maintain traditional tensions well known to students of Chinese society in the past. Hence, what we are witnessing at the level of social relations and subjectivity is an *incomplete modernity*. By this term, I do not mean that China is too slow in the process of modernization. On the one hand, China has become quite modernized; on the other hand, Chinese modernization is accompanied by profound moral conflicts and emotional struggles, which make people in modern China unable to feel at home or content. The more modernized China is—in technological, institutional, and economic ways—the sharper such conflicts become. In order to make modern Chinese civilization more comfortable and less conflicted, China needs to complete modernization at the level of relationships, subjectivity, and moral experience. As long as the process of modernization in this sense is unfinished for ordinary Chinese people, it is an "incomplete modernity."

When I tried to study family politics that led to suicide, many villagers said, "It [suicide] is for trivial matters. How can there be great conflicts between family members?" It is true that the reasons for many suicides appear quite trivial. The fact that so many trivial matters are pushing people to commit suicide, however, shows that this is by no means a trivial phenomenon. In newspapers, on television, or on the Internet, we frequently read suicide stories of famous people, young students, peasants, workers, or others who protest public politics. But when I was doing my fieldwork, I found that this kind of suicide is by no means the major type. Though they are more numerous, the suicides that take place in the domestic realm and in connection with family politics do not attract mass media attention. No reporter seems interested in a peasant woman's suicide following a trivial quarrel with her husband. This is why people seldom considered suicide in peasant families to be a big problem before Michael Phillips published data showing the high suicide rate in China.

Different types of family relationships produce different problems. Traditionally in China, relationships between parents and children, husband and wife, and brothers were considered the most important family relationships. In today's China, both filial and conjugal conflicts, as well as in-law relationships, can lead to suicide, whereas conflicts between brothers are seldom reasons for suicide. Ninety percent of all suicides in China occur in rural areas. For this reason, suicide cases in rural China tell us the most about suicide in China, and suicide can tell us about strained familial bonds and other experiential effects of modernization for ordinary Chinese.

CONJUGAL CONFLICTS

Yunxiang Yan remarks in his *Private Life under Socialism* that a significant change in China today is that the conjugal relationship has replaced the patriarchal relationship as the central axis of the Chinese family (2003: 109). Happiness in family life largely depends on the conjugal relationship. Conflicts between a couple in the West lead to many things, from unhappiness to divorce. But in China such conflicts can lead to suicide.

There are several main types of conjugal conflicts; two of these—domestic violence and sexual affairs—are readily understandable. But another kind of conjugal conflict, trivial quarrels, which are far more frequent and usually innocuous, can remarkably lead to suicide. At such moments, family members appear to commit suicide quite impulsively. For instance, Yang Benqing committed suicide after a trivial quarrel with her husband. A tractor from a neighbor's village powered through Yang's wheat field and destroyed some of the crop. The driver apologized to her husband, who forgave him. When Yang returned home, she discovered that the wheat had been destroyed, and reproached her husband for being a coward and not protesting their loss more forcefully. After this quarrel, Yang drank pesticide and died.[2] Another case is that of Yu Guo and his wife. At first, there was no serious conflict between the couple; their relationship was good. But neither Yu Guo nor his wife were on good terms with Yu's brothers. Both became depressed over being angry at the brothers and, as a result, often quarreled with each other. Yu's wife was very aggressive on one occasion, and so he drank pesticide as they quarreled.[3] While the arguments that precipitated these suicides seem minor and the suicidal act itself seems impulsive, there are deep structural, emotional, and moral stakes to motivate them.

The minimum moral requirement of a couple in rural China is that they treat each other on equal terms and be faithful to each other. But even in a family where there is no domestic violence or extramarital affair, and even when the couple enjoys a good relationship, suicide can occur. This appears due to a fundamental problem concerning contemporary Chinese people's ideas about, and experiences of, marriage and family.

Usually a couple in rural China gets to know one another in one of two ways: matchmaking is still the most frequent, but romantic love—popular in cities—is sometimes found in rural areas. Although matchmaking is most prevalent, it does not play the central role it once did in traditional marriages. In such marriages, parents and matchmakers were involved throughout and had the final word; now, a matchmaker only introduces a young man to a young woman. Once the two have met, they are on their own, and will usually spend a long time becoming familiar with one another. Hence, the couple decides if they are a good match and shall marry; neither the matchmaker nor parents has decisive authority. In spite of its ancient provenance, rural folk still prefer matchmaking because it seems a more rational way to learn enough about each other quickly before deciding to proceed with a relationship.

At the same time, romantic love is gradually gaining popularity. But older people worry when their children fall in love first. They believe that people in love are simply too romantic to assess the real characteristics of their potential partner. Members of the older generations frequently warn young people: "Be careful and follow your parents' advice when looking for your partners. Romantic love cannot bring good fortune to you." In spite of these warnings, more and more young people are falling in love, getting married, and facing uncertain fortunes in their family lives. Now, even the most stubborn parents seldom openly oppose their children's romantic love, although they worry about the possible consequences.

In one village, the marriage of one couple, Hefang and Kang Hui, is a well-known case of romantic love (Wu 2009: 33–37). Hefang, an actress in a theatrical troupe, got to know Kang Hui, an electrician in the same troupe. Although Kang Hui was much older than Hefang, he was kind to her and she was really touched. They married after the troupe disbanded, despite Hefang's mother's strong objection. She did not return to her natal family until several years later. Kang Hui was kind to her at first and said, "Just beat me when you are angry." In the beginning, Hefang only tapped him gently, but after she gave birth to a son, she sometimes really wanted to beat him. Hefang thought Kang Hui was not good at earning money. He was fond of smoking and always bought expensive cigarettes, which made Hefang uncomfortable. Once Kang Hui drank too much alcohol and fell asleep, and when Hefang returned home after playing mahjong, she found chicken droppings in the room. She was very angry and beat him. He jumped up, also enraged. Holding her hair, he beat Hefang violently. Hefang grasped a bottle of sleeping pills and swallowed them. Scared, Kang Hui rushed her to the hospital. He promised that he would never fight back again, even if Hefang beat him.

A fellow villager commented on Hefang's dilemma,

People in love are blind, but family is something very different from being in love. They have to face many trivial things and complex interpersonal relationships in everyday life. In the case of matchmaking, however, one is more reasonable and thinks carefully about the background, personalities, and defects of the spouse, so it is easier for one to find a good match. When Hefang fell in love with Kang Hui, everyone else knew they were extremely different from each other and could not live together; but Hefang was in love and totally blind. She could not think about it at all.

Many people agree that romantic love blinded Hefang and contributed to the problems in their family. Their analysis appears to make sense because Hefang's attitude toward Kang Hui changed considerably after they got married. In order to get to the heart of this issue, we need to understand how romantic love affected their game of power.

The power structure in this family struck me as one in which both husband and wife had a certain amount of moral capital and neither was in an obviously disadvantaged position. Because Hefang married Kang Hui in spite of her family's objections, she thought she was doing a great favor to him. Kang Hui let her down because he did not live up to her expectations for earning a good living. Kang Hui's inability to provide a good life granted Hefang the right to blame him. That said, Kang Hui treated Hefang well and even granted her the right to beat him when she was angry. The more Hefang beat him, the greater the right he had to fight back. Hence, Kang Hui accumulated moral capital by tolerating Hefang's wrath and physical assaults.

Kang Hui finally burst out in anger. He had accumulated sufficient moral capital so that he felt he was justified in fighting back. Hefang did not expect him to do so because she felt she had a good reason to criticize him. In this case, neither of them accumulated moral capital. Instead, they were engaged in an intense moral competition for dignity. Attempting suicide, as extreme as it sounds, was Hefang's strategy to win this emotional, micropolitical, and moral game of power. This logic is embedded in passion and sensitivity to what is considered right, but it is still rational: I see it as a moral sensibility.

It was their love for each other that won moral capital for both. Nevertheless, love did not decrease their conflicts, but intensified them. It was love that made an otherwise trivial conflict so unbearable as to provoke a suicide attempt.

Critics of romantic love in China worry about young lovers' blindness to each other's negative attributes, because that blindness could undermine the harmony of the future family. These worries are based on the critics' understanding of the games of power in the family. Villagers usually evaluate several factors of the spouse-to-be in matchmaking: family background, ability, personality, and appearance. The determining principle is that the basic characteristics of the individuals should match. A man should marry a woman from a family of similar socioeconomic means, and vice versa. Too much of a difference in family background is likely to create an imbalance in the couple's power structure. For instance, if a wealthy woman marries a poor man, the man will enter the marriage holding a risky disadvantage in power. Nothing can guarantee that a future couple will maintain a power balance, but prudent villagers try to match these objective qualities and reduce the probability of a serious imbalance. Those who hold these principles in high esteem are not ignorant of the role of affection in family life. They know that a couple should also get along well and truly care about each other. Their logic is that the objective qualities will be the basis for both an equitable power distribution and happiness because of long-lasting affection. However, affection is generally held to be predicated on an equitable power balance—a couple cannot have a harmonious family unless the two strike that balance across social and moral status. Only then can love be long lasting. "What is love?" an old woman once commented to me, "If you stay together and live well, you will finally love each other. You can never establish a family based on love."

However, those who believe in romantic love usually follow a different logic. For them, the family begins with affection and aims to maintain and expand that sentiment. Love is not seen as the basis of family life, but something important in itself. With the family revolution in modern China and the growth of individualism, the freedom to love is integrated into the idea of autonomy. To love is now a critical requirement for building and maintaining one's dignity. Suicide stemming from the misalignment of an arranged marriage or failure of love is seen as a powerful attack against the traditional family system. I also know of two girls from my fieldwork who committed suicide when their parents denied them freedom to pursue romantic love. Despite the objections of Hefang's parents, she managed to marry Kang Hui. Choosing this independence is seen by many young people as a way to maintain face and freedom (Croll 1981: 80–106).

Hefang's dilemma was based neither on her mistake in choosing the wrong husband nor on her unreasonableness, but on the cultural conflict between love and family life. The Chinese family revolution has provided more freedom and dignity to people, but it has not guaranteed their happiness as a family. Chinese people in the modern era are subject to the influences of both tradition and modernity. On the one hand, young people still commit suicide because of arranged marriages; on the other hand, many people suffer from the freedom to love. This relatively new freedom is not accompanied by a parallel transformation in family relations that represents the full modernization of the family as is seen in Western societies. Hence, incomplete modernization is at fault here.

FILIAL PIETY

There is a popular expression in China: "Filial piety is the primary virtue, but a heartfelt feeling of filial piety counts, not filial acts; otherwise a poor man cannot be filial." This adage carries two basic insights into traditional family values: that filial piety is seen as the most important virtue (Fei 1975), and that, regarding how to be filial, most important is the feeling state. If one does not behave well, but expresses the proper feeling, it is sufficient to meet one's filial duty. In today's China, however, both meanings of this expression are being challenged as moral experience shifts toward something new and different.

Nobody can deny the positive meaning of filial piety in China. Children are obliged to take care of their parents. Not only is this the basic moral duty, but it is also emphasized in Chinese law. However, when we come to concrete behavior, it is no longer so simple. With the spreading of individualism, parents no longer have absolute control over their children and they are not able to intervene in their marriage and everyday life. Children are quite autonomous. Can a child who is disobedient be filial?

During interviews, many old people said, "Now women's social status is not low, but old people's is low." The power relationships in the modern Chinese family have changed significantly. For example, old people often live in small run-down houses, while young people live in better ones. This appears on the surface to be a complete reversal of filiality. For some children, filial piety only requires economic support. Even Confucius remarked on the society of his day, "Nowadays filial piety merely means being able to feed one's parents. Even dogs and horses are being fed. Without reverence, how can you tell the difference?" (Confucius 1997: 53) In fact, many parents commit or attempt suicide not because their children fail to take material care of them, but because they do not show proper respect. In my survey, most elders agree that filial impiety is a big problem in contemporary China. However, young people do not agree. They still consider filial piety important and don't think of themselves as unfilial, however, their conception of filial piety is different from that of their elders. Yet, elderly parents are not satisfied with the respect and care received from children; sometimes, this can lead to suicide. Suicide of this type involves different understandings of filial piety; it is a tragedy of generational change.

An example is Dongxue, an old woman who committed suicide in 2005. She had a very complex relationship with her children. After the death of her husband, each of her three sons and three daughters wanted to take care of her, but her temper became volatile, she began to act strangely, and she often quarreled with them. She hung herself following what they regarded as a small quarrel with them. Although the children thought they had tried their best, they were not able to satisfy their elderly mother.[4]

In such a case, we cannot simply blame the children, but must further reflect on how Chinese today interpret the significance of filial piety. Children still feel the cultural obligation to support their parents financially, but for their parents, the children also must go beyond material assistance to provide emotional and moral care. Add possible early dementia into the mix and the consequence is not so difficult to understand.

Jiaolan attempted suicide owing to problems with her son. Following her attempt, she had a long talk with me, and provided this narrative fragment:

Last year I felt quite unhappy and did not want to live any longer. I bought some sleeping pills and wanted to take them. My son is too difficult to cope with. I am sixty-six years old. I did all the work in the field and became very strong. Even now I do all the work in the field, and nobody else takes care of it. I have one son and one daughter, but they simply do not respect me.

My relationship with my children is not good because they do not treat me as their mother. I never tell this to the villagers. Unlike his father, my son does not drink alcohol. In several respects he is similar to me, but his temper is as bad as anyone else's in his father's family. I have spoiled him, and he does not concern himself with me at all. He never gives me a penny. I am unlike other old people who ask money from their children. I only want them to give me money voluntarily. You know, the money that I ask from them is different from the money they give me. I wish that my work and concern for them can finally move them, but all my efforts are futile.

Sometimes I really feel that I cannot live like this any more, that there is no hope in this life. I am working for the sake of my son and my daughter day and night, but I never please them. They do not understand what I think and what I aim at. One day last year I worked in the field for a whole day and came home. They already had dinner, but I had eaten nothing that day. I could not find any food in the house and wanted to cook something. I began to work in the kitchen while my son was taking care of the foxes that we cultivate. Seeing that I was about to cook, he asked angrily, "Did you not eat enough?" My tears immediately flowed. I had worked for a day and returned home without eating anything. They did not wait for me to have dinner; that is fine. I also could forgive them if they did not cook for me; but why did they forbid me to cook my own food? I really could not bear what he had said and wept for a whole night. "Let us see whether your life will be better after my death," I said. I decided to commit suicide.

The next morning I went to the county seat and bought three bottles of sleeping pills. Suicide is like this: when one has made a decision and commits suicide without hesitation, it is completed; if one hesitates for a while, perhaps he will not do it and throw away the pills when the moment has passed. I was really angry when buying the sleeping pills, but when I got back to the village and met the villagers, we talked happily, and I forgot all my sadness. I put aside the three bottles and did not attempt suicide this time. (Wu 2009: 112–117)

When I talked with Jiaolan's son, he did not seem to be uncaring toward his mother. Jiaolan's words disclose why she was really dissatisfied with him: "I am unlike other parents who directly ask money from their children. I only want them to give me money voluntarily. You know, the money that I ask from them is different from the money they give me." If she asked for money from her son, she put herself in a humiliating position, as if she were begging. If her son would voluntarily give her money, the situation would be different, and he would show his respect and filial piety. Although the material benefit would be the same, its significance in family politics and moral experience is different. Villagers often teach young people that though their parents do not really lack money, they should still provide financial support in order to show filial piety and thereby to please their parents. Giving money often has more symbolic meaning as a filial gift than economic importance.

Jiaolan complained that her children did not treat her as their mother. A villager commented on her son: "That young man is sometimes confused." He did not really mistreat his mother, as Jiaolan seemed to imply, but he could not find a suitable way to please her. What Jiaolan meant, by criticizing him for not treating her well, was that he did not fulfill his moral duty to show due respect through acts of filial piety. Thus, she could not enjoy her moral capital in the game of power with her son, and this disappointed her greatly.

Jiaolan became depressed because she could not make use of her moral capital and enjoy the respect of her son in family politics. All her efforts to manage the family did not give her an advantageous position in their moral game of power. This depression and frustration both amplified and found expression in the anger she felt upon returning home from the field to find that her son and daughter-in-law had not cooked dinner for her. A good son, as she implied, would wait to have dinner or cook for her. She had been working for a whole day, exhausted and hungry, for the sake of the family. Hence, she had moral capital to ask her son to cook. Nevertheless, not only was he reluctant to cook for her, but he also criticized her. His attitude here is strange; there must have been some misunderstanding. Perhaps he thought Jiaolan already had dinner or forgot that she had not eaten. Whatever the reason, his angry response was not the proper way to speak to his mother. Jiaolan felt indignant and righteously wronged to be scolded by her son after a day of hard work on behalf of their family. She decided to show him that he could not survive without her. Her suicide attempt was her resistance against her son's harsh attitude and a cry for justice.

Food appears to be a trivial matter, but in fact it is symbolically loaded in the family's core exchange relationships and can lead to tragedies. Jiaolan is not the only parent who has attempted or committed suicide on account of a conflict over food. An elderly man from Jianli hung himself because his son and daughter-in-law had hidden steamed bread and instead fed him rancid food. Another elderly man in Gouyi hung himself when he found there was no egg in his soup while everyone else at the table had one. Eryao, an old woman from Shuizhou, drank pesticide when she found her daughter-in-law had not cooked for her. All these parents felt disrespected, ignored, or morally "put down" (Wu 2009: 117–118).

IN-LAWS

Eryao's story is quite similar to Jiaolan's. She usually cooked for the whole family. One day Eryao did not make lunch. Her daughter-in-law, in turn, only made enough food for her husband and herself. When Eryao found there was no food left for her, she committed suicide. Although her daughter-in-law had a bad reputation afterward, she tearfully said to me, "I am not such a silly woman. My relationship with my mother-in-law was very good, and we often joked with each other. Well, now I know that I am a woman notorious for impiety. I do not know why, but I was especially uneasy those days, and hence did not say good words to my mother-in-law. Who knows why she could not think it through this time?" Instead of criticizing her for a lack of piety, most villagers who knew the details said she was very "confused," similar to what people said about Jiaolan's son. By "confusion," they meant that the person was not morally bad, but had no idea about how to please and was simply inept in showing filial respect.

I do not know precisely why Eryao complained about her daughter-in-law, but I suspect it might be similar to why Jiaolan complained about her son. For these parents or parents-in-law, filial piety is not a matter of intention, but a matter of proper manners. In other words, one is not filial merely by stating the desire or will to be. The younger person has to behave properly to show filial piety. Parents cannot force their children to obey or respect them. With the growing emphasis on freedom, autonomy, and equality in the Chinese family revolution, traditional hierarchical and patriarchal systems are broken; yet harmony in the family is still crucial, and it rests on the morally appropriate resolution of the familial game of power I have described. Here, both family dynamics and moral life demonstrate the consequences of incomplete modernity: the Chinese family today is unsettled, neither traditional nor modern, but something unstably in-between.

Although Eryao's story is very similar to Jiaolan's, it turned on a conflict with her daughter-in-law. The relationship between mothers-in-law and daughters-in-law has structurally been a fraught relationship for Chinese. Because it is the meeting point between conjugal and patriarchal ties, it strains both. On the one hand, a conjugal conflict can be transformed into a conflict between the wife and the entire family of her husband, especially her mother-in-law; on the other hand, the problem of filial piety can also be a conflicted relationship between the parents and the families of the children, especially the daughter-in-law, as in Eryao's story. Because of this complexity, not only can conflicts between mothers-in-law and daughters-in-law lead to attempted suicides, but such strife can motivate husbands and sons to do so as well.

I came across many cases of daughter-in-law suicides. For instance, a young woman from Zhengding County committed suicide apparently because her mother-in-law reproached her for losing in a mahjong game. There are also many cases of mother-in-law suicide. One mother-in-law committed suicide simply because she found her lunch was a little different from that of other family members.[5] Changzhai, a man in Haixing County, was married to a woman who had a bad relationship with his parents. Whenever they quarreled, they blamed Changzhai. He finally committed suicide owing to the unbearableness of this constant conflict.[6] What seems on the surface trivial represents at a deeper level of moral experience and individual subjectivity serious issues of what is at stake in social relationships and personal affect.

Zilan's story yields a deeper understanding of the in-law relationship in a family. When I first heard that she once attempted suicide after a quarrel with her husband, she told me that it was entirely due to a trivial matter. Several days before New Year's Day, she asked her husband to open the gate of their yard when she heard someone knocking. Since he refused, they quarreled with each other, and her husband beat her violently. When her husband left in anger, Zilan attempted suicide by drinking pesticide.

The story seemed very straightforward; this is what often gets reported in a newspaper account or clinical report. But after I investigated further in the village, I learned that it was much more complex. Zilan's husband had a very big family. She had not only parents-in-law, but also grandparents-in-law. Zilan's husband had a brother who was in jail. Because his wife and two children had a hard time without the brother being present, Zilan's parents-in-law helped them more than they helped Zilan, which made her unhappy because she also had two children, and her husband was not at home either, owing to his work as a driver. She was resentful and often quarreled with her in-laws for that reason.

A villager said, "Once when I was passing their door, I saw Zilan's father-in-law was holding her hair and slapping her violently. Zilan was crying loudly. I went to stop him. Even if she behaved badly, her father-in-law was not supposed to beat her. This happened several days before her husband came back. I guess her husband was angry when his parents told him of this. The real reason for her quarrel with her husband and her suicide attempt was her quarrel with her father-in-law."

Zilan's aunt also married into this village. After her attempted suicide, Zilan's aunt went to Zilan's grandfather-in-law's house to ask about it. The old man said, "If I were her husband, I would have beaten her to death." Her aunt burst out immediately: "How could you beat her? How can you say such stupid words?" Ever since then, the aunt has stopped talking to the grandfather.

Zilan complained about her husband's reluctance to help her, but these complaints were far less serious than her complaints about her in-laws. Without her many-sided and troubled relationships with her aggregate family, Zilan almost certainly would neither have quarreled so strenuously with her husband nor have attempted suicide (Wu 2009: 63–69).

An aggregate family, as Ellen Judd defines it, is "a family that has divided into more than one household but retains close economic cooperation and sociopolitical relations" (1994: xiv). Although they did not live in the same house, the several nuclear families had very close relations with each other.

When Zilan was quarreling with her parents-in-law, even if she were unreasonable, her father-in-law should not have beaten her. As my guide said, a father-in-law is not supposed to beat his daughter-in-law, for two reasons. First, parents-in-law in the family of today's China no longer have absolute authority over daughters-in-law, although daughters-in-law are supposed to be obedient to them. Second, even if mothers-in-law are often in direct conflict with their daughters-in-law, fathers-in-law are not supposed to get involved. As men, they should neither be too intimate with nor too harsh to their daughters-in-law. In the contemporary Chinese countryside, it is very difficult to maintain a good relationship between in-laws. As Chen Feinian points out, in families where husbands work outside the village like Zilan's, a mother-in-law is often in a more disadvantageous position than her daughter-in-law (2001: 52). Both parents-in-law and daughters-in-law are found to commit suicide because of domestic conflicts. The size of her aggregate family might have been why Zilan was in a disadvantageous position. However, it is hard to assess whether she was really in such a position. Whatever Zilan said or did, her father-in-law's violent beating violated the basic rules for in-laws, and this prompted the villagers to lose respect for him.

Another instance of her in-laws' social inappropriateness is Zilan's grandfather-in-law's words to her aunt: "If I were her husband, I should have beaten her to death." Even if Zilan had been at fault repeatedly, as a senior in the family, the grandfather-in-law was not supposed to say such harsh words, especially to Zilan's aunt. The old woman's visit to the old man was a friendly gesture. As a senior member of Zilan's natal family and the matchmaker, she felt responsible for Zilan's fortune in the village and was of course concerned about her attempted suicide. Perhaps she sided with Zilan, but her visit at least showed her intention to mediate. The old man's harsh words, however, dissolved all her good feelings before they could have a serious talk. He offended Zilan's aunt, the best person in the village to mediate between Zilan and her in-laws, and made it more difficult for Zilan to mend the discord with her in-laws.

Zilan's in-laws' behavior hurt Zilan, but this did not really break the power balance. When Zilan was arguing with her parents-in-law, she did not expect to be treated very well by them. She knew that they would be engaged in a sharp conflict. Hence, Zilan did not think about suicide when her father-in-law was beating her. It was only when her husband quarreled with her that she drank the pesticide. That was the balance of power most at stake for her. This power balance in the nuclear family is key to understanding her attempted suicide.

When Zilan was arguing with her parents-in-law, from her point of view she was struggling not only for herself and her children, but also for the nuclear family including her husband. Her husband was supposed to support her and argue with his sister-in-law and his parents. When her husband failed to calm and comfort her over his parents' mistreatment, but instead beat her, she became extremely sad over his lack of compassion and felt an urge to resist. Unlike her parents-in-law, her husband shared her same interest to protect the nuclear family. His attitude toward her was more important to her than that of her parents-in-law, because her fortune in life was bound to his.

With regard to one's personal happiness, the nuclear family today weighs much more than the aggregate family, and the power balance between a husband and a wife is more important than that between the couple and the husband's parents. A woman is more frustrated when her dignity is threatened within the nuclear family. The conflict between in-laws is especially dangerous when it is transformed into a conflict with the husband.

Zilan's husband was in a more difficult dilemma. On the one hand, he had more responsibilities to his parents than Zilan did; on the other hand, he knew that Zilan was suffering for the nuclear family. It was not a good solution for him to side with either party. In such a case, a wise husband might criticize his wife in public and smooth things over in private. Such a strategy demands skill and patience. If he sided too much with his wife, he would get a reputation for lacking filial respect, a risk that most men dare not take. Therefore, to punish Zilan was a more acceptable solution, though not an ideal one. Hence his wife became the victim of his strategy to harmonize the aggregate family.

Local people comment, "The key figure in mediating between the parents-in-law and the daughter-in-law is the husband." The husband, as the son of his mother, is also seen as a member of the nuclear family of his parents. As a member of both nuclear families, he is responsible for the harmony of both. A mother commented about the husband's position: "When his mother is not satisfied with his wife, she is likely to complain to him, and his wife also complains to him about his mother. If he is wise enough, he should know how to satisfy both women and make the whole family harmonious. A silly husband, however, might make things worse by intensifying the conflicts between the two women." What is at stake here is the cultural emphasis on sustaining the harmony of the family as a balancing of power. Increasingly, the intrusion of major changes in the local worlds of rural people, such as migration and the changing status of women, makes that task more complicated and the likelihood of its failure more real.

An example will illustrate how a husband can worsen the situation. A young woman from one of the villages I studied once complained to her husband about her mother-in-law and said, "I will divorce you if she always does that." She was not serious when saying so, but when her husband tried persuading his mother to treat his wife better, he told her his wife threatened to divorce him if she did not stop. Enraged, his mother said, "Let her get a divorce if she wants." She also did not actually mean this. But the man repeated it to his wife without qualification. A trivial argument eventually became a huge conflict, and the young couple had to move to the house of the wife's parents. This husband wanted to make both women treat each other better, yet his efforts not only proved futile, but actually made things worse. In this sense, the silence of Zilan's husband was better than the loquacity of this husband.[7]

Daughters-in-law and parents-in-law do not live in the same nuclear family and they frequently are not dependent upon each other; yet, the daughter-in-law relies on her husband, and the parents-in-law on their son. It is through this same man that the personal happiness of the two parties is linked. It is also through him that they maintain a power balance. When a daughter-in-law is mistreated by her parents-in-law, the domestic injustice usually is not so serious as to lead to her suicide unless her husband also treats her badly. When a mother-in-law is mistreated by her daughter-in-law, she is also unlikely to commit suicide unless her son favors his wife or she thinks he does. Although the conflict between in-laws is often a thorny issue in the contemporary Chinese family, and can be a cause for suicide, it worsens especially after being transformed into a conflict within the nuclear family. I am suggesting that this transformation is occurring more and more commonly because of the intensification of these deep structural tensions owing to changing gender status, rural to urban migration, and the new emphasis on the expression of individual interests. Here again, I think of this as an incomplete modernity.

MENTAL DISORDER

These cases show that domestic conflicts are often direct reasons for suicide. This does not mean, however, that mental disorder never contributes to suicide. In many cases, mental disorder also appears in people who are deeply involved in family problems. For instance, Jiaolan shows some symptoms of depression, though inconstant and not severe. In her case, however, mental disorder does not appear to be the direct reason for her suicide, but rather another consequence of her family problem. That is to say, suicide and depression can result from the same familial conflicts and are not necessarily causally linked to each other.

There are also suicides directly caused by or closely related to mental illnesses. According to Michael Phillips (Phillips et al. 2002), who has carried out the relevant research, about 63 percent of Chinese suicides have had symptoms of mental disorders. Though it is far less than in most Western countries, where the estimates are as high as 90 percent, still more than half of all suicidal people in China appear to have mental illnesses. It seems to me, however, the key issue is not how many people have a related mental illness, but what their mental illness means to them and whether it is the source of the suicidal act. The next case might help us with this.

A man from Langao told me about several cases, but was a little reluctant to tell me about the suicide of his cousin, an individual with a serious cognitive disability. I begged him to describe the case, and he briefly told me the following story:[8]

My cousin Chaoyuan was a "fool." [This highly pejorative term is widely used in rural areas to describe both mentally handicapped and psychotic individuals.] He was very polite when first meeting someone. He could say hello and other greetings at first, but became lost as you talked more with him. He was more than twenty years old, but unable to work, and he spent his days playing so that he was readily recognized by neighbors as abnormal. He was not considered to be a full person, but rather, a "fool." [Again, this highly pejorative expression of nonpersonhood is widely used in China and is a major source of stigma and discrimination against those with serious psychological and psychiatric problems.] Sometimes he rode a bike on the road. Whenever he saw a pretty girl along the street, he shouted to her and even followed her. One day he repeated some meaningless words. Because he appeared so foolish, I slapped him in front of several people. He returned home and drank pesticide and died. His mother and brother were also fools.

I was astonished to see my interviewee smiling when he talked about his role in Chaoyuan's death. He "confirmed" that Chaoyuan was really a "fool" by telling me both his mother and brother were also "fools." When emphasizing that Chaoyuan was a "fool," he implied that this case was valueless and could be dismissed. Although I had begged him several times to describe it, he thought he was not really telling me a story of suicide, but was showing me that this case actually didn't count. That is to say, because the suicide had a mental health problem, he was not a full person, and only a full person could, in this widespread view, commit suicide.

Another villager told me about Chaoyuan's suicide in more detail:

> Chaoyuan and some other young men had done some work for the village committee and they were supposed to be paid by a cadre, who was Chaoyuan's cousin. His cousin knew that Chaoyuan would not use the money to live a life of fortune and feared that he might soon waste the money. He said, "I will keep the money for you. When it is time to irrigate or buy some fertilizer, I will give it to you. Otherwise, I am afraid you will waste it." His cousin was also concerned about Chaoyuan's life. Seeing that everyone else was paid but he was not, Chaoyuan did not consent and debated with him. His cousin was angry. Chaoyuan could not understand him and even quarreled with him. He then slapped Chaoyuan, and Chaoyuan drank the pesticide after returning home.

According to this villager, Chaoyuan's cousin was not as cruel as he had made himself out to be. His cousin even smiled when telling me the story not because he was especially cruel, but because Chaoyuan was not supposed to be respected as a person. His cousin said, "Nobody considers him to be a person." He was held to be a "nonperson," and thus nobody should be held responsible for his death. "Nonpersons" can be teased, made fun of, shouted at, or shamed without any bad consequences for the aggressors. All these acts are seen as ways to play with them. If nonpersons become angry, people will laugh as if they enjoy their anger. Some people said, "People treat them as if they are kids." "Nonpersons" share a main feature with children—they do not marry and have their own families and are not considered full persons. Children, however, will eventually become full persons, but nonpersons are socially excluded from becoming full persons. Some villagers implied that Chaoyuan would not have been considered a "fool" if he were educated. Because he was not cultivated into an adult through education, he could not grow up and thus behaved like a child. (See chapter 7 by Guo and Kleinman in this volume for further development of this point.)

Chaoyuan's was one of several suicides that were not counted by locals as "suicides." When talking about them, people would say, "He is a fool, and you do not need to study him," or "His suicide is not a suicide, because that is a madman." Suicide is seen by the local people as a form, though imperfect, of resistance that can only result from actions of normal people. For people like Jiaolan, who became depressed due to family conflicts, suicide is still seen as a positive resistance caused by family problems, and her depression is regarded as only another consequence of these problems. Rural Chinese do not see suicide caused directly by mental illness as typical, because the mentally ill are not seen as being qualified to commit suicide as a moral act.

OTHER TYPES OF SUICIDE

There are three other common types of suicide that can tell us other things about China today.

YOUTH SUICIDE

In recent years, youth suicide has become a serious problem both in the countryside and in urban areas. Academic pressure, parental biases, social fashion, psychological problems, and sexual problems all can lead young people to commit suicide. As in other types of suicide, domestic problems also greatly contribute to this issue. Education is an increasingly crucial component of family life. The educational failure of youth often means the failure of a whole family because it greatly limits life chances for all.

Academic pressure is an important reason for suicides among students. For instance, Xiaoqin of Qinglong County could not stay in school because her parents could not afford her tuition. She drank pesticide and died. Shiqing of Qinglong County could not go to school because of an illness and committed suicide.[9]

Like the examples of suicide owing to family problems, family conflicts sometimes cause young people to commit suicide. Xiaoxiao of Haixing County was the second child of her parents, who were both officials in the county government. Because her birth violated the one-child policy, her parents hid her in her grandmother's house; otherwise, they would be seriously criticized or even lose their jobs. She could not return to her parents' house even after growing up. On one occasion her mother did not wish to recognize her; this upset Xiaoxiao greatly. She drank pesticide and died.[10] Luosheng, a twenty-one-year-old man, was at his grandfather's house when the old man lost eight hundred yuan. His grandfather thought it was Luosheng who had stolen the money and reproached him. Without further investigation, Luosheng's father blamed him also. Unable to bear the injustice, Luosheng stood in front of a train and killed himself (Wu 2009: 10).

Sexual relationships represent another reason for youth suicide. For instance, Sanli, a young high school teacher from Xinle County, had a boyfriend who her parents did not like. Her sister helped her to persuade their parents to accept this young man. Several days after they succeeded with this, however, Sanli broke up with him. Her sister blamed her, "I took such an effort to help you. How can you break up with him so soon?" Sanli responded by committing suicide.[11] In cases like this we have to come to terms with the dawning, and deeply troubling, realization that suicide has become a coping strategy in rural China. And though an extreme action, it is, it seems, one of the means by which family members deal with each other.

These youth problems represent the key issues in the family in China today. Liberty and individualism have been the central themes of the modern family revolution; yet people cannot merely pursue liberty without a moral concern. This makes it especially difficult to educate young people. They treasure liberty and autonomy very much and are very sensitive to their parents' interventions. But the parents' responsibilities are complicated by the fact that they must not only respect the liberty of their children, but also educate them to be moral adults. The conflicts between these two concerns are often reasons for suicide.

SUICIDE BECAUSE OF POVERTY

Although suicide is not necessarily related to poverty, there are still cases in which people clearly committed suicide because of economic pressure. For instance, Shuying of Qinglong County was part of a large family. Her mother-in-law was sixty years old and her grandparents-in-law were more than ninety years old. Her husband still had three younger brothers and one younger sister. It was very difficult to support all nine family members. Finally she and her spouse moved to another house. But they were still very poor. When their children went to school, they had to borrow money for their tuition. When her first daughter was about to marry, she found that she could not afford her dowry and committed suicide. Whether the affect associated with this act was humiliation, resentment, or demoralization, the financial influence was great.[12]

Although such cases are related to economic pressure, they are not simply due to economic problems. In the suicide of Shuying, the quarrels between the couple also played an important role. Even if we understand it from the perspective of economics, it is not only about money. An important part of family life is to raise resources that support family members to cultivate a common hope for the future and an improved family lifestyle. Living a successful family life requires diligence, hard work, and the material and symbolic capacity to support family aspirations. When economic problems make these impossible, the failure of family life might lead to suicide.

SUICIDE FOLLOWING A SERIOUS DISEASE

In such a case, a patient might commit suicide because of overwhelming and uncontrolled physical pain, a hopeless clinical situation, such as terminal cancer, or an unendurable economic burden owing to health care expenditures. For the elderly especially, this is an important reason behind suicide (Jing 2007; Li et al. 2009).

Although not as frequent as other major types, we not uncommonly see suicides of these three types in rural China. Every type of suicide represents one aspect of moral experience. And yet, since suicide is a complex thing everywhere, we can never exhaust typologies of suicide.

Nevertheless, the high suicide rate in China—especially in rural areas—shows us that as China undergoes social development at the most rapid of rates, its long cultural tradition is in acute tension with modernity in complex ways. The moral experiences of Chinese people are also becoming extremely complicated and my research documents that this is the major reason for suicide in today's rural China. Modern ideas have infiltrated millions of Chinese families and offered the promise of liberty and happiness; but they have also intensified many family tensions. The growing awareness of individualism is endangering the structure of many families, but this is not making family politics simpler. On the contrary, because family members can no longer necessarily rely on hierarchical structures to cope with each other, they need more subtle strategies to make a family harmonious. For instance, women are not only vulnerable to patriarchal systems, but are also subject to the complex relationships they are trapped in. In order to have a peaceful family life, a young wife must be clever enough to cope with her husband, her parents-in-law, and her children at the same time. Women commit suicide more frequently because their situation is more complex and more tension ridden; and perhaps also because the greater competence required to deal with these realities is not easily acquired or perfected by many. When a husband is trapped in a complicated situation between his wife and his parents, suicide might also occur to him as a final resort. When educational problems, economic pressure, or a health crisis endanger family life, suicide might also be a consequence.

RESEARCH AND PREVENTION

When Chinese people talked about Yu Hong's notorious suicide, some scholars were already aware of the prevalence of suicide in China. Though suicides among the cultural elite are not infrequent, they are by no means representative of the main trend of suicide in China.

I contend, based on years of research, that most suicides in rural China are a form of resistance to family politics and domestic injustice. With the growth of individualism in the modern era, rural Chinese people have begun to treasure their dignity, autonomy, and freedom; however, they are still in want of consistent and robust modern family ethics. That is to say, the moral experience of rural Chinese families is alive with tensions and problems, such as ones I have described. To adequately address these, China needs to develop a strong and influential family ethics that takes seriously the changes that modernity has created for the family. In order to accomplish this, we require deeper study of how Chinese culture is responding to modernity. At the same time, efforts at suicide prevention are also crucial.

Fortunately, some prevention programs have already been launched. Rural Women, an NGO, identified the problem of suicide as early as 1996. After a long period of research and pilot trials, it finally implemented a substantial prevention program in 2002. By 2008, Rural Women had established "Suicide Prevention Groups" in six counties. Because its program is concretely rooted in the experiential realities of ordinary Chinese, it does not copy prevention programs from the West. As organizers explained during an interview, Rural Women's idea of suicide prevention is to "make the family harmonious and life happy." In all the villages where it has launched programs, there have been, remarkably, no completed suicides, and only three cases of attempted suicide. These impressive results demonstrate that this program has the right focus (the family) and is making progress. It is to be hoped that similar programs can be developed in more places in China in order to try to contain a problem that ethnographic research now shows is mostly about what is happening to moral experience within the family in the new China.

Suicide in rural areas is inseparable from the clash of altered expectations, persistent cultural structures, inadequate coping alternatives, and a highly lethal method. The internal politics of the family are in part similar to the past, yet also reflect a changed moral world. It is an incomplete modernity at the same time that it is also an incomplete tradition. Modernity has destroyed many traditional institutions and endangered traditional moralities in China. While people still identify with some ideas in traditional Confucianism, such ideas are not sufficient to provide a good life for them. If such a traditional morality cannot rebuild itself in a modern world, it cannot be complete. China has entered a new reality, but the past continues to weigh heavily on the present. Without rebuilding its cultural tradition, China cannot have a complete modernity; without responding to the modern challenges, it cannot have a complete tradition either.

NOTES

1. This chapter summarizes my main argument in the book *Suicide and Justice* (Routledge 2009). I thank Routledge for permitting me to reprint some materials here. In addition, I thank *China Journal* for allowing me to reprint some case materials that were first published in my article "Gambling for Qi."

2. This case is from my field notes.

3. This case is from my field notes.

4. This case is from my field notes.

5. This case is from my field notes.

6. This case is from my field notes.

7. This case is from my field notes.

8. This case is from my field notes.

9. Both cases are from my field notes.

10. This case is from my field notes.

11. This case is from my field notes.

12. This case is from my field notes.

REFERENCES

Chen, F. 2001. "Family Structures, Familial Relationships, and Socioeconomic Changes in China and Russia." PhD dissertation, Department of Sociology, University of North Carolina.

Confucius. 1997. *The Analects of Confucius (Lun Yu): A Literal Translation*. Translated by Chichung Huang. New York: Oxford University Press.

Croll, E. 1981. *The Politics of Marriage in Contemporary China*. Cambridge: Cambridge University Press.

Fei, X. 1975. *Earthbound China*. Chicago: University of Chicago Press.

Freedman, M. 1971. *Chinese Lineage and Society*. London: Athlone Press.

Jing, J. 2007. "State Comrades and an Elderly Woman's Suicide." *Critique of Anthropology* 27, no. 2:147–163.

Judd, E. 1994. *Gender and Power in Rural North China*. Palo Alto, CA: Stanford University Press.

Li, X., Z. Xiao, and S. Xiao. 2009. "Suicide among the Elderly in Mainland China." *Psychogeriatrics* 9, no. 2:62–66.

Lu, Z. 2005. "An Interpretation of the Inner Story of Ge Mai's Suicide." *Yinshan Academic Journal* 18, no. 4:78–81.

Phillips, M., X. Li, and Y. Zhang. 2002. "Suicide Rate in China: 1995–1999." *The Lancet* 359, no. 9309:835–840.

Rural Women. 2008. Suicide Prevention Programs. Unpublished.

Wu, F. 2004. "Gambling for Qi." *China Journal* 53, no. 1:7–27.

———. 2009. *Suicide and Justice*. London: Routledge.

Yan, Y. 2003. *Private Life under Socialism*. Palo Alto, CA: Stanford University Press.

Yu, X. 2004. *Haizi: A Biography*. Nanjing: Art Press of Jiangsu.

CHAPTER SEVEN · Stigma
HIV/AIDS, Mental Illness,
and China's Nonpersons

Guo Jinhua and Arthur Kleinman

Stigma—the psychological and interpersonal experiences of being discredited and discriminated against because of a particular condition—comes as close to a universal reality of being human as any human quality studied by social scientists and psychiatrists (Yang et al. 2007). So the study of stigma should tell us something about what is particular to Chinese culture as well as how the huge changes in social life that Chinese have lived through are affecting a core human condition. Having spent years studying stigma in China, we have come to see it as a window through which we gain a different view of individuals, families, and networks, along with their interactions with health care and welfare institutions. We get to see a different side of the Chinese.

In particular we are interested in the stigma associated with mental illness and HIV/AIDS. While other health conditions—notably leprosy and epilepsy—have a long history of stigma in China (as they do in the West), mental illness and HIV/ AIDS are leading examples of stigmatized conditions today (See Leung 2009; Kleinman 1995; Kaufman et al. 2006). All over the world, stigmatized individuals are neglected, abused, and marginalized. Their desperate experiences express something of the universal tragedies of social life, but also, as we shall see, they speak to particular ways of being human: ways of being American, Indian, South African, and, in this instance, Chinese. In the Chinese case, experiences of stigma (and of those who stigmatize) are caught up in a deep cultural and psychological logic that defines normal adult persons against those who are categorized *and* treated as nonentities, nonpersons, even nonhumans (Guo 2008). This sad and saddening moral dynamic is most redolent of Chinese life experiences for the mentally ill and those with HIV/AIDS. In his long influential treatise, *The Normal and the Pathological,* the French historian and philosopher of medicine Georges Canguilhem ([1943] 1991) claimed that over the long European tradition this borderline between the normal and the abnormal became the grounds for social discrimination in the treatment of people not only by the profession of medicine but also as an existential reality in society at large. Much the same can be observed among the Chinese. But in the Chinese case, the remaking of a sick individual as a nonperson is both a telling instance of extreme stigma and a reverse mirror for better understanding what a person is in Chinese culture.

MENTAL ILLNESS

Although data released from the Chinese Health Ministry count sixteen million people in the country as sufferers of mental illness, Sing Lee's chapter in this volume explains that depending on the criteria applied, tens and tens of millions of Chinese may be suffering from a mental health condition. While the number of cases of depression has continued to rise, estimates of cases of schizophrenia, the most serious psychotic disorder, have remained more or less constant at around six million people afflicted.[1] By 2001, there were roughly one hundred and fifty thousand beds devoted to patients with this chronic condition in Chinese mental hospitals and psychiatry sections in general hospitals. Of the over twenty thousand doctors in these facilities, fewer than three thousand are trained psychiatrists (Cohen 2001).[2] So, there is a huge gap between the demand for mental health care and the available care resources, and an equally large gap in the availability of high-quality services. As a result, fewer than 10 percent of people with mental illnesses are receiving treatment. In addition to the shortage of mental health care resources, the stigma associated with mental illness forms another obstruction both for patients to seek effective help and for the mental health care system to deliver services. Stigma related to mental illness makes the current limited mental-health-care resources unavailable for those who need help; hence, people with mental illness often live in worse conditions than those caused by the illness itself. In China, among the reports related to mental illness available in the public media, people with psychosis play a leading role with pejorative overtones and violent events, in which either mentally ill persons attacked or killed others or were killed themselves. People with mental illness are routinely described as dangerous (and while there is increased risk of violence among the mentally ill, that risk is modest and nowhere near what is portrayed in the media), and their alleged threat to society is still the leading concern of the state and the health care system. That is to say, instead of focusing on patient needs and rights, Chinese governmental institutions focus on protecting society from patients, whose potential for violence is greatly exaggerated.

The tendency in traditional Chinese medicine to somatize mental disorders and consider them physical diseases or symptoms of physical disorders has a profound influence on both the public and medical professionals' view of mental illnesses in China (Kleinman 1988). This cultural view undermines the need for a special care system dealing with mental illness, and shunts patients to clinics of general medicine, neurology, and traditional Chinese medicine. Buddhist, Taoist, and other folk healers still play a role, but there is no evidence they are effective against psychosis. In the late nineteenth century, Western missionaries introduced professional mental health care to China. After 1949, when the Chinese Communist Party (CCP) took over the country, mental illnesses were politicized and considered a leftover from *jiu shehui* (old society), which, along with drug abuse and prostitution, was assumed to be produced by the evils of feudalism and capitalism. It was thought that in the *xin shehui* (new society) established by the CCP there would be no more mental illnesses, and even those mentally ill persons left by the old regime would automatically recover because of the establishment of a new socialist regime.[3] This politicized view of mental illness directly led to the denial of the existence of mental illness and exclusion of mental illnesses from the concern of public health. This point of view also explains why mental health care was virtually suspended after 1949.

During the Cultural Revolution, mental illness was connected with wrong political thinking (Pearson 1995); the label of mental illnesses was used as a weapon to delegitimize and attack political dissidents. After the Cultural Revolution, mental health care started to develop but at a slow pace and only in large cities. Clearly, the somatization of mental illnesses in traditional Chinese medicine theories combined with the political construction of mental illnesses under the Communist regime to contribute to the public view of mental illness in today's China: taking care of mentally ill persons is basically a family duty, rather than a medical responsibility of the state. In contemporary China, mental health care for psychosis retains the classical polarity between asylum warehousing and home care. Rehabilitation is limited. Once the knowledge that a person has chronic psychosis is disclosed, patients have great difficulty marrying, finding a job, attending school, or becoming independent.

HIV/AIDS EPIDEMIC

The first HIV/AIDS case in China was documented in 1985. The patient was an Argentine-American tourist who died of AIDS at Xiehe (Peking Union) Hospital in Beijing. In the following several years, the Infectious Diseases Prevention Center tested 310 blood samples collected across the country among hemophilia patients who had used imported blood products. It turned out that three of them were HIV positive. In addition, an international student was found to be HIV positive. In 1987, another HIV case was found in Fujian Province. The patient was a native but had been living in Hong Kong and the United States for over ten years before he returned to China for medical help. In China before the 1990s, HIV/AIDS had been deemed a foreign (capitalist) disease that could not exist in a socialist society like China. "The corrupted Western bourgeois lifestyle" was believed to have provided the impetus for what were labeled as social evils, such as prostitution, drug use, and homosexuality, which resulted in various diseases including HIV/AIDS. At the time, the Chinese government asserted that the absence of HIV/AIDS in socialist China constituted substantial evidence for the superiority of socialism over capitalism.

In 1985, the Ministry of Health submitted a report (Chinese Ministry of Health, 1985) to the State Council, remarking that sexual intercourse is a major HIV infection route and calling on the medical system to monitor the health condition of foreigners who were traveling in China and prostitutes who have sex with foreigners. In 1986, the Ministry of Health issued a notice on strengthening national surveillance of the HIV/AIDS epidemic (Chinese Ministry of Health, 1986) and urged government offices at all levels to take strong control over the information related to HIV/AIDS in order to prevent panic and "bad influences." In 1987, the Ministry of Health submitted another report (Chinese Ministry of Health, 1987) to the State Council and pointed out that there were four major sources of HIV infection in China: 1) foreigners; 2) prostitutes and gay men; 3) imported blood products; and 4) infection within hospitals due to the reuse of needles and surgical instruments. In this report, the Ministry of Health suggested that the Ministry of Public Security take serious actions to crack down on underground prostitution. It stated, "Recently, owing to the influence of corrupted capitalist thoughts and lifestyle, prostitution is spreading across the country, more and more people are infected with venereal diseases. Specifically, a minority of prostitutes like to hang out and sleep with foreigners. Moreover, a number of gay men are also found in Tianjin and Harbin. Even Hong Kong newspapers named Guangzhou a 'paradise for gay men.'"

At the time, epidemiology directed by political ideology had come to dominate the Chinese government's policies on how to deal with the early epidemic of HIV/AIDS. Based on the idea that HIV/AIDS originates in foreign countries, the government's policies were mainly aimed at preventing it from entering China. All of these policies and related practices also reinforced the impression already formed among the general Chinese population that HIV/AIDS is a foreign disease that did not exist in China.

By the end of the 1980s, facts began conflicting with the political ideology and propaganda the Chinese government had long fostered. The first wave of infection stormed Yunnan, a province located in China's southwest, bordering such Southeast Asian countries as Thailand and Burma. Drug abuse and sex tourism were held responsible; minority populations were at high risk. Since the mid-1990s, China has entered a phase of rapidly increasing HIV/AIDS infection. A 2003 report released by the Chinese Health Ministry estimated the country's historical number of HIV/AIDS cases to be one million and the approximate number of Chinese living with HIV/AIDS at the time to be eight hundred and fifty thousand. Of them, approximately 95 percent had not been diagnosed and so were unaware that they were infected. Blood transfusion, drug abuse, and commercial sex were recognized as major infection routes (Chinese Health Ministry 2003). Until recently, the state denied that men having sex with men was a serious risk factor.

Infection routes play a role in determining how and when HIV/AIDS patients experience stigmatization (Kaufman et al. 2006). Drug users, commercial sex workers, and gay men generally hesitate to seek help because of the strong stigma and discrimination against them, while people who contract AIDS during blood selling and blood transfusion often consider themselves innocent victims. They are likely to speak out in public and seek compensation and medical help. Hence, their HIV/AIDS identity is more easily exposed. In this sense, these "innocent" victims often have a more painful life experience than other patients. Most of these patients are from the poorest rural areas of China, especially in Henan Province. Research showed that stigma remained even after fellow villagers possessed accurate medical knowledge of HIV/AIDS and that stigma related to HIV/AIDS often spread from patients to their families, and even the entire village (Gao et al. 2004). According to media reports, many families with HIV-positive members were either locked up behind walls constructed by villagers or kicked out of the village, and their children were forced to quit school. In some cases, the entire village was stigmatized and isolated, and people from other villages refused to visit or do business with that village (Tang 2004; Wang 2008). Stigma related to HIV/AIDS also exists in health care institutions in China. General hospitals often refuse to receive people who have contracted HIV/AIDS (Wang and Zhang 2006; Li et al. 2007). Among the medical professionals working with mental illness and HIV/AIDS, there is a noticeable disparity between attitude and practices (Peng et al. 2006): not surprisingly, then, doctors and nurses seem to nurture the stigma associated with HIV/AIDS.

It is noteworthy that the Chinese government's initial responses to the HIV/AIDS epidemic to some extent maintained and even strengthened stigma related to the illness. By classifying patients into several subgroups in terms of infection routes (blood selling, blood transfusing, drug abuse, and commercial sex), the Chinese government divided HIV/AIDS patients into different social groups with different levels of social status. In the beginning, the state only provided free HIV tests and medication to "innocent patients" who were infected through blood selling and transfusion, in which the state itself had a causal role (see chapter 2 by Jing Jun in this volume); later they changed the policy to cover the entire HIV/AIDS group. In a sense, stigma has been legitimized by the state's policy, even though the same government is also supporting antistigma campaigns. In fact, the government's differential treatment of HIV/AIDS patients, based on transmission routes, reflects the logic of stigmatization rooted in broader Chinese society.

In fighting against the HIV/AIDS epidemic, government officials at all levels in China often apply the strategy of scaring people away from contracting the illness, which further strengthens stigma related to HIV/AIDS among the general population. In a context of fear, both HIV/AIDS patients and others tend to exploit HIV/AIDS-related stigma. Public reports show that, in some cities, thieves have claimed to be HIV positive when caught by the police, or intentionally have had themselves infected, in order to escape from the law. Their use of HIV/AIDS as a scare tactic is based on two facts: first, the police are afraid of HIV/AIDS patients; and second, the justice system is not yet ready for the new situation brought about by HIV/AIDS and does not have the institutional arrangements for criminals with HIV/AIDS (Feng and Li 2007). In some places, HIV/AIDS patients are said to have been hired to do debt collecting because no one dares to defy them. There were also rumors going around in several cities during the period of 2001 through 2005 (Beijing, Shanghai, Tianjin, and Guangzhou in 2002; Shanghai, Nanjing, and Hangzhou in 2005) that HIV/AIDS patients were trying to attack other people with contaminated syringes to have more and more people infected with HIV in order to get revenge on society. These rumors have not been confirmed, yet they showed the pervasive "moral panic and crisis of trust" in Chinese society in the face of its HIV/AIDS epidemic (Jing 2006).

ETHNOGRAPHY

This chapter is chiefly based on fieldwork aimed at researching stigma associated with mental illness and HIV/AIDS, which was conducted by Guo Jinhua in China from January 2005 to June 2007. The research included: one year in Jingmen City, Hubei Province, studying the chronically mentally ill; and one year in Beijing and six months in Dali, Yunnan Province, studying people with HIV/AIDS. The ethnography included hospitals, free standing clinics, NGOs, families, and networks of patients. Over the past several decades, Arthur Kleinman (1986; 1995; Lee et al. 2005a, 2005b) has studied stigma among people coping with mental illness, epilepsy, leprosy, and SARS; that work informs our interpretations as well. Through the field-work, we found that stigma related to HIV/AIDS and mental illness has much to do with the basic moral common sense concerning what makes a person in the local Chinese context, while the culturally grounded governmental policies and institu-tionalized practices help maintain and strengthen the stigma.

MORAL COMMON SENSE IN THE CONTEXT OF CHINA: WHAT MAKES A PERSON?

In the Chinese view, no one is born a full person. That is to say, no one is born with the right to be a person; instead, one has to learn to be a person and also to act as a person to prove his or her personhood. Being an adult person can only be achieved through *zuo ren* (acting as a person), which means one has to show others that he or she is a person by acting as a person. Being a person implies an obligation to engage appropriately in interpersonal exchange relationships, build social networks, and maintain a moral status (face) (Fei 1992; Tu 1987). Acting as a person is to fulfill this obligation. Whether or not one should be treated as a person with rights is based on whether or not one has fulfilled the obligation of acting as a person. Rights come after obligations. One has to exchange the fulfillment of social obligation for the claim of personhood and the rights of being treated as a person. Acting as a person helps an individual establish social relationships, build social networks, earn social face, as well as receive acknowledgement as a moral agent.

In this sense, an individual who is considered unable to fulfill this social obliga-tion will be seen as a nonperson. Nonpersons do not receive social recognition nor are they acknowledged to be moral agents. Hence they have no social support or social protection. People without social face or acknowledgement of their moral sta-tus belong nowhere, which is the very reason that they can be ignored, humiliated, and treated as nonpersons. Stigma has much to do with losing personhood.

In the context of China, then, what exactly makes those with mental illness or HIV/AIDS assume the status of nonpersons in the eyes of their communities? What happens when they take on this status? And what does being a nonperson tell us about Chinese personhood more generally? Several cases illustrate our findings and their significance.

STIGMA RELATED TO MENTAL ILLNESS

GUIYING, A RURAL WOMAN WITH SCHIZOPHRENIA

Guiying, who lives in a village in central China, had been working as a tailor before she married in 1984.[4] After marrying, Guiying quit her job and stayed at home, devoting most of her time to farming and housework. Guiying and her husband built themselves a new house, which made the family stand out from the rest of the families in the village. They were both admired and envied by their neighbors.

In 1993, Guiying's father-in-law died in an accident. That night Guiying began acting psychotic, and after that she was hospitalized for a month. Subsequently, her illness recurred several times. Whenever something bad happened to her family, her illness reappeared. Guiying's most recent illness relapse was caused by her son's court trial. At the time, her son was working as a handicraftsman. Unfortunately, he happened to be hired by an exploitive boss, who unjustly refused to pay him after he had worked for a month.[5] The young boy became angry and stole his boss's cell phone. He was arrested by the police when he tried to sell the cell phone. At trial, the judge ordered the boy to be put on probation with a fine of three thousand yuan. Guiying became acutely psychotic when she heard this news.

Guiying's mental illness imposed a heavy financial burden on her family, including increased medical fees and loss of manpower in housework and farming. But her illness also challenged the family owing to the shame it brought them in the village.

Guiying and her relatives used to visit each other frequently, but after she developed schizophrenia, her relatives seldom came by. As for her relationships with neighbors and other villagers, Guiying complained that some of them often made fun of her after they found out about her mental illness. Guiying's overtly psychotic behavior eventually made her mental illness apparent to everyone in the village. Sometimes when she ran into other villagers "they would stop and stare at me, saying that someone in my family is in trouble. They know I am likely to go crazy if I hear such bad news concerning my family. They just like to watch how scared I become and then start laughing at me," said Guiying. For the rest of the villagers, she said, "I can feel that they intend to avoid me. I did not feel that way right after

I got sick, but later on I found out that things had changed a lot. The way they look at and talk to me both make me feel that I am different in their eyes. Sometimes when I saw they were chatting together, I felt like joining them, but once I was there, standing or sitting next to them, they would stop talking. I can immediately feel the tension coming out all of a sudden, which also makes me nervous and not know what to say."

Guiying was also excluded from family events in the village, such as weddings and funerals. The other families would no longer notify or invite her to attend these events as they did earlier:

We used to help each other on these things. For example, when your family has a wedding or funeral, you just let me know and I will be happy to go over to help with everything, such as receiving guests, cooking meals, and washing utensils. It is very common in the village. People feel they are honored when they are asked for help, even though the work could be exhausting; if you were not notified, it would be a shame on you. It means that the host family looks down on you and does not care about your social face. In my case, I guess that they think my presence would ruin the events and make themselves feel ashamed. They used to ask me for help before I got sick; but after that, they tend to ignore or avoid me. A person with mental illness like me simply loses social face. You are no longer a normal person; nobody cares how you feel. None would care about your social face, which is why they are not afraid to shame you. Even so, you have no right to argue or complain about the way you are being treated. You have to accept it.

The fact that Guiying was no longer invited to attend those ceremonies owing to her mental illness indicated that she no longer was socially sanctioned: meaning, her personhood was no longer recognized by the village community. Guiying's social death resulted from the fact that she was considered to have lost her ability to make *guanxi* (social relationships) because of her psychosis. Therefore, in the villagers' opinion, Guiying was not able to be a person anymore, and for that reason she was excluded from the social life of the village. Guiying's mental illness transformed her into a nonperson by shutting down her social relations and breaking her social network. As a nonperson, she could be teased, disdained, and avoided; her feelings as a human being, her social standing (social face), and her moral reputation (moral face) were no longer recognized or acknowledged. She was, from the perspective of her social world, no longer a full human being—no longer an adult with rights, responsibilities, and autonomy.

Although Guiying still is socially excluded in her village, most of the time she is able to live her own way. Unlike Guiying, many people with schizophrenia, especially those who have behaved violently, are chained and locked up at home.

FUQUAN, A MENTALLY ILL PERSON WHO WAS CHAINED AND LOCKED UP AT HOME FOR SIXTEEN YEARS

When he was sixteen, Fuquan started acting psychotic.[6] One day when his father and sister were trying to stop him from smashing furniture, Fuquan injured them badly with a kitchen knife. The villagers began calling him *fengzi* (crazy). Under great pressure and out of concern for the safety of other villagers, Fuquan's father used an iron chain to bind his son and locked him up at home. Fuquan was chained and locked up for the following sixteen years. During that period, he escaped twice. The first time was in 1998. He ran away when he was unlocked because of the coming Spring Festival. The following day he was found in a town about ten kilometers away. He lost six fingers because of the freezing weather. After the festival, he ran away again and had been missing for nearly one year when he was found by a villager. This time, he lost five teeth.

Fuquan once told his sister that he would rather die than live in such a painful way. He attempted suicide twice but failed. The first time, he poisoned himself, but he was taken to the hospital in time; the second time, he tried to hang himself with wire and was saved by his family. Fuquan said to his sister, "I make you all in the family suffer. If I die, you do not have to waste your time on me."

Each year, Fuquan's illness recurred at least four times, which cost his family more than ten thousand yuan to pay his medical fees. Both Fuquan and his family were living under great pressure in the village. Compared to Guiying who was socially excluded, Fuquan was physically and socially isolated. He was made invisible in his village because he was chained and locked in his home all the time.

The public media in China sensationally and constantly broadcast reports of violent behavior and even killings committed by the mentally ill. Reports also emphasize *wu fengzi* (violent mentally ill persons) being killed by their families. Without the intervention of the state and governmental institutions to counteract public misperception and media distortion of mental illness, many families' painful journey of fighting mental illness ends in tragedy. Families often find blame hard to accept; indeed, anyone who witnesses this journey can hardly blame these families.

A YOUNG MAN WITH MENTAL ILLNESS MURDERED BY HIS FAMILY

A murder was reported from a village in Yunnan Province in 2007.[7] A father, with the help of his brother and oldest son, killed another son who had been suffering from schizophrenia since 2006. As the report showed, the victim had given his family a terribly hard time. He raced around all the time, did not sleep at night, stole livestock from both his own family and neighbors and then sold the animals, beat up his father, and put poison in a neighbor's food. The family had been in a poor financial situation even before the son was diagnosed with schizophrenia. They could not afford outpatient treatment or hospitalization. The entire family was under great pressure from neighbors who blamed and criticized them for their son's behavior. Out of the intense shame and unbearable suffering, the father killed his mentally ill son with the help of his brother and oldest son. They used an iron chain to bind the victim, and then strangled him to death. In the end, the three murderers were each sentenced to ten years in prison. Neither the state nor any governmental institution showed up during the process in which the family needed help, but appeared as the judge and punisher only after the family resorted to murder to end the suffering caused by the son's disease and local responses to it.

A GIRL WITH SCHIZOPHRENIA
SUFFOCATED TO DEATH BY HER OLDER SISTER

Another case illustrates the nonpersonhood of a psychotic Chinese woman through the popular response to her murder.[8] Juanjuan, the second oldest in an urban family with three daughters, started acting strangely in 2001, when she was just eleven years old. She would periodically and unpredictably break out into violence. She poked her father in the eye with a chopstick, which nearly made him blind in that eye; she slashed her sister, Tingting, with a kitchen knife, leaving a long facial scar; she hit her mother on the head; she stabbed neighbors with scissors; and she pushed an eighty-year-old woman into a ditch. The family was blamed by the police for not controlling her behavior, because in Chinese family law, they are responsible for the behavior of their members. Out of desperation, the family chained Juanjuan at home, and Tingting dropped out of school to watch over her. The family spent over one hundred thousand yuan (a huge sum for them) seeking help for Juanjuan. Finally in 2007, the family committed her to a mental hospital for two thousand yuan each month—a sum that placed the family at the edge of bankruptcy. Several months later, the family found Juanjuan in a terrible condition: thin because she refused to eat, dirty with feces caked on her body, and wearing nothing but a coat with bloody scars on her wrists left by handcuffs. Tingting volunteered to stay with her and care for her in the hospital. That same night, Tingting used a pillow to suffocate Juanjuan. Tingting admitted what she had done and explained that she wanted to end the family's misery.

After the arrest, more·than two hundred neighbors sent a letter to the court testifying that Tingting was a good person who should only receive a minor penalty for her action. Tingting was sentenced to probation. The killing followed years of caregiving and was justified by the family as ending their unbearable burden. The public response provoked a fierce controversy. On the one hand, a minority debated whether it was right to kill a family member; on the other, most defended the event as nothing more than a family tragedy that had been resolved within the family. The unspoken understanding seemed to be that this was not the murder of a person; rather, it was the terrible but ultimately necessary means of controlling a dangerous nonperson. Nor was the health care system blamed for its failure in caregiving and in preventing violence. The expectation of many seemed to be that the agencies of the state had no responsibility here: neither for preventing the tragedy nor for judging its consequences, because the victim herself did not possess the rights of a full person, whose death would normally be an issue of justice and responsibility.

In the case of mental illness, patients are considered nonpersons because they are believed to have lost the ability to fulfill the social obligations of being full persons. They are said not to be able to act as competent adults. Their social positions are no longer recognized or acknowledged; their social relationships are cut off and their social networks are shut down. They are excluded from the social world where they live. No social support is available for them. In short, they suffer a social death, the consequences of which can be dire—in the unusual cases just described, social death can even lead to the failure to protect life itself.

People stigmatize mentally ill patients because they consider these patients nonpersons who are unable to be normal adults and, therefore, do not deserve to be treated with face and dignity. That is to say, stigma follows and results from nonpersonhood in China, and not the other way around as stigma theorists contend (Yang and Kleinman 2008). By treating such patients with disrespect, humiliation, and discrimination, people also protect and advance their own social and moral status. Pushed to the wall to protect what is most at stake—namely, the family and its full-fledged members—the mentally ill nonperson can even cease to exist.

STIGMA RELATED TO HIV/AIDS

Although the Chinese government appeared to deny and ignore the HIV/AIDS epidemic until the late 1990s, it changed its attitude dramatically after the SARS crisis (2002–2003). Owing to increasing international criticism, the desire for full membership in the global community, and perhaps feelings of guilt by leaders of many local governmental institutions for their involvement in HIV/AIDS cases caused by blood selling, the central government began to take a relatively open stance toward the release of relevant information and offers of international aid. Through cooperation with the WHO and many foreign organizations (including the American CDC), the state's institutions at all levels became active in this epidemic. In 2003, the Chinese government introduced its "Four Free and One Care" policy for AIDS control, which was not only a promise but a serious on-the-ground involvement of the Chinese government in fighting the HIV/AIDS epidemic. This policy, which provides free treatment, has been welcomed globally and is greatly appreciated by HIV/AIDS patients in China; nonetheless, problems like stigma related to HIV/AIDS remain real and pressing.

SHUFEN, A TEACHER WHO CONTRACTED HIV THROUGH BLOOD TRANSFUSION

Shufen and her husband both had been working as middle-school teachers for ten years in a county of Shanxi Province.[9] In 1996, Shufen received a blood transfusion right before she gave birth to her second child. In 2000, Shufen and her four-year-old daughter both tested HIV positive.

"We felt fearful, hopeless, and desperate. We were fearful that other people would know about our HIV situation. We began living our lives like thieves, always looking over our shoulders. Once other people found out our secret, my whole family would become *wenshen* [the evil of plague] in their eyes." Years later, Shufen still appeared shaken when she recalled those nightmarish days. Despite her efforts at secrecy, the family's HIV status was exposed in 2001. Soon thereafter, a rumor spread across the small town, saying that all of Shufen's family members had AIDS. "Wherever we went, there were always some people pointing at us from behind. If we ran into someone, the person would immediately shun us while covering mouth and nose with a hand. When we went shopping, the bosses of stores would become fearful and start waving to us as we got close, shouting, 'Don't touch my stuff! Go away!' They waved us away like they were driving away flies. That was not the life a normal person deserves to live. My family became monsters and beasts in other people's eyes," Shufen recalled.

Shufen remarked that her family started bearing a new special identity in the local community. The new identity placed her family in a most awkward situation when they were facing other families in daily life. In the past, when her coworkers, friends, and neighbors were hosting ceremonial occasions, such as weddings, funerals, or births, she always attended, bringing *liqian* (gift money) and staying for the banquet offered by the hosts, but after her family's HIV status was revealed to the community, she often had difficulty deciding whether she should go to these parties.

Because of her family's HIV/AIDS situation, Shufen and her family members were unwelcome in their small town. They were no longer invited to attend any ceremonial events. They were no longer acknowledged as full persons; they were ignored, shunned, and avoided by the local community. In other people's eyes, they did not deserve to be invited to the ceremonies held in the local community. The absence of some families at such ceremonial events goes unremarked and disguises the critical breakdown of the interpersonal relationships and social networks of those families who do not fit the local moral image of the socially included. This social invisibility hides the social suffering caused by social exclusion. In the Chinese context, stigma breaks down social relationships and reveals the boundary of social networks. The excluded exist beyond the boundary of friendship, kinship, and community.

HIV also ruined Shufen's and her husband's teaching careers. After Shufen's colleagues found out about her AIDS status, they would no longer allow themselves to get close to her or talk to her face to face. Her office became a prohibited area; coworkers sharing the space with her began moving out one by one. Meanwhile, Shufen noticed that even her students also started shunning her. Whenever she stepped into the classroom, her students immediately covered their mouths with their hands. Shufen said, "I felt a pain in my heart when I saw my students doing this to me. The pride and dignity of being a teacher I used to have are all gone. But I had to stand it. I just could not imagine what it was going to be like if I lost my job." Several months later, the school forced Shufen to quit her job. Soon her husband also quit for the same reason, though he was not HIV positive. Shufen's son was also forced to quit the kindergarten he attended at the time, though he was a healthy child, free of HIV. The other families complained that they could not let their own children stay with a child from an HIV family and they even threatened the director of the kindergarten, saying that if Shufen's son stayed they were going to have their own children transferred to other schools. Under pressure, the director had to ask Shufen to take her son home. After that, her son had to stay at home all the time. None of the other local kindergartens would accept him. He also lost all of his friendships; nobody would play with him. Consequently, Shufen made the difficult choice to send her four-year-old son away to live with a relative in another town where their story was not known.

Shufen's whole family was stigmatized and excluded from the local community. The social mechanism underlying stigmatization changed from the stigmatizers' shunning and avoiding the stigmatized to the stigmatized's avoiding stigmatizers; that is to say, the stigmatizers' fear of the stigmatized is replaced by the stigmatized's fear of stigmatizers. The threat and danger posed by the public to the stigmatized replaces that posed by the stigmatized to the public. We might call this process self-stigmatization.

HAITIAN, A GAY MAN WHO CONTRACTED HIV

Haitian had been a government employee in Beijing.[10] He was married for twenty years, but he was gay. Chinese literature citing homosexuality dates back to ancient times. After the Chinese Communist Party took over the country in 1949, homosexuality was deemed a sexual crime until 1997 and then classified as a mental disorder until 2001.

In today's China, homosexuality is no longer regarded as a category of mental illness or a crime, and society also seems increasingly tolerant of it. Yet, homosexuality, in fact, has gone underground; it has been absent from and intentionally ignored in public discourse. Gay men had never been paid public attention until the HIV/AIDS epidemic began shedding light on this group. In China, homosexuality started to draw public attention because it constitutes a major infectious route for HIV/AIDS, and preventing the spread of HIV became the main way to talk about homosexuality in public discourse. Thus, official acknowledgment of the existence of homosexuality did not lead to social acceptance. Strong stigma is still associated with homosexuality in China; in daily life, many Chinese consider homosexuality to be abnormal and immoral. It not only arouses disgust and disdain among the general population, but also poses what is seen as a serious challenge and threat to family values and creates frustration and despair within families who have gay family members. The situation caused by having a gay family member is very much similar to the one resulting from having a mentally ill person at home. Many gay men decide to hide the truth from their families because they feel ashamed; moreover, they are fearful that their parents will be unable to endure the truth. They often deem telling the truth and revealing their homosexual identity to their parents as "unfilial" behavior that will break their parents' hearts and make them question how they have raised their children. Two decades ago, Haitian married a woman because he himself did not recognize his sexual identity at the time. Among the young generation of gay men in today's China, under the social pressure of stigma associated with homosexuality, most still tend to hide the truth from their families and marry women, though they are all too well aware of their homosexuality.

In 1999, Haitian tested HIV positive. Later, his work unit found out about his illness and informed him that he would be able to keep his work position and continue to receive his wage as well as other benefits, but he would not have to work anymore. Hence, Haitian "retired." Commenting on how his work unit responded to his AIDS status, Haitian said, "They told me that they did this for my own good, and also for other workmates. They said, 'That way you don't have to come to your office and feel uncomfortable in front of your workmates, and your workmates won't panic either. Otherwise, there is no way to keep the work running. So it is good for all of us.' "

Shortly after he tested positive for HIV, Haitian told his wife that he was gay and had contracted AIDS:

That was like a bolt from the blue. She was shocked, frustrated, and angry because I had been hiding my gay identity from her over those years, and then she panicked about my AIDS status. I suggested that we'd better get divorced, but later she refused my suggestion. She was afraid to tell her parents the truth, considering her parents' age and unstable health condition. In fact, I didn't tell my own parents either. My wife was fearful that everyone, including her parents, friends, and workmates, would find out I had AIDS if we got divorced. That would be a big shame. So we didn't go for divorce. So we just pretend to live together and hide my AIDS status from everyone else. In fact, we are still living together in the same apartment as we had been before. My wife bought herself a new set of furniture and utensils, including cookware, dining utensils, storage equipment, washing machine, and bathroom items. Basically, we are still living in the same apartment but we are not sharing anything. Even the space we are using at home and the period of time we are spending at home has come to be marked and classified. We both remind ourselves not to go beyond the boundary. There are some spaces I will never go, and some things I will never touch. We avoid seeing each other at home and always try to leave when the other is coming home. In general, I stay at home during daytime while my wife is away for work; in the evening, before the time she comes home, I go out, leaving the whole apartment for her, and then I come back late at night. Only when our parents or friends come to visit us, we have to stay together and pretend to be husband and wife.

Haitian and his wife had been living like this for six years at the time of this interview. Concealing HIV/AIDS status, ranging from removing the tags on medication bottles to not disclosing their HIV/AIDS status to anyone else, is a common management strategy among HIV/AIDS patients in China. In general, they hide the disease from people outside the family; within the family, most patients tend to hide it from family members other than spouses, and a few of them even hide it from their spouses. They conceal their disease for fear that their AIDS status might be revealed to the public, resulting in their stigmatization and social exclusion. They also conceal it out of concern for their family members, especially their parents. Many put it this way, "I am afraid to tell my parents about this. How can I tell them that I am gay and now I have AIDS? I believe that this is going to give them a heart attack, and they simply cannot stand this attack. Moreover, I don't want to see that they are going to be humiliated this way at their age."

DAWEI, A DRUG USER WHO CONTRACTED HIV/AIDS

Dawei had been a drug user in Yunnan for ten years at the time of the interview excerpted here.[11] Dawei always attributed his social failure to the injury to his right leg, caused by an accident twenty years earlier. He felt that his life was completely changed by the accident.

In 1994, at age fifteen, Dawei dropped out of high school. He could not find a job mostly because of his disability. Gradually, he met several friends and started using drugs when he would spend time with them. "Finally I found somewhere I belonged and someone I could talk to," Dawei said, "it was not like what you think. We were sharing needles not because we could not afford extra needles or we were so eager to get the drug injection that we did not have time to get a new needle. It was not like that. We shared needles because we meant to do it. That was how we were supposed to do it. We were brothers. We used drugs together and shared needles with each other. It was nothing but brotherhood. That is what brothers should do."

Later, Dawei was caught using drugs by the police and he was sent to a local detox center for compulsory detoxification. The detox centers are controlled and managed by the public security bureaus (i.e., the police). Soon the message that Dawei was caught using drugs and sent to the detox center was officially delivered to his family and also his parents' work units. His father and mother were both criticized at their work units. What does the parents' work unit have to do with their son's drug problem? It must be understood in the context of the Chinese *danwei* (work unit) system. In China, a work unit is the name given to a state-owned enterprise. During the planned economy period prior to market economic reforms, a work unit acted as a total system that was controlled by the Communist Party's branch secretary and monitored every aspect of its members' lives. Each *danwei* provided housing, food, child care, schooling, and hospitalization for its members. A work unit had a substantial and profound influence on the lives of its members, who had to obtain permission from the work unit for marriage and pregnancy, and sometimes even for small things like buying a bicycle. A work unit was managed not only as a place of employment and living, but also as the principal site where Party policies and moral education were implemented. Members who did not comply with Party policies could be punished by their work units; the leaders of a *danwei* might teach them a lesson via private talk or criticize them in public in an open meeting, decrease their salary, withhold the incentives they were promised, and even remove their positions.

When market economic reforms were launched in China in the late 1980s, many social services provided within the danwei were discontinued. The control of work units over their members was greatly weakened. However, the work unit still can exert some power in contemporary China. The effort that the government has made to maintain its control of individuals through the danwei has been attenuated but has not ended. That is why Dawei's parents were criticized by their work units for their son's drug abuse.

"It was so embarrassing." Dawei's mother said when she recalled the meeting. The Party secretary who led her work unit mentioned her name in front of all of her workmates and blamed her for failing to teach her son to be a respectable person. She recounted the interaction:

> He said that it was my husband and I who should be blamed for the fact that my son became an addict and that my family must take all the responsibilities. He questioned me in front of all the people in the meeting. He asked me how I could let it happen. I didn't know what to say. It was so embarrassing. And then he went on to say that my family brought shame to this work unit and damaged the work unit's good image and reputation, and it was all because of my son. I felt so ashamed at the moment; I really hoped that there was a hole in the ground so I could hide myself inside or escape from there. It was *diu si ren le* [literally, losing face to the point of death].

Dawei's father was criticized too during a meeting in his work unit. In addition, the leaders demanded that he write a *jiantao* (a self-criticism report) and then submit it to the Party secretary.[12]

Public criticism is the historical remainder of struggle sessions. Struggle sessions were well known as one of the methods applied to foster class warfare during the Cultural Revolution (1966–76). Humiliation, accusation, and ad hominem attack were the major techniques applied in struggle sessions. In China today, the extremely radical and violent form of struggle sessions is gone, but the state continues to support the idea behind this political technique and to implement milder methods, such as humiliation and criticism, in order to consolidate social control. That is what happened to Dawei's parents. The detox center informed the family and their work units about Dawei's drug problem, and then the parents were both criticized at the work units' meetings. Informing the family and the work unit shows the absence of the idea of personal privacy in China. The key to understanding this official procedure lies in recognizing that it is meant to make one's misconduct known to others, to stigmatize the offender and his family, thus damaging their moral status, and therewith to punish them socially. It is meant to discourage others from behaving in a similar way.

In Dawei's case, humiliation was used to punish and stigmatize this drug user and his family in order to mobilize and promote the public antidrug campaign, called "The People's Antidrug War." As a matter of fact, humiliation and stigmatization have been used as major methods in fighting drug use and the HIV/AIDS epidemic in China. Stigmatization has been widely applied in many areas for social control, and it is almost universally believed to be an effective prevention measure. That is, using humiliation and stigmatization to socially punish the misdoer is believed to be a powerful tactic for warning other people not to engage in socially defined misconduct, such as sexual deviance and illicit drug use.

Among the general population in China, HIV/AIDS is basically considered a dirty disease caused by sexual deviance and drug abuse. Although many patients contracted HIV/AIDS through the transfusion and sale of blood in China, Chinese people still instantly link HIV/AIDS to sexual deviance or drug abuse. Therefore, it is hard to deny that the stigma associated with HIV/AIDS in China has a lot to do with the stigma of sexual deviance and drug abuse. In the Chinese context, both sexual deviance and drug abuse are not just considered issues related to personal lifestyle or individual morality; instead, they both signal betrayal of the family. This association also applies in the case of HIV/AIDS. In the Chinese view, contracting HIV/AIDS itself suggests that a person has already betrayed his or her family and, consequently, leads to the patient no longer being considered a family member. Based on this thinking, HIV/AIDS patients are considered to have failed to act as moral persons; without family recognition and protection, they soon lose their personhood and are considered nonpersons.

In contrast to its passivity and failure to intervene in the social course of mental illness, the Chinese government has actively engaged in fighting against the HIV/AIDS epidemic. Based on research (Jin 2005) conducted in Beijing, the reason is not that policy makers in China have a less stigmatizing attitude toward HIV/AIDS than toward mental illness. The truth is, from the perspective of the Chinese government, the danger posed by the HIV/AIDS epidemic to the regime and the entire country is much greater than that posed by mental illness. HIV/AIDS is considered an epidemic dangerous to public health, a moral danger that disgraces the country, and a threat that delegitimizes the country's membership in the global community, so it really matters more. Underlying these concerns is the basic perception that HIV/AIDS is a danger to societal security and stability, the preservation of which has always been the first and foremost concern of the Chinese government. Mental illness is perceived to be an individual or family problem that does not threaten societal security and stability in any serious way. Although mentally ill persons are routinely treated as a danger to public safety, this danger is assumed to remain in local communities and has never presented itself as a threat to the whole of society. Thus, in China the HIV/AIDS epidemic constitutes a serious danger to what matters most to the state, while mental illness does not—or at least not yet—which explains the state's relative indifference to mental illness and the mentally ill.

Stigma has been widely used by the state as a political and moral tool for social control in China. Stigma against rural workers prevents them from achieving social mobility. Rural laborers who have worked for years in cities nevertheless are not granted urban *hukou* (household registration) and the benefits that follow from it; their children are not allowed to attend the schools in the cities where they are working. Instead, rural workers are considered a population that could seriously compromise societal security and stability. Stigma drives gays, sex workers, and drug users underground and discourages them from seeking medical care—a particularly troubling consequence in light of the fact that these groups are associated with heightened risk of falling victim to infectious disease.

CONCLUSION

Stigma constitutes a critical site for observing the profound social impact of the nation's transformation to a market economy: the unbearable social exclusion of various marginalized groups and pervasive feelings of insecurity among the general population. Stigma reveals social injustice and social suffering imposed on marginalized groups by the entire society; conversely, stigma demonstrates the widespread apprehension in society at large. In today's China, social injustice and suffering are tolerated, accepted, and even legitimized as if they are the price the country has to pay for becoming a richer and stronger modern nation. In the face of such radical social transformation, the state, to some extent, is sacrificing its legitimacy. It no longer stands for social justice. In order to regain some of that legitimacy, the state must deny or ignore certain disadvantaged groups' claims to the protections and benefits that accrue to the status of full, socially sanctioned personhood when meeting those claims would put the state in conflict with mainstream interests and concerns. These two facts constitute an ironic and painful image in contrast to the more widely promoted one of flourishing modernization and economic growth in China.

As we have described in the ethnography, stigma is a totalizing social phenomenon. It is created, shaped, maintained, and strengthened by the joint forces of government policies, institutions, and daily local moral practices. Accordingly, the government, work units, the health care system, schools, local communities, and families are all involved in the process of stigmatization. Stigma is neither a problem of the stigmatized nor a problem of stigmatizers; instead, it is a problem of the whole of society.

In China, stigma related to mental illness and HIV/AIDS has much to do with moral common sense: what makes a person and what makes a nonperson. People stigmatize not because they are ignorant or they lack sympathy, as is assumed by many. Rather, stigma is about the basic moral common sense and fundamental social values on which a society is based and managed. Stigma related to mental illness and HIV/AIDS is not just the generalized public perception of health risk posed by these diseases; instead, it implies a strong, emotionally charged evaluation of the moral status of patients, their families, and even the local communities to which they belong. Patients are judged by the local moral meanings of the actions believed to have caused their disease as well as for seemingly imperiling their families and communities by bringing disease into privileged social spaces. This judgment directly leads to another moral judgment about the identity of the patients and their families: namely, that because they have done these things to their families and communities, they are no longer persons. Hence, stigmatization is a moral response toward what really matters to people who have been threatened by illness. To stigmatize means to apply local moral meaning to judge and punish patients, their families, and even their local communities for threatening values central to social life. Doing so is an effort to recognize, acknowledge, and protect what really matters, and this in essence means protecting what is core to people's lives and defending their local culture. Stigma shows us that what really matters in Chinese society today is security. People stigmatize because they sense their individual security has been threatened by illnesses perceived to be especially dangerous; and governmental institutions stigmatize out of the concern that societal security has been compromised by the HIV/AIDS epidemic.

Stigma implies social exclusion of socially sanctioned nonpersons, meaning that these persons belong nowhere, have no rights, and possess no protections. Many patients have a long history of experience with stigma, which was not exclusively related to the two illnesses we discussed in this chapter. They often consider their entire life a continuum of being stigmatized rather than different phases constituted by different kinds of stigma. For them, there was no way to differentiate one stigma (say that of social class or, in the case of ethnic minority group members who have been especially hard hit by AIDS, racial stereotyping) from another. Being stigmatized is a pervasive and endless life experience of being socially excluded and treated as nonpersons. This fact suggests that mental illness and HIV/AIDS are not the only factors that can make a person into a nonperson or nonhuman. Rather, mental illness and HIV/AIDS are just examples of various carriers of stigma. Hence, the key to understanding stigma associated with mental illness and HIV/ AIDS goes beyond the diseases themselves and has to be located in the formation of social exclusion—a universal human condition. This universal condition, however, has been purposefully fostered by the Chinese government as one of its most powerful means of social control. For example, Mao ruled via the stigmatization of entire classes of people as class enemies and enemies of the people. Even in the era of reform, Chinese governing practices still rely on excluding entire groups of people, especially those focused on in this chapter. Hence, antistigma work in China must challenge the moral and political method of controlling society via the social creation of nonpersons.

Around the world, stigma appears to be stronger where there is an absence of programs and practices that enshrine humanitarian ethics and human rights. This is true in China where particularism is still more valued than universalism and social values are still centered on community and society rather than the individual. There is no cure for stigma since there is no cure for social distinction. Yet, adding humanitarian ethics to moral common sense certainly can at least make fewer people suffer and make them suffer less. In China, both government officials and the general public used to believe that the idea of human rights is nothing other than a weapon that Western countries use to denigrate China. There has been a change in recent years in the way the Chinese government responded to international criticism of its human rights conditions. The Chinese government has now turned to refute criticism by questioning other countries' qualifications and right to criticize China, which indicates that the Chinese government has started to acknowledge the idea of human rights. More recently, in early November 2008, the State Council formulated a draft of a "National Human Rights Action Plan." One of its goals is to raise awareness of human rights issues throughout Chinese society. Therefore, the current broad social context in China makes it possible and promising to discuss and act on the issues that hit disadvantaged groups the hardest, including perhaps the role stigma plays in isolating, excluding, and dangerously disadvantaging particular categories of Chinese people. The explosive transformation of China into a modern society has happened so fast and so unevenly that the still pervasive use and abuse of stigma can be thought of as a cultural remnant that individuals will no longer tolerate, that society no longer needs, and that the state in its evolution toward modern forms of governing must, and perhaps now does, recognize is inappropriate and unjust.

NOTES

1. The Chinese Health Ministry reported in 2001 that more than 7.8 million people in China suffered from schizophrenia. In May 2010, perhaps prompted in part by a series of school killings that had begun two months earlier in March, the National Center for Mental Health at China's Center for Disease Control issued a revised estimate of the incidence of mental illness in China. The Center concluded that more than one hundred million persons are afflicted by some form of mental illness, of whom sixteen million are believed to suffer from serious psychotic disorders. These figures reflect dramatic increases over past estimates.

2. Data released by the Chinese Health Ministry in 2001 indicate that at that time there were one hundred and ten thousand beds in 575 psychiatric facilities in China; and of the seventy-seven thousand doctors and nurses in those facilities, thirteen thousand were fully trained.

3. In Chinese communist ideology, "old society" refers to the society before 1949, while "new society" refers to the socialist society after 1949. In sharp contrast to the old society, portrayed as corrupt, exploitative, and supportive of inequality, the new society is construed as promoting beauty, equality, and perfection. Broadly speaking, the old society implies evil while the new one suggests good.

4. Guo Jinhua learned the details of this case through fieldwork that began in 2005 in the psychiatry clinic at a general hospital in Jingmen, Hubei Province, China. There, the researcher met the patient's husband when the latter came to the clinic to refill the patient's prescription. Subsequently, with the husband's consent, the researcher visited the family and interviewed the patient on several occasions.

5. There are frequent reports in contemporary China of business owners who refuse to pay employees for work performed. These reports indicate that workers—especially migrant laborers—in both private and public industry are vulnerable to exploitation by dishonest employers. Due to the marginalization of their interests relative to those of powerful employers and the lack of legal protection, workers often find that they have

few options for recovering withheld wages, and must resort to holding rallies, protests, and even appealing to higher authority. The term *taoxin* ("begging for salary") is frequently cited when it comes to the difficult journey workers must make in order to receive back pay from corrupt business owners. In 2003, when the Chinese prime minister Wen Jiabao visited a village in Chongqing, a rural woman appealed to him for help recovering wages owed to her family. With Mr. Wen's help, the family received full payment on the same day.

6. This case comes from fieldnotes taken by Guo in 2005 at a mental hospital in Jingzhou, Hubei Province, China, where he conducted research on stigma related to mental illness.

7. See www.chinacourt.org, accessed May 14, 2008.

8. See *Guangzhou Daily*, July 24, 2008.

9. This case comes from fieldnotes taken by Guo in 2006 in the STD clinic of an infectious disease hospital in Beijing, China, where he conducted research on stigma related to HIV/AIDS among people who were infected through blood transfusion.

10. This case comes from fieldnotes taken by Guo in 2006 in the STD clinic of an infectious disease hospital in Beijing, China, where he conducted research on stigma related to HIV/AIDS among gay men.

11. This case comes from fieldnotes taken by Guo in 2007 in the dermatology clinic of a general hospital in Dali, Yunnan Province, China, where he conducted research on stigma related to HIV/AIDS among drug users.

12. *Jiantao* literally means "self-examination and criticism." It is a common genre of writing that nearly every Chinese person begins to learn in elementary school. Teachers often assign *jiantao* to students as punishment for misbehavior—being late to school, missing class, failing to finish homework, violating classroom rules, fighting with each other, and so forth. Generally, a *jiantao* comprises four parts: in the first, the author must describe his or her wrongdoing; in the second, he or she must analyze why it is wrong (in this section, it is important to acknowledge that the offending behavior could seriously undermine the honor and stability of the author's peer social group); in the third, he or she must show contrition by apologizing to teachers and classmates and expressing regret and self-hatred; in the final section, he or she must pledge not to misbehave in the future and vow instead to do good always. Once a *jiantao* is written, the student must submit it to his or her teacher, who may request that the student read it to the class.

REFERENCES

Canguilhem, G. [1943] 1991. *The Normal and the Pathological*. Translated by C. Fawcett. Cambridge: Zone Books.

Chinese Ministry of Health. 1985. "Guanyu jiaqiang jiance, yanfang aizibing chuanru de baogao" [Reports on Strengthening, Monitoring, and Preventing AIDS Transmission from Foreign Countries to China]. Weibaofangzi, no. 78. December 10.

Chinese Ministry of Health. 1986. "Guanyu jiaqiang aizibing yiqing guanli de tongzhi" [Notification on Strengthening AIDS Epidemic Control]. Weifangzi, no. 1. January 3.

Chinese Ministry of Health. 1987. "Guanyu jiaqiang aizibing yufang gongzuo de qingshi" [Report on Strengthening AIDS Prevention]. Weibaofangzi, no. 30. March 26.

Chinese Ministry of Health. 2003. "Zhongguo aizibing fangzhi lianhe pinggu baogao" [A Joint Assessment of HIV/AIDS Prevention, Treatment, and Care in China].

Cohen, A. 2001. *The Effectiveness of Mental Health Services in Primary Care: The View from the Developing World*. Mental Health Policy and Service Department, World Health Organization.

Fei X. T. 1992. *From the Soil: The Foundations of Chinese Society*. Translated by G. G. Hamilton and Wang Z. Berkeley: University of California Press.

Feng L. and Y. Li. 2007. "Speculations on Some Issues in Drug Control Behavioral Intervention by Public Security Organs Applied in HIV/AIDS Prevention Affairs." *Yunnan jingguan xueyuan xuebao* [Journal of Yunnan Police Officer Academy] 2:54–56.

Gao J. et al. 2004. "Survey on HIV/AIDS-Related Stigma and Discrimination among Residents in a Rural Community with a Past History of Paid Blood Donation." *Zhongguo aizibing xingbing* [Chinese Journal of AIDS & STD] 10, no. 3:175–177.

Guo J. 2008. "Stigma: Social Suffering for Social Exclusion and Social Insecurity from Mental illness to HIV/AIDS in China." PhD dissertation, Department of Anthropology, Harvard University.

Jin W. 2005. "Analysis of the Finding of a Survey Regarding Discrimination against HIV/AIDS among Government and Party Officials." *Zhongguo aizibing xingbing* [Chinese Journal of AIDS & STD] 11, no. 2:88–90.

Jing J. 2006. "The Social Origins of AIDS Panics in China." In *AIDS and Social Policy in China*, edited by J. Kaufman, A. Kleinman, and T. Saich, 152–169. Cambridge, MA: HIV/AIDS Public Policy Project, Kennedy School of Government, Harvard University.

Kaufman, J., A. Kleinman, and T. Saich, eds. 2006. *AIDS and Social Policy in China*. Cambridge, MA: HIV/AIDS Public Policy Project, Kennedy School of Government, Harvard University.

Kleinman, A. 1986. *The Social Origins of Distress and Disease: Depression and Neurasthenia in Modern China*. New Haven, CT: Yale University Press.

———. 1988. *Rethinking Psychiatry: From Cultural Category to Personal Experience*. New York: Free Press.

————. 1995. "The Social Course of Epilepsy: Chronic Illness as Social Experience in Interior China." In *Writing at the Margin*, 147–172. Berkeley: University of California Press.

Lee, S., L. Chan, A. Chau, K. Kwok, and A. Kleinman. 2005a. "The Experience of SARS-Related Stigma at Amoy Gardens." *Social Science and Medicine* 61:2038–2046.

Lee, S., M. T. Y. Lee, M. Chiu, and A. Kleinman. 2005b. "Experience of Social Stigma by People with Schizophrenia in Hong Kong." *British Journal of Psychiatry* 186, no. A6:153–157.

Leung, A. K. C. 2009. *Leprosy in China: A History*. New York: Columbia University Press.

Li, L., et al. 2007. "Using Case Vignettes to Measure HIV-Related Stigma among Health Professionals in China." *International Journal of Epidemiology* 36, no. 1:178–84.

Pearson, V. 1995. *Mental Health Care in China*. London: Royal College of Psychiatrists.

Peng, Z., et al. 2006. "Knowledge, Attitude, and Practice about HIV/AIDS of Public Health Professionals in Some Area of China." *Zhongguo yaowu yilaixing zazhi* [Chinese Journal of Drug Dependence] 15, no. 1:49–52.

Tang, Y. 2004. "An Investigation on Knowledge and Attitude of AIDS among Rural Residents." *Shiyong yufang yixue* [Practical Preventive Medicine] 11, no. 2:266–268.

Tu, W. M. 1987. "Confucian Humanism in a Modern Perspective." In *Confucianism and Modernization: A Symposium*, edited by J. P. L. Jiang, 59–75. Taipei: Freedom Council.

Wang, F. 2008. "Analysis on the Factors Influencing Attitudes and Practices Related to HIV/AIDS Discrimination among Rural Inhabitants." *Zhongguo jiankang jiaoyu* [Chinese Journal of Health Education] 24, no. 8:569–571.

Wang, Y., and K. Zhang. 2006. "HIV/AIDS Stigma and Discrimination in Health Care Services." *Shengzhi yixue zazhi* [Journal of Reproductive Medicine] 15, no. 1:67–70.

Yang, L. H., and A. Kleinman. 2008. " 'Face' and the Embodiment of Stigma in China: The Cases of Schizophrenia and AIDS." *Social Science and Medicine* 67:398–408.

Yang, L. H., A. Kleinman, B. G. Link, J. C. Phelan, S. Lee, and B. Good. 2007. "Culture and Stigma: Adding Moral Experience to Stigma Theory." *Social Science and Medicine* 64, no. 7:1524–1535.

CHAPTER EIGHT · Quests for Meaning

Arthur Kleinman

This is the forty-first year since I began my research in a Chinese community (Taipei, Taiwan, 1969), and it is a little over thirty years since I started up studies on the China mainland (Changsha, Hunan, 1978). In the six and a half years that Joan Kleinman (my wife and collaborator, a trained sinologist who died in March 2011 after living with Alzheimer's Disease for a decade) and I lived in Chinese society, I personally carried out or was a collaborator on studies of the health care system, including professional, folk, and family-based care. I also have conducted research on depression, neurasthenia, chronic pain, epilepsy, schizophrenia, suicide, end-of-life conditions in the elderly, SARS, AIDS, pandemic flu, the health of rural-urban migrants, the psychiatric profession, and the traumatic impact of the Cultural Revolution on survivors who experienced serious violence. The themes may sound greatly different, yet underlying and connecting them is an abiding vital interest in people's quest for meaning (Kleinman 1986, 1988, 2006). Faced with the dangers and uncertainties of their own embodied suffering and the insecurities and seemingly endless changes in their cultural worlds, how do ordinary Chinese make sense of their experiences? Or do they make sense? What kind of quests for meaning do they embark on? And where do those inner journeys lead them? Furthermore, what do quests for meaning have to tell us, beyond personal biographies, of what is happening to Chinese culture? And how is that connection between the person and the context, the emotional and the moral, best studied?

My projects have involved ethnographic observation, clinical interviews, small group discussions, questionnaires, epidemiological surveys, life histories, analysis of critical events, archival research, and cross-cultural comparisons. But mostly I have talked with individuals and their friends and family members—sometimes on just one brief occasion, but often in depth and over long stretches of time. I have listened intensively, asked probing questions, talked about myself, responded to questions, and, after getting to know people, teased out narratives about who they are and where they see themselves headed. Listening to personal stories so as to hear within them themes that resonate with collective experience is what I can claim as expertise. I also have tried to keep up with the academic literature in this area as well as watch movies and documentaries, read novels, study artistic creations, and converse with ordinary people and elites over what it all means. And as a clinician I have had the special privilege of seeing numerous Chinese patients in evaluations, hospital settings, and psychotherapy.

Frankly put, my work in Chinese society has had more than academic value for me. My family has grown up and developed with Chinese friends, the Chinese language, Chinese books, Chinese food, Chinese art, Chinese furniture, Chinese experiences. My son and daughter attended Chinese schools, and my daughter went on to major in East Asian Studies, take a PhD in the politics of China, marry a Chinese-American, and raise two Chinese-American children. My wife and I found that the values that resonated most with us were about family, reciprocity, the moral basis of interpersonal connections, self-cultivation, vital energy, and moral emotions. Chinese cultural values (largely neo-Confucian) helped center our lives and have greatly assisted me in recent years in dealing with my wife's Alzheimer's disease. Hence, I am not an objective observer and neutral participant in new developments in Chinese society. These people and their world matter greatly to me.

As a teacher at Harvard for thirty-five years (and the University of Washington for six), I have taught and advised hundreds of Chinese and Chinese-American students: undergraduates, medical students, doctoral students, postdoctoral fellows. And I have also had teaching experiences at the University of Hong Kong, Chinese University of Hong Kong, National Taiwan University, Academia Sinica (Taiwan), Hunan Medical College, Fudan University, Shanghai Mental Health Center, and Peking University, among other Chinese institutions. These experiences include rich and extensive interactions with Chinese academic colleagues in medicine, mental health, and social science. Not least of the relationships that have informed my understanding about things Chinese are the ties I have developed with the coauthors of this book, each of whom is a former student and all of whom are valued colleagues.

With this as prologue, let me turn now to the quests for meaning of Chinese friends, patients, and research interviewees. I employ the term *quests* in the plural because the first thing I need to say is that there is no such thing as a single, culture-wide quest for meaning. That is the stuff of newspaper and television stereotypes. China is as plural and complex as the United States and any other major society. Meanings may arise from cultural texts and traditions and relate to society-wide events, but it is always the individual who remakes those collective values and explanations into the special combinations of ideas, feelings, and practices that matter. That search to make sense of the world, and one's special place in it, rarely is a solitary act, but gets embodied in interactions with others who hold importance in our lives. The upshot is that the quest for meaning is simultaneously our own and our world's. And that's why I have always felt that getting it right when we talk to individual Chinese tells us as much about their local worlds as it does about them.

THE VARIETIES OF QUESTS FOR MEANING

For ordinary Chinese, there is a highly practical orientation to the world.[1] That world has presented itself for a long time as dangerous and uncertain. Concrete issues, from household finances to tensions at work and including the myriad of small-scale details that define the expediency of life lived among others, require practical and often urgent responses. A great deal of affect, attention, and action is required that exhausts energy and constrains other limited resources. Politics on the grand scale have only intensified this sense of material issues that must be quickly addressed and handled locally. The infrapolitics of the family and work must keep even the most experienced and socially adept of people on their toes and ready to act. Sickness and misfortune of a variety of kinds are so commonplace that no one can regard life as secure and fail to heed everyday alarms (Kleinman 2006).

Hence, when Chinese go to religious shrines to pray and ask for the intervention of gods and ancestors, they are most commonly concerned about narrow concrete problems: for example, whether a child will succeed in school and pass a key exam; if there is enough money available to pay off a loan; how to placate an irate in-law; what level of gift to give at a local cadre's daughter's wedding; or how to help an elderly parent recover from a stroke. This is what I believe is meant when Chinese admonish that they have no time for anything beyond the serious, practical problems of the workaday world. Yet, even in the setting of mobilizing resources to deal with the aftermath of serious problems like a severe accident, ordinary people are also often engaged in a quest for meaning. They search diligently for evidence that, not withstanding a terrible misfortune, the world is still predictable and manageable; that their lives are significant; that the things that really do matter to them and their families—things like resources, status, key relationships, and all sorts of culturally particular practices—are secure. This is the most ordinary quest for meaning. It is the effort to build a life for oneself and for one's family. And it is all about strategies of searching, enduring, and getting on with things that are immediately (or soon to be) at stake. For the poor, the ancient emphasis on things that must be tolerated and endured is still present; yet for the burgeoning middle class and many others, this cultural common sense is giving way to the idea that things as they are can be improved and altered, and therefore the idea of the efficacy of individual agency and collective action is increasing a sense of happiness; if not for oneself (and it often is for oneself) then for one's children and grandchildren. Closely related to this ubiquitous odyssey are struggles for meaning that may be more particular, even if broadly shared, and that reflect differences in education, income, gender, age-cohort, and local setting. The quests for meaning that I will now examine are the ones that have come to the fore in my conversations with people.

THE QUEST FOR HAPPINESS

At the Beijing Summer Olympics (and later at the Shanghai World Expo), it was widely reported that no one watching the crowds and observing people in the street could fail to be impressed by two emotions: *pride* at what China had achieved as a rising power and *happiness*. People were having a good time. They were relaxed, smiling, and enjoying the fanfare, the ceremonies, the events, and just being out and about. In Athens, Atlanta, and other cities where the Summer Games have been held, this observation would hardly raise an eyebrow, yet for China it is nothing short of momentous.

To understand why, think of what a Chinese man or woman in their eighties has lived through: the chaos of the warlord period and the uncertainty of the early years of the Nationalist government's efforts to reunify a fractured country; the long war with Japan during which hundreds of millions of people were uprooted and twenty million were killed; the turmoil and disintegration during China's civil war; the brutal excesses of the early days of the Chinese Communist Party's efforts to exterminate class enemies, with perhaps a million landlords killed; the deep tragedy of the Great Leap Forward, which produced the most deadly famine in history with thirty million deaths; the whirlwind of destruction called the Cultural Revolution, when intellectuals, cadres, and ordinary urban dwellers got caught up in the fire of mass political campaigns, brutal struggle sessions in every work unit, and the meltdown of government and civil institutions. Add in the Korean War, when China suffered a million casualties, and all the paranoia-generating political campaigns against rightists, counter-revolutionaries, and others labeled enemies of the people. Then consider the early days of the great transformation to a market economy, when uncertainty was so substantial people didn't know which direction would bring safety and security. Against this troubled and troubling historical background, isn't the audacity of simply being happy and enjoying life the most remarkable of collective and personal changes?

The quest for happiness is one of the most important stories in China today. In 1978, when I first visited China, the Chinese I encountered were fearful, watchful, exhausted from the ferocity of the past, dizzy with the instability and turmoil of the transition from radical Maoism to the new market economy, and still experiencing the pain and suffering, intensified by the Cultural Revolution, that had more or less become the accepted reality of everyday life for Chinese in the twentieth century. Thirty years on, the situation for ordinary Chinese is so very different that we can say without exaggerating that the psychology of the Chinese people has undergone arguably its most dramatic transformation since the decline of the Qing dynasty in the late nineteenth century. What was once available only to the rich and powerful has become an everyday reality for ordinary people, who can go out to restaurants, shop for all kinds of goods, take in the latest movies, use leisure time to exercise and travel, and just plain enjoy themselves. Or, put differently, hunger for food, which had beset Chinese for centuries and become a fixture of their cultural imagination, was no longer (for most) either a reality or a fear. Now it was replaced by a hunger for those good things in life that were flooding the market and the imagination.

Much of social science has carried with it an implicit critique of middle-class enjoyments that represents both the revolutionary aspirations of its founders and the resentments of academics against bourgeois society. Rightly, social studies of China have emphasized the plight of marginal groups, the growing social and health disparities between the poor and those who are better off, and social problems like corruption, uncontrolled development with environmental degradation, and failure of regulatory systems. And these critical views are also apparent in this book's preceding chapters. Yet, it is crucially important to balance our sense of China with an understanding of the great achievements in poverty reduction, the growth of what will shortly become the world's largest middle class, and the transformation of ordinary life for most Chinese. What has been achieved is nothing short of making possible for many a good life. And the quest for meaning for hundreds of millions of Chinese is the search to build and sustain a good life: a life filled with simple pleasures; a life that is relatively and modestly secure in a dangerous and unpredictable world; a life that offers better chances for children and grandchildren; a good life that represents a new normal. And "good" here means for many doing good for others, as can be seen in the public discussions unleashed by the Sichuan earthquake in the media and on the Internet, which turned on the meaning of life and the importance of volunteering to assist others. This is China's true cultural revolution. We have already noted in this book the increasing popularity of psychology and practical self-help manuals. For many, it is a *positive* psychology that matters. The purpose of these works is often quite explicitly stated to be increasing people's happiness. "This quest for inner happiness goes side by side with the quest for material gain and social entitlement" writes one of the Press's China scholars who reviewed this volume.

So it is not at all surprising that the quest for happiness is a common narrative in interviews with ordinary Chinese. It is a narrative that regards the current political reality as acceptable because it has made possible the opportunity to live a good life. And it is also a narrative that tends to deemphasize the troubles of the past and to sublimate resentment and remorse into more pragmatic emotional responses that can advance personal interests. This collective emotional response is highly pragmatic in its effort to serve those interests that are believed to bring about a good life, to deny (or, at least, postpone) the wages of trauma and humiliation, and to avoid obsessing over memories that can't be changed. Many Chinese, from different social strata, have told me that the quest for happiness (or fortune and good life) is the meaning first and foremost in their lives.

A thirty-five-year-old Beijinger, a married academic with a young child, put it this way in 2007: "My wife and I want to live a good life. Be successful, enjoy things! We want our daughter to succeed, but we also want her to be happy. My parents are enjoying themselves; yet I think they regard us as a little selfish. We want to take advantage of new opportunities, have a good time. Every day I realize how unusual that is when you consider what our families had to endure in the past." A fifty-year-old Cantonese-speaking physician had this to say in 2006: "I like to be happy. I enjoy myself. So does my husband. I want to dine out, shop, travel. We work hard. We are not rich. But we can still have a good time. In that way, I sometimes feel closer to the young generation and to foreigners than I do to my parents. They still seem suspicious of life." A seventy-five-year-old Shanghainese grandmother, whom I met at a traditional Chinese medicine clinic, concluded with the self-reassuring sense that she and her husband had, against the odds and perhaps against even their own expectations, crossed over to safety: "I meditate. I practice qigong. My husband and I like to do [ballroom] dancing. We are happy. We don't often look back. Why do it? It's better to enjoy ourselves now. We are old and we are happy." The eighteen-year-old daughter of a Chinese entrepreneur in Shanghai was talking to me in Hong Kong about the experience of being a university student (in Shanghai in 2007): "My generation is different. We all see that. We can be serious. But we want also to be relaxed, have a good time. There is so much out there for us. We feel that life should go well for us. I like to do things, get out with my friends, have a good time."

Maybe the most impressive instance I have come across of the individualistic search for happiness is Lee Guancao, a dynamic, young-looking fifty-year-old visiting fellow in a leadership program at a leading American university. He told me that he had given up an extremely promising political career to join the political science faculty at a major Chinese university from which he was currently on leave for several months. In response to his decision, his superiors and colleagues in the government bureaucracy told him that he was destroying a very bright future and needed to regain his senses and return to his post as a high-ranking cadre in Shanghai. He refused and they accused him of being selfish. His response, he told me, was that he knew he was being selfish and rather than bothering him, his selfishness made him feel that he was finally doing what he had always wanted to: namely, build an academic career on his own terms. And that made him feel good and that was what mattered. This story was confirmed for me by several Chinese visitors who knew Mr. Lee. They thought he had taken a chance—he would never again be a political powerhouse—but he had so often proved himself to be effective, they both said he would do fine as an academic. I talked about this case, under a pseudonym, with a group of fifteen or so graduate students from China who were studying at a U.S. research university. All recognized Mr. Lee's selfishness, but most were unwilling to challenge his decision and actually said that as long as it made him feel good, it was an appropriate choice. One even said to me, "What's wrong with being selfish? Isn't that the only way to get what you want and feel fulfilled and feel good too?"

THE QUEST FOR JUSTICE

Among a minority of informants, there is an alternative quest for meaning that turns on narratives of recrimination and the enduring quest for justice. In his chapter on suicide in this volume, Wu Fei delineates a deep sense of domestic injustice in the suicide of rural women who kill themselves as an act of complaint, revenge, or re-sistance. Wu Fei also notes, as have others before him, that Chinese history is filled with models of moral suicides in the public sphere—such as that of Qu Yuan[2]—that are intended to be powerful examples of criticism of injustice and the demand for the provision of justice (Lee and Kleinman 2003). Petitioners, who travel to Bei-jing and live in uncertain circumstances in the hope of buttonholing an official who will listen to their stories of local wrongs and redress the abuses, embody this moral quest; their frequently shared experiences of failure underline the tragic inefficacy and quixotic despair this quest so often ends in.

The literature on the consequences of the Cultural Revolution, including my own research, is replete with illustrations of the persistence of deep affects of disquiet, anger, guilt, recrimination, and retribution that underlie the everyday thoughts and feelings of Chinese who see themselves either as victims or victimizers owing to misplaced loyalty (see, for example, Feng 1996; Liang and Shapiro 1983; Kleinman 1986; Thaxton 2008; Thurston 1987). But Chinese novels, movies, and documen-taries suggest that such raw and unresolved emotions are present in individuals who experienced other political catastrophes under Chinese communism. These sad nar-ratives seem even more common among Chinese who have left China for other coun-tries, where they feel free to publicly express their powerful memories, troubling questions, and frequent rejection of China's political status quo: redemption deferred is stamped on their faces. Today, one also reads accounts of brutal treatment by lo-cal officials leading to lifelong quests for justice. One of my students has studied ru-ral peasant women in a remote village that in former times was a model commune (Chang in preparation). What was portrayed as voluntary hard work is now bit-terly represented and resented as forced labor. And among those who have been imprisoned, these stories of the abuse of power still burn with the white heat of unresolved hatred. Ralph Thaxton (2008) has described an entire rural community in Henan that keeps alive the bitter memories, history of resistance, and coping strategies for dealing with the abuses of state power.

I have had many interviews in China and with Chinese in the United States in which the experience of suffering from injustice is what seems most at stake in people's lives. The quest for making sense of political injustice, especially, looms large. Although a few of my informants admit that they cannot make sense of what has injured them and their close family members and friends, most do come up with life-sustaining interpretations. These, in my experience, are less likely to draw on traditional cultural resources than to be highly context-specific understandings of why bad things were done to good people like them. Referring to these personal accounts of the tragic effects of public injustice as "social suffering," colleagues and I have emphasized that not only are their causes social, but the experience itself—painful, suffocating, demoralizing, anger provoking—is often shared by members of the same family and network (Kleinman, Das, and Lock 1997).

The physician I call Dr. Yan Zhongshu, whose words are cited in this volume's introduction as a reminder that older Chinese carry with them the memories and social reflexes that helped them cope with the mass violence of Maoist political movements, had this to say about his nemesis during the Cultural Revolution: "We never spoke again about that time. We worked together for years. There was a superficial return to speaking terms. We joked together oftentimes and we even took a few meals together. But whenever I thought of my poor wife, or my sons and me drinking that sickening brackish water, I felt ice in my heart. I could not forgive him. I did not trust him" (Kleinman 2006: 105). Dr. Yan went on to describe how the new changes in China have left unaffected his bitter and irresolvable feelings about the past injustices and his uncertainty about the present era:

I can remember the past as if it were here right now, but I have no sense of what the future will be like. My feelings and values belong to the past. Even in the worst days I could still sense that I knew what I should do. Now I'm very unclear. What once was good is now bad; what once was bad is now good. And still we live on. Some days I feel dizzy, as if I couldn't find my place on the ground. It's not the same ground. What matters now doesn't appeal to me, and, having finally gotten out of China, it doesn't have to appeal to me. (Kleinman 2006: 117–118)

Dr. Yan, like other Chinese of his generation whom I have interviewed, who suffered the worst of the Maoist political campaigns, is unable to leave the past behind. The present holds little attraction for him, though he realizes it is a much different and better time in material terms for him and for his children and grandchildren. This state of mind, in which the bitter past is not only unforgettable but still lives on in the cruel reality that shaped the present, this persistence of dark memories as a judgment, is also visible in an experience I had in the 1980s with one of the senior Chinese psychiatrists whom I first encountered in Hunan in 1978 and whom I have come to know and admire over the years. We were, as I recall, walking down a street in Changsha engaged in a lively conversation about the past, not far from the hospital where he worked, when he became agitated and pointed at a nearby building. He almost shouted that that building was where the political cadres had their special store. He shook with distain for the hypocrisy of the Communist ruling class, who advanced utopian idealism about equality while maintaining special stores where only they could have access to the highest-quality food. And then he continued on to criticize the cadres' other special privileges, their special schools and their special ward in the hospital. This usually quiet and contained colleague exploded with anger over the injustice and the falsehood. Yet over the past decades, I have heard fewer and fewer such expressions of violent memory and resentment. The feelings have not all disappeared but they are weakening. The loss of intensity is noticeable in the voices of numerous Chinese I know who refused to return to China after the brutal crackdown of June 4, 1989. They are coming to terms with a life of exile that includes the sense that the China of today is simply a different China from the one they were raised in. One told me that while today's China was still politically oppressive, "it no longer has people by the scruff of the neck." This businessman in his forties from Shandong Province also told me that while he and his friends would never give up the cause of justice for the great abuses of the past, the feeling of resentment and the desire for revenge were weakening and no longer mobilized the same passionate energy they once had. He also expressed the feeling that he and his generation had to deal with the promising reality of a new China that had accomplished many positive things that deserved acknowledgement.

Counterbalancing this picture are the thousands of local protests in rural and urban areas and the many petitioners to the central government whose demands for the righting of local wrongs stay clear of critiquing the leadership of the party-state or questioning its legitimacy, but which target despised party secretaries and other local bureaucrats who are blamed for corruption, malfeasance, and failure of exercising responsible governance. Their acute and chronic grievances speak to both the new willingness of the party-state to tolerate some criticisms as well as the still widespread sense that behind the façade of forbearance there remains the dark shadow of repression on behalf of authoritarian political control. The right to sue local governments for wrongful doings has contributed (as has investigative journalism, again focused on local cases) to this emergence of a contemporary quest for local justice as a legitimate and even occasionally successful mode of living a moral life in contemporary China. Colleagues of mine who conduct research among rural Chinese and rural migrants to Chinese cities comment that resentment, even deep resentment that borders on resistance to the agents of the state, seems to be increasingly balanced by hope for the next generation (see Zhang, Kleinman, and Tu 2011).

THE QUEST FOR RELIGIOUS MEANING

China watchers have repeatedly noted a rejuvenation of religion in contemporary China. Buddhist temples have been rebuilt and are filled with people conducting rituals like burning incense, drawing joss sticks, throwing divination shells, and participating in group chanting. Taoist temples also are attracting many devotees. Christian churches are packed with worshippers. Indeed, there are now estimated to be between seventy and one hundred million Christians. Mosques are also well attended, and Islam may also have fifty million adherents, especially among Uyghur, Hui, Mongolian, and other ethnic minorities. Popular Chinese exercises, martial arts, and traditional medical practices—like qigong, a huge movement in the 1980s and 1990s, later discredited—often take on the appearance of spiritual quests. Indeed, the traditional Chinese activities of nourishing life, ensuring good health, and increasing longevity through bodily practices have also added a sense of finding spiritual meaning in cultural practice.

There is a popular hunger for religious values and sentiments. These are sought after to confront a secular world that is increasingly seen to be hypermaterialistic and wildly commercial, a world bereft of moral authority, aesthetic significance, and a spiritual center. The hyperpragmatism of everyday political life is also a stimulus for this quest. Communist ideology has had its effect, and now there is also a blowback against official atheism and what is widely regarded to be a delegitimated Communist credo that not even high-ranking cadres seem to believe in any longer. The same corrosive cynicism that has tarnished Confucian conventions and Communism has undermined traditional Chinese moral values. Religion offers special sanctioning for values, along with a feeling of sharing in a community of believers and finding a framework to make sense of the dangers and uncertainties that are a normal aspect of everyday life. Loss, suffering, and threat are the classic reasons for individuals to seek *theodicy* or *sociodicy*—a sanctioned understanding of why bad things happen to good people and how to justify the goodness of god or society in the face of misfortune. These have been as central to the Chinese tradition as to the other great religions of the world. To the surprise of some, six decades of Communism has not erased their presence in China.

The Falun Gong movement, as David Palmer (2007) has charted its course, is but one notorious illustration of the rise and fall of popular religious movements and their tendency to be perceived by Chinese authorities as a potential political challenge. Again, there is a long history of such movements taking on political significance in China. Hence what is especially notable about the current religious revival is that a great deal of it seems to be occurring in the private space of the individual and the family. This protestantization of religion occurs through the narratives of a personal journey to find meaning in life, and not surprisingly we find it among middle-class professionals and business people, including those who have spent time abroad and have been influenced by the religious renewal that is integral to our era's globalization. As a sociologist from Shanghai told me: "People say they are spiritually lost, but are not sure what religion is suitable for them. Yet they need some spiritual home."

A thirty-six-year-old medical researcher from Hangzhou with whom I had a series of personal talks in 2009 explained her religious journey as a return to roots: "I grew up in a family network that included grandparents and granduncles and aunts who had an old Christian background. Religion skipped my parents' generation and my childhood. Then when I spent a year in New York I felt myself drawn to church. Now I regard myself as a Christian and I want my son to share that feeling. It is as if I have come back to my family's lost tradition and been found and saved." A sixty-year-old businessman from Shanghai whom I met for the first time in Boston in 2009 had this to say: "China, you know, has no moral compass today. Some people, maybe lots of people, are not bothered too much by that, but I am and so are many of my friends. I don't get all that enthusiastic about going to church. And the same holds for Buddhism. But I believe in a kind of fusion religion, you know. Half reverence for ancestors, half a kind of theism. God is in small things. Life is sacred. My friends and I read a lot of books on religion." Cai Youxin, a twenty-eight-year-old cadre whom I spoke with in Shenzhen in 2007, pointed out that he came from a small town in Guangdong Province where his family had practiced Buddhism for generations, even during the worst years of collectivization: "We practiced secretly then. Now, has religion come back! There are so many temples and shrines in my hometown, it is a constant religious festival. I pray and do ritual practices before big decisions or when I start something new and important. A lot of my colleagues do the same. I don't see any problem in doing the work of a cadre." Finally, a visiting academic colleague from China in his sixties had this to say on the question of the religious quest for meaning:

My family came from a small city in east China. We have always worshipped the ancestors. And we continue to do so. From my experience of ordinary Chinese I'd have to conclude that ancestor worship is alive and well. If you are looking for religion in China, you must start with this family-based practice. It is the practice that counts. I doubt most Chinese could discuss a theory of religion, but practicing ancestor worship in its most concrete way is what their religious quest for meaning, using your expression, is about. So maybe, I don't know, practicing religion—I mean doing rituals—is what meaning is about for me.

There is something happening in the realm of religion in China today—institutional, personal, secret—that few China watchers have adequately addressed. There is a movement underway—part endogenous, part global—and it is unclear what its consequences at the individual and collective levels will be. But no one should underestimate the potential to produce change.

THE QUEST FOR RESPECT

I first stepped off the plane in Beijing on a warm April day in 1978 and, together with the other members of a government-to-government rural health delegation, spent the next month traveling to remote areas in China's north, west, and south observing clinical and public health facilities (Committee on Scholarly Communication with PRC 1980). At one point, we passed through Changsha, the provincial capital of Hunan. With several American colleagues, I visited Hunan Medical College, formerly the Yale-in-China Medical School. Meeting with a faculty that had such a long and distinguished connection with America, I was taken aback that so few spoke English. I struggled in Chinese to ask technical questions about branches of medicine that were quite distant from my own expertise. Absent technical vocabulary, I used tortured circumlocutions to make sense of what was going on in medical specialties two years after the official end of the Cultural Revolution. When I finally got around to my own clinical discipline—psychiatry—I was annoyed to hear repeated what I had been told almost everywhere our group had visited: namely, that China had almost no mental illness because it was a socialist country and did not suffer from the capitalist ills that create alienation and mental illness. Because I had been introduced to three professors of psychiatry, it was disappointing that they went along with the party line and denied that mental illness was a problem. When we finally got to our hotel, it went from a steamy hot night to a tropical downpour, and my colleagues and I were further disappointed to learn that our evening flight to Guilin had been grounded until the following morning.

I was in the process of getting ready to go to bed, when my roommate, the medical sociologist David Mechanic, who shared my frustrated interest in mental health, answered a knock on the door, and ushered in the three psychiatrists we had had such an unproductive introduction to earlier in the day. They literally crept into a lounge area beside our room, as if they were scared of doing something illegal—which in fact they were, because in 1978 ordinary Chinese were not allowed into the hotels that housed foreigners, unless they had special permission, which our guests apparently didn't have. During the day, the youngest member of the group, Professor Shen Qijie, had acted as their head; now he stepped back and the oldest member, Ling Mingyou, did the talking. In elegant, American-accented English, he introduced himself as the founding chair of the Department of Psychiatry and the former dean of the Medical School. Professor Ling was wearing ancient eyeglasses—horn rimmed, circular, with one of the lenses broken into several pieces. After overcoming my surprise and irritation that I had sweated so hard to translate earlier in the day, when in fact there was a perfect person to translate, who knew all the fields of medicine, I expressed my dismay that the conversation had been so uninformative. Professor Ling smiled and commiserated with me, adding that virtually everyone in the audience spoke English, but was unwilling to do so because during the Cultural Revolution this had been considered a negative sign that one might not just be a "smelly old intellectual" but a rightist or even a counterrevolutionary with foreign ties. He then described the existing mental health care system, the kinds of patients they were seeing, and the woeful condition of the psychiatric profession. At the end of our talk, I mentioned that I had collaborated with the Taiwanese psychiatrist, Lin Tsungyi, who had initiated the WHO's International Pilot Study of Schizophrenia, arguably the first really important study in global mental health. Professor Ling had heard of Dr. Lin and the study, but knew little about either. Indeed, in the main he and his colleagues were depending on journals and texts from the 1940s and '50s. Ling Mingyou begged me not to forget them. He asked me to agree to develop a relationship with their department that would foster clinical research and clinical research training and thereby help develop psychiatry in China. And so moved was I by this experience that I did just as he requested.

I tell this story to set a personal background to understand the search for respect. Professor Ling and his colleagues felt disrespected, lacking dignity, and how could they not have, given the systematic demeaning of intellectuals and academics under radical Maoism. But their eloquent expression of making Chinese psychiatry more worthy of respect was addressed to Westerners who represented not just a world level of academic and clinical expertise unavailable in China at the time. There was also the deep cultural trauma of the nineteenth and twentieth centuries in China of feeling left behind by modernity. Westerners had helped to break China and overshadow its glorious past. True, its Communist revolution had strengthened China, transforming it from the "sick man of Asia" to a healthier and more robust society. But in 1978, China was still very poor and its level of science, technology, professionalization, and academic achievements was, for Chinese intellectuals, unacceptably low. Professor Ling and his colleagues, like thousands of other researchers and teachers, felt that they had no status (face) in a world that they knew was increasingly defined by new forms of knowledge generation and application. It was humiliating for them to acknowledge the primitive condition of psychiatry, the rest of medicine, and science in China. And their quest for upgrading their university, hospital, and academic work was a quest for modernization, and it was also a quest for the respect China's modernization would bring to an ancient society and a proud people who felt the sting and choke of others' pity and their own disappointment.

Over the past three decades, I have talked with hundreds of Chinese students and faculty members who have organized thoughts about their future within a story line centered on the search for respect, both collective and individual. In those accounts, there is usually slippage from talking about oneself to talking about one's field in China and from there on to China itself. It is easy to detect in this story line nationalist pride in China's achievements—economic, technological, scientific, professional—over the recent past. Doubtless respect for self and country feeds into nationalistic aspirations and dreams. Yet, the issue of "respect" seems to center more on professional competence and achievement, so that it is the particular discipline or specialty at hand, and the experts in it, that matters most.

The search for respect as a quest for meaning in life binds together personal identity, professional status, and Chinese collective status. The message is: we have accomplished enough to show our competence at the world level—personal, professional, collective—and that means we deserve respect. The corollary goes: if you fail to show us respect, if we feel disrespected, you will hear about it.

When I first published my findings on neurasthenia in Hunan in the early 1980s (Kleinman 1986), I didn't fully appreciate how sensitive my senior Chinese colleagues would be over whether their diagnosis of neurasthenia indicated, first, that they didn't possess the diagnostic acumen to identify depression, and, second, that they were not competent in modern psychiatry. My intention was neither; but the controversy that ensued taught me a lesson for a lifetime: in affairs academic, as in life affairs generally, begin with the acknowledgement of others and affirm your respect for their ideas and practices. Nowadays, a new generation of leaders in China's psychiatry profession, who seem much more secure in their professional identity, have become considerably less touchy about the limits and outright problems in professional practice and also more willing to see themselves as members of a global specialty. Among them and many others, one also hears, more and more frequently, the clamorous quest for self-respect drown out the search for collective respect. Recently, a young Chinese psychiatrist told me that for his generation it was legitimate to make demands for career development that were completely selfish. He went on to tell me that his agemates often upset their senior colleagues by openly expressing the view that they counted more than their work units.

Over the past decade, however, the cultural and personal sides of the quest for respect have been manipulated by the state to encourage outright nationalism and ethnic chauvinism. Fueled by China's extraordinary economic achievements as much as by the party-state's rhetoric and propaganda, nationalism has emerged as the cultural glue that holds together the increasingly diverse interests and plural perspectives of the Chinese. The dangers of ethnic nationalism are all-too-visible in the increasingly tense relations with ethnic minorities, in the periodic explosions of anger at the West, usually stoked by the party-state, and in the military build-up that is seen as threatening by China's neighbors. Its grounding in the subjective experiences of Chinese makes it even more dangerous, because once personal emotions are mobilized, a force is unleashed that is not easily controlled. This is a lesson the Chinese government is learning the hard way in Xinjiang and Tibet. And yet, as Martin Jacques (2009) shows in his polemical and flawed yet provocative book *When China Rules the World*, this century-long collective quest for respect and dignity animates the gathering sense that China is finally regaining its rightful place at the very center of the world system.

WOMEN'S QUEST FOR A VALUED STATUS

The Chinese revolution, in principle, overthrew the millennial patriarchal structure of power. Women were told they were responsible for holding up half the sky. As in so many other areas, socialist pronouncements and legislation said all the right things, yet were neither fully honored nor widely applied. Even today, women's search for meaning includes a struggle for a valued identity and status: but the question of value for women is fraught as they must weigh their traditional economic and reproductive "value" to others as daughters, wives, and mothers, against the newly visible individualist values of aspiration, accomplishment, and pleasure in their own personal lives. This conflict between women as "valuable" and women feeling "valued" in industrial and industrializing countries is not new, but the intense and long-standing emphasis on patriarchy and filial piety in Chinese society combined with the unbelievable speed of social, political, and economic change and the complex interplay of urban and rural social worlds has made this a particularly difficult historical moment for Chinese women.

As Wu Fei shows in chapter 6, rural women in China are often under great pressure as caregivers for children and in-laws, as peasant-farmers, as wives whose husbands have migrated to the cities, and as members of communities that, in a past they can often still remember, devalued their gender from birth to death; and, under a Confucian system of values held obedience—to their fathers, then husbands, and then sons—to be their highest sanctioned aspiration. Whereas the study of suicide in rural China leads to a more disappointing picture of the advances that women have made, the findings on divorce may provide cause for optimism.

As my colleagues and I have reviewed in the introduction, divorce is another realm in which women are demonstrating their dissatisfaction with their status. Between 1979 and 2008 the divorce rate in China grew from 4 percent to 21.8 percent, a massive increase. Interestingly, even in rural China 70 to 80 percent of divorces today are initiated by women. This striking statistic is destroying assumptions that women are more dependent on marriage than men—in fact, the reverse seems to be true: divorced women seem to have greater success remarrying than divorced men. As the research of Liu Yanwu (2009), a Chinese rural sociologist, illustrates, the desire for divorce combines a resistance against traditional family structures with a powerful quest for personal fulfillment: in his study of thirteen rural women who had divorced their husbands, only one described the traditional conflict with her mother-in-law as the primary motivation for her actions. The rest cited extramarital affairs or lack of satisfaction with their husbands as the cause. No longer content with a subservient role in the households, many are leaving marriage in "the pursuit of happiness," disturbing the stereotype of the wife as the selfless and devoted caregiver.

In the professional world, women's increased opportunities as factory workers, students, and small business owners have improved their position, but they must still work extra hard and count on favorable circumstances to secure a valued status. Women's success in wresting significance from society and in building lives that combine a valued domestic and career status is remaking the map of gender relations in China. Now, almost for the first time, many parents regard their daughters, not their sons, as their future security. Husbands' behavior increasingly signifies recognition that marriage is about shared opportunities and responsibilities. And yet, other evidence counters this more positive impression suggesting that women still face significant barriers. For example, research is only now documenting serious levels of physical abuse of women that we have every reason to believe is very long standing (Cao et al. 2006; Hicks 2003; Tsui et al. 2006; Xu et al. 2005).[3] The development of concern for gender issues in the media and in schools is promising, but the ways in which women are valued, affirmed, and glorified are rarely neutral, and rarely simplify the daily search for meaning for ordinary Chinese women.

During the 1960s as part of Mao's initiatives to develop the "iron rice bowl" of rural labor productivity, "iron girl brigades" were formed that were supposed to be representative of the equality that women were granted under Chinese socialism. Women as agricultural workers were represented as strong and focused, and as key players in the communist project (Hanser 2005). But as Amy Hanser discusses, this elevation of women's strength and importance has since been devalued and made an object of scorn, seen as illustrative of the failures and excesses of communist development. Now, as she shows, "the admired woman worker is likely to be a model—a fashion model" (2005: 282). Rather than drawing on the strength and vitality represented by their contribution to "iron rice bowl" and the nation, women are expected to draw on "the rice bowl of youth," and parlay their beauty and sexuality into professional success. This has consequences not only for young women searching for life paths (Hanser shows how even female retail employees in high-end boutiques can expect to have their careers end at age thirty), but also for the ways that the bodies of older women are being recast as useless and low class because they are associated with physical labor.

These conflicts are most visible and acute for women who are escaping the traditional constraints and drudgeries of marriage and work in rural areas, and following their dream of a better life to work in urban China. Tamara Jacka (2006) has movingly documented these women's quests for a better life in her ethnography *Rural Women in Urban China*. Women from rural China migrate to the cities with many goals; to go to school, to experience new things, to escape marriage and the rural life, to "blaze a path" (2006: 149) in the world, or simply, as one of Jacka's informants noted, to follow "the beautiful dream" (2006: 139). These migrant workers, with little money or support, rarely find what they are looking for and instead settle for lives of endless, difficult labor, often under economically and sexually exploitative conditions. Still, few of the women that Jacka interviewed expressed a desire to return to rural areas because the independent drudgery of the city, even with few prospects for employment after age thirty or forty, seemed to them preferable to rural drudgery confined by the traditional family social system. Those who did return to the village, often with entrepreneurial ambitions of applying what they had learned in the city toward improving their families' conditions, are often ridiculed. As one woman recounted:

I thought I'd go home and go into business with members of my family. I thought I could plant fruit trees or else seedlings. I've had a look at the market. Everyone cursed at me. Then they sent me away. They wouldn't agree. . . . So I thought I'd sign a contract [with the local government] to run an orchard. But I'm not the head of a household so I couldn't do that independently. That is to say, even if you have money, you can't necessarily be the one to make the decisions. Girls can't do anything in the countryside. You can only become independent of your family once you're married, but then you must do as your husband says. If my family had been willing for me to stay at home, they could have let me take my portion of land. But they wouldn't let me, they believed I was just a dependent. (2006: 156)

As in this case, women's plans, and even financial means, may quickly outstrip their perceived social role, leading to intense frustration, at least in the short term.

Yet despite the many complexities and trials of this changing, and yet still in many ways traditional, China, women still seem to feel a strong sense of hope, and many female migrants to the city remain there out of a simple sense of excitement; excitement about the dynamism of the present and the opportunities of the future. Another woman Jacka interviewed noted "I definitely won't go back [home to the village] in the short term. In Beijing I have things I want to do . . . because now Beijing has entered the world and it's won the bid for the Olympic Games. . . . Even though working outside is full of suffering—you go to work at seven in the morning and you don't finish till nine in the evening, and in the evenings it's cold and you feel very tired—but, still, it's interesting" (2006: 149).

As a number of contributions to this volume have noted, China's many changes have weighed especially heavily on women, but have also had real and surprising emancipatory effects. The equality, if only in name, of women under communism has allowed for the development of a strong feminist movement in urban China, and the one-child policy, while robbing women of a traditional source of personal and social value—children—has also freed up their bodies and attentions for other pursuits and ambitions. These ambitions do not always match available opportunity; even today, women's voices can be drowned out in public without setting off much notice and their status remains constrained in institutions such as larger businesses, research centers, universities, and bureaucracies.

However, the upshot is that the informed social movement to secure more valued positions for women in Chinese society may be one of the more promising sources of reform. There is evidence that this movement is gaining force and popularity. Hence, it is not surprising to hear women challenge real constraints and barriers, and seek remedies from society's leading institutions. In clinical interviews and small group discussions, I have been impressed by the increasing substitution of a narrative of active struggle, excitement, and anticipated success, particularly among the younger generations, for one of passive resistance and expectant failure.

THE QUEST TO DO GOOD IN THE WORLD

While global institutions of humanitarian assistance pretty clearly grow out of the Western tradition of religious philanthropy and secular welfare assistance, both ancient Chinese society and the neo-Confucian tradition fostered ideas and practices of improving the world (Puett 2001; Tu 1985). In Taiwan and Thailand, Buddhist charities have been active in disaster relief and in responding to the social epidemic of drug abuse. Yet, in the People's Republic of China, until very recently, all efforts at humanitarian assistance were controlled by the state and private volunteerism was discouraged. As noted earlier in this book, this changed with the 2008 Sichuan earthquake. In its aftermath, the Chinese government permitted individual volunteerism and the work of NGOs that were not under state control. While there are different interpretations for why this happened, surely one of the reasons must have been sensitivity to the wave of global social movements of humanitarian aid and volunteerism that respond to natural and man-made disasters, a wave that is increasingly seen by ordinary Chinese in the media, including the Internet, and is mobilizing their interest. Another reason surely is based in the ideological emphasis of Maoism on the role of the Party in serving the people and in the actual campaigns to address such public issues as poor hygiene and sanitation, infestations with disease-causing carriers, vaccination, and child survival that followed closely upon one another in the 1950s and '60s.

In this volume, Jing Jun's chapter documents the impressive development of voluntary blood donation in Chinese cities. He attributes this remarkable development to the growth of altruism in China. Other examples of individual efforts to improve the world include the emergence of support groups for patients and their families who are facing particular health problems like schizophrenia, autism in children, epilepsy, lung cancer, and so on. The development of popular concern about controlling pollution and protecting the environment is another example, as is the new interest of China's super-wealthy in giving through private rather than state-controlled channels.

From my own experience, I can narrate the development of a family support group in Shanghai. This group came together with the assistance of local psychiatrists to improve communication about how to deal with psychotic symptoms and behaviors and how to educate neighbors to be more tolerant and less stigmatizing. It was viewed by professionals as a powerful illustration of the importance of empowering families and patients through knowledge and outreach activities, and was seen, therefore, as a potentially important way to increase recognition and treatment of mental health problems. Other such groups have come together around preventing suicide and protecting women from abuse (Wu 2011).

Zhou Haiwen, a forty-five-year-old architect in Nanjing, complained to me about how little attention is paid in China to obvious dangers like inadequate protection of pedestrians crossing major streets where cars are driven as if the purpose were to scatter those trying to make it across; building sites with rebar projecting out onto the sidewalk and concrete slabs balanced precariously on cross-beams over people's heads; work units with sink holes that are unrepaired and unprotected; and so on. She and her professional colleagues were creating a list of local dangers to present to local bureaucrats with the expectation that they might be controlled and improved so that others would not get hurt. She regarded this as a sign of how middle-class expectations might change the inattention of authorities and ordinary people to a degree of danger no longer acceptable. She saw her profession, her colleagues, and herself as doing good for their city and other urban settings.

But the impulse to do good in the world is wider still. The new environmental consciousness, interest in human rights, consumer protection efforts, volunteering, as well as concern with improving regulation more generally and with ending corruption—all are illustrative of prosocial ideas and collective practices that could have a large effect on social life and personal choices. Nowhere is there a more impressive example than in student associations that abound on university campuses and aim to enrich student life and introduce some degree of self-governance.

Side by side with materialist and selfish concerns, one hears, especially among young people, tales about experiences and experiments with efforts at encouraging an ecology of flourishing, improving local living conditions, working for environmental improvements, reforming educational institutions, and getting caught up in cyber communications about global problems like climate change, global health, and women's issues. Doubtless, youth are sensitive to political constraints on how far these experiments can go without provoking surveillance and repression; yet there is something afoot among educated Chinese youth that indicates idealistic impulses to assist others and improve conditions are revivifying—and taking on a global perspective—with uncertain consequences. Indeed, in the public sphere, this nascent movement to do good for others runs up against an authoritarian regime that does not allow that public sphere to be free and open. The potential for conflict grows as Chinese society becomes more mobile, pluralistic, and connected to the outside world. But I see no evidence that this youth movement will morph into a political uprising that resembles what happened in Tunisia, Egypt, and Libya as this book went to press, though doubtless this is on the minds of China's leaders.

THE QUEST FOR STABILITY AND ORDER

Another quest for meaning is the result of the disorienting changes of the past decades, especially among older Chinese. Even for Americans and Europeans who travel to China frequently, and who have done so for several decades, the pace and nature of change can be difficult to put into a coherent picture. Reality, at least at the surface, is a constant blur of change. So much more is the confusion and unsettling sense of life becoming uninterpretable for Chinese who have lived through the transition to communism, the turn into radical revolutionary Maoism, later still the pivot to market socialism, and now the current transition to a shaky mix of global liberal and local authoritarian cultural scenarios.

Chinese businesspeople have complained to me about having to adjust to the systematic application of standards and rules for the first time as the government becomes truly serious about laws governing business practices. Yet at the same time, other Chinese have complained of the failure of regulation in food safety and standards for medications. The newspapers speak of consumers who are hesitant to trust the reliability of products, and yet want to purchase things that put them at a higher standard. The behavior of the young is looked on with a combination of envy and dismay by older Chinese, several of whom in a Shanghai club for the elderly told me they felt like they were watching the creation of a new world: one they neither fully comprehended nor felt comfortable with. They and others complain of a sense of insecurity; they are no longer at ease in the world around them. The social order seems to be undergoing a tectonic shift. (See the chapter by Yan in this volume on the changing moral landscape.)

One Chinese intellectual, a retired professor at a leading university, grumbled that "I always looked forward to things getting better, and they really have. So why am I upset with this new age? It's everything of value melting away. It's the extent and rapidity of change. I can't recognize my neighborhood. All the new buildings. New buildings, new streets, new styles, new ideas. . . . Sometimes I feel like I am lost. I get dizzy just thinking about all the changes. It's not a good feeling. Where's the stability?"

This elderly acquaintance is not alone in feeling disoriented; other elderly men and women have conveyed the same message, only without the grumpiness and negativity. Indeed, others manage to worry about instability while portraying a much warmer and happier sense of their lives.

THE DIVIDED SELF

These are only a few of the varieties of quests-for-meaning experiences that have impressed me over the years. Their development in part relates to the flourishing of individualism that Yunxiang Yan describes in his chapter in *Deep China*, and in part they offer further illustration of the refashioning of the moral context and the moral person in Chinese society that my colleagues and I have outlined in the introduction. The fact that real lives encompass more than one such quest, and that personal struggles to fashion meanings that matter may intensify meanings that are contradictory, supports our sense that the divided self is a useful metaphor for the Chinese experience. Huang Yongyu, the famous elderly Hunanese artist whose painting of an owl with one eye closed became the subject of state criticism during the Cultural Revolution (see the introduction in this volume), somewhere noted that his painting was not a blink or a wink, but the way he had heard owls sleep. While this tongue-in-cheek theory is unlikely to be ornithologically accurate, the sense of necessary alertness even in periods of quiet rest is not, as we have noted, an inappropriate metaphor for the sensibility to danger and uncertainty that has long been part of Chinese culture and that was intensified to a fever pitch during the days of radical Maoism. How valid is it as an image for China today?

In my personal opinion, it is still a valid depiction of the human condition in China. The divided self (or double consciousness) of the Chinese turns on the unsettling realization that things can get worse (much worse) in a hurry and that the moral context in Chinese society can be and frequently is divided against the moral person. The state that has been so successful at creating prosperity (albeit with worsening social inequality) is also repressive and can be dangerously so. The moral context created by the party-state is as much a place of collusion and collaboration with ruthlessly pragmatic power as it is a place of aspiration for and achievement of a better life for many of its citizens. The individual as a political subject experiences misplaced loyalty and dreams deferred as well as surveillance and control. Yet, that same individual is the beneficiary of poverty reduction, food security, social stability, and a health status unimaginable for most Chinese before 1949. The terrible excesses and abuses of the collectivist era are gone. There are village-level elections; the urban work unit no longer dominates the lives of its employees. There are numerous freedoms in everyday life. And yet each individual is socialized indirectly by the state and directly by the family to understand the very real limits of those small freedoms as well as the responsibility to live a divided life with great alertness to the boundaries that one does not trespass, no matter what is at stake. My point is that those boundaries are not just in the external world, but have been internalized by the self as self-censorship, self-control, and self-discipline; but also, and most problematically, self-division. That is to say, the divided self is how China is governed, not just experienced. When James C. Scott (1990) wrote of an individual's hidden transcript in authoritarian societies standing against the government's public transcript, he had in mind the acts of resistance that ordinary people master to delay, deflect, and defeat state power. I use the image of the divided self to suggest that personal "transcripts" in China are not only or primarily about acts of resistance; they are also acts of accommodation and collaboration that enable ordinary people to negotiate China's social reality in such a way as to open or protect the individual's space while getting on with life lived in an authoritarian society. These acts of accommodation, however, place a particular moral burden on the inner world of the Chinese just as they complicate the local moral world those individuals inhabit. That is a burden of contradiction, compromise, and irony that each Chinese person experiences and negotiates in his or her own way. Yet just as a moral world can be remade, so too can the divided self be refashioned, even if it is the consequence of the operation of biopower (see Foucault 1990), once it is clear to the person what is really at stake for him or her. In fact, when generalized to whole communities, working out how to resolve the tensions of the divided self even carries with it the potential to remake China's moral worlds.

Wu Zhenyu is a fifty-three-year-old engineer with considerable foreign experience who now works for a multinational firm in Beijing and with whom I have been acquainted for more than twenty years. In 2006, during a visit to Boston, Wu and I had a long conversation about the idea that the consequence of China's fraught moral context had been a divided Chinese self.

"I find the idea an attractive one," Wu said to me with a sad smile. Wu was silent for a while, and then carefully continued:

Maybe it's particularly appropriate as a way of understanding Chinese of my generation and those who are older. But the more I think about it, it's relevant for younger Chinese too. What I like about this idea is that it corresponds with how I feel inside. It's something my friends and I have talked about. There is a feeling of an inner self that you can express to others, and another part that you can't, or you feel you shouldn't. There is also a sense of contradiction. What you can't say sometimes contradicts what you do say. That's true about political affairs. But it also holds for ethics. The values we express are the ones you are supposed to claim you believe in; those aren't what you actually value. What I mean is you can't openly talk about things that go against the grain. It used to be you couldn't talk about self-interest: you know, building a career, making money, and the like. That has all changed. But you still can't talk about what really bothers you about what's going on around you.

I keep secret my criticism of the hypocrisy in government pronouncements; the inequalities that challenge the very idea of a communist or socialist society; the collusion between powerful people: cadres and businessmen. Once you go public, your words come back to affect what you do. I once criticized a business deal that I thought was not in my company's interest and certainly not in the public interest. Afterward, I was frozen out of just about everything having to do with that deal. On the surface everything seems like the U.S. or Europe, but it isn't. The Party is in there with other powerful interests, working backstage. So, by the time things are presented for official comment or negotiation, the whole thing has been decided. Corruption is structural; it's in the system. Same with the influence of the Party in other fields, things are not what they seem to be. And people know that. So they internalize it. If you are going to get ahead, you accept all that: the lies, the hypocrisy. The Party doesn't just win. It needs to show it has taken the moral high ground. So that makes the moral high ground suspicious. It really isn't a high ground. So what happens when you corrupt the moral system, it corrupts everyone. You can't trust your own feelings. You lose your idea of what is right and what is wrong. So inside yourself, even, maybe you keep one eye open on advancing your self-interest but the other eye is closed to your pain, the feeling you have that it is wrong and you should not be part of it. That's the contradiction, the division inside.

Seen one way, the divided self is but the subjective equivalent of the moral-political resistance of Chinese communities to the policies and programs of an authoritarian party-state. Here, insecurity in the relation of individuals to the state and social mistrust intensify the sense of division in the self and in society. Yet, seen in quite a different way, this inner division is evidence of a deepening and complexifying of the interiority of the person. Subjectivity in today's China is expanding. The space of the self is being more richly furnished in emotion, memory, and sensibility. Perhaps in a spiritual sense as well. At the core of this transmutation is a divided self that increasingly can multitask, feel comfortable with contradiction and imagine a new and different China.

The divided self qualifies these quests for meaning. Chinese individuals can't easily separate the moral and the emotional from the political; yet unlike the past, where the dividing line was clear, everything today has blurred the line between the private and the public. Within the self, the line is also blurred between what is deeply personal and what is an intrusion of the authoritarian state into speech and behavior. It is this uncertainty and even confusion that is simultaneously troubling and promising. In a sense, the divided self of individual Chinese is a simulacrum of the divided nature of Chinese society and the Chinese state. How the state will respond to greater civic and subjective diversity and openness is still not settled (Zhang, Kleinman, and Tu 2011). It could mean more authoritarianism. But the longer it remains divided, the greater the room for innovation and even liberation of self and society. That is why so much depends on understanding the Chinese people as experiencing moral division deep within and also in the divided worlds of China today.

NOTES

1. With the exception of my personal accounts of conversations in Hunan in the 1970s and '80s, I have altered details about the individuals whose words are quoted in this chapter in order to conceal their identity and to protect their anonymity.

2. Qu Yuan (ca. 340–273 BCE) was a Chinese scholar and minister to the king of the southern state of Chu during the Warring States period, who drowned himself in the Miluo River in what is now Hunan Province as an act of criticizing the emperor for bad governance and injustice. Qu Yuan's Confucian suicide is celebrated each year on the fifth day of the fifth moon by dragon boat races and by throwing sticky rice wrapped in lotus leaves into the river to feed his ghost.

3. Some of this research is with Chinese immigrants in the United States, where the topic itself is receiving increased attention. While research in China is limited, memoirs, novels, films, and personal accounts suggest that violence toward women is a serious family issue.

REFERENCES

Cao Y. P., et al. 2006. "Hunansheng jiating baoli de liuxingbingxue diaocha zongti bao-gao" [An Epidemiological Study on Domestic Violence in Hunan, China]. *Zhonghua liuxingbingxue zazhi* [Chinese Journal of Epidemiology] 27, no. 3:200–203.

Chang, S. In preparation. "Study of Dazhai Village in Xiyang Township, Shaanxi, China." PhD dissertation, Department of Anthropology, Harvard University.

Committee on Scholarly Communication with PRC. 1980. *Rural Health in the People's Republic of China: Report of a Visit by the Rural Health Systems Delegation, June 1978.* Bethesda, MD: U.S. Dept. of Health and Human Services, November 1980, NIH Publication No. 81–2124.

Feng, C. 1996. *Ten Years of Madness: Oral Histories of China's Cultural Revolution.* San Francisco: China Books.

Foucault, M. 1990. *The Will to Knowledge.* Vol. 1 of *The History of Sexuality.* Translated by R. Hurley. London: Penguin Books.

Hanser, A. 2005. "The Gendered Rice Bowl: The Sexual Politics of Service Work in Urban China." *Gender and Society* 19, no. 5:581–600.

Hicks, M. H. R. 2003. "Prevalence and Characteristics of Intimate Partner Violence in a Community Study of Chinese American Women." *Journal of Interpersonal Violence* 21, no. 10:1249–1269.

Jacka, T. 2006. *Rural Women in Urban China: Gender, Migration, and Social Change.* New York: M. E. Sharpe.

Jacques, M. 2009. *When China Rules the World: The Rise of the Middle Kingdom and the End of the Western World.* London: Penguin Books.

Kleinman, A. 1986. *Social Origins of Distress and Disease: Neurasthenia, Depression, and Pain in Modern China.* New Haven, CT: Yale University Press.

———. 1988. *The Illness Narratives: Suffering, Healing, and the Human Condition.* New York: Basic Books.

———. 2006. *What Really Matters: Living a Moral Life amidst Uncertainty and Danger.* New York: Oxford University Press.

Kleinman, A., V. Das, and M. Lock. 1997. *Social Suffering.* Berkeley: University of California Press.

Lee, S., and A. Kleinman. 2003. "Suicide as Resistance." In *Chinese Society: Change, Conflict and Resistance,* 2nd ed., edited by E. Perry and M. Seldon, 289–311. London: Routledge.

Liang, H., and J. Shapiro. 1983. *Son of the Revolution.* New York: Alfred A. Knopf.

Liu Yanwu. 2009. "Nongcun fuqiguanxi yu jiatingjiegou de biandong" [From Nuclear-

Family-Based to Individual-Based: A Study of Rural Conjugal Relationship and the Changes in Family Structure]. *Xinan Shiyou Daxue xuebao* [Bulletin of the Southwestern University of Petroleum], no. 2.

Palmer, D. 2007. *Qigong Fever.* New York: Columbia University Press.

Puett, M. 2001. *The Ambivalence of Creation.* Palo Alto, CA: Stanford University Press.

Scott, J. C. 1990. *Domination and the Arts of Resistance: Hidden Transcripts.* New Haven, CT: Yale University Press.

Thaxton, R. 2008. *Catastrophe and Contention in Rural China: Mao's Great Leap Forward, Famine and the Origins of Righteous Resistance in Da Fo.* Cambridge: Cambridge University Press.

Thurston, A. F. 1987. *Enemies of the People: The Ordeal of the Intellectuals in China's Great Cultural Revolution.* New York: Alfred A. Knopf.

Tsui K. L. et al. 2006. "Risk Factors for Injury to Married Women from Domestic Violence in Hong Kong." *Hong Kong Medical Journal* 12, no. 4:289–293.

Tu, W. M. 1985. *Confucian Thought: Selfhood as Creative Transformation.* Albany: State University of New York Press.

Xu, X., et al. 2005. "Prevalence of and Risk Factors for Intimate Partner Violence in China." *American Journal of Public Health* 95, no. 1:78–85.

Wu, F. 2011. "Governing Suicide: An Ethnological Study of Rural Women's Program of Suicide Intervention." In *Governance of Life in Chinese Moral Experience: The Quest for an Adequate Life,* edited by E. Zhang, A. Kleinman, and W. M. Tu, 182–196. New York: Routledge.

Zhang, E., A. Kleinman, and W. M. Tu, eds. 2011. *Governance of Life in Chinese Moral Experience: The Quest for an Adequate Life.* New York: Routledge.

GLOSSARY OF CHINESE
TERMS AND NAMES

CHAPTER 1 (YAN)

Chinese Characters	Pinyin Transliteration	Meaning
《北京文艺》	Beijing wenyi	Beijing Literature
逼捐	bi juan	aggressive and ungrateful push for donation
大公无私	dagong wusi	complete impartiality and selflessness
德治	dezhi	rule by virtue
干折	ganzhe	converting
个人自由	geren ziyou	personal freedom
公德	gongde	public morality
公房	gongfang	residential unit allocated by the state
关系	guanxi	social relationships
毫不利己, 专门利人	hao bu liji, zhuanmen liren	seeking no advantage for oneself, pursuing benefits only for others
老实	laoshi	honesty and obedience
乐百事集团	Lebaishi jituan	a Chinese soft drink company
雷锋	Lei Feng	the name of a model soldier
商品房	shangpinfang	a commercial flat purchased after the housing reform
私房	sifang	family housing with a pre-1950s private ownership

温柔	wenrou	gentleness
协议	xieyi	agreement
养老	yanglao	elderly support
义务劳动	yiwu laodong	volunteer work
有个性	you gexing	having individuality
《中国青年》	*Zhongguo qingnian*	*China Youth*
《中国青年报》	*Zhongguo qingnianbao*	*China Youth Daily*

CHAPTER 2 (JING)

Chinese Characters	*Pinyin Transliteration*	*Meaning*
艾滋村	Aizi cun	AIDS village
八路军	Ba Lu Jun	Eighth Route Army
共青团	Gong Qing Tuan	Communist Youth League
好吃懒做	haochi lanzuo	gluttonous and lazy
快速分血机	kuaisu fenxue ji	high-speed spinner
献血法	Xian Xue Fa	Blood Donation Law
血头	xue tou	blood contractor

CHAPTER 3 (ZHANG)

Chinese Characters	*Pinyin Transliteration*	*Meaning*
爱	ai	love; can refer to romantic love
爱情	aiqing	romantic love
包二奶	bao ernai	"to have a second pair of breasts," meaning to have a regularly paid mistress or concubine
吹箫	chuixiao	fellatio
打飞机	da feiji	to receive manual stimulation of the penis
婚外恋	hun wai lian	extramarital love
结伴不结婚	jieban bu jiehun	cohabiting
男科	nanke	men's medicine
情	qing	sentiment or affect
情爱	qing'ai	sentimental, romantic love
扫黄	sao huang	"sweeping yellow," referring to striking against the sex industry and pornography
色	se	lust
爽	shuang	ecstatically pleasurable due to having good sex

同性恋	tongxing lian	same-sex love
同志	tongzhi	"comrade," borrowed from vocabulary of the communist revolution to denote gays and lesbians
小姐	xiaojie	"little elder sister" or "young lady," now meaning a sex worker
性	xing	sex
"性"	"xing"	sexuality
性爱	xing'ai	sexual love
养生	yangsheng	nurturing life, or the cultivation of life
养小蜜	yangxiaomi	"to have a little sweetie," meaning to have a subordinate as a mistress
一夜情	yiye qing	one-night stand

CHAPTER 4 (PAN)

Chinese Characters	Pinyin Transliteration	Meaning
单位人	danwei ren	a "work unit person"
纺嫂	fang sao	"textile sisters"; laid-off workers from the textile factories
风水	fengshui	geomancy
复兴	fuxing	revitalization
工人新村	Gongren Xincun	Workers' New Village
户口	hukou	household registration
街道	jiedao	streets; street offices
南巡	Nan Xun	Inspection Tour of the South
棚户	penghu	shacks; slum
平民村	Pingmin Cun	Commoner's Village
上只角	shang zhi jiao	upper quarters; uptown
社会人	shehui ren	a "society person"
苏北	Subei	Northern Jiangsu
湾桥	Wan Qiao	Bay Bridge
文明社区	wenming shequ	a "civilized community"; model community
下岗	xiagang	someone who has been laid off or is unemployed
下只角	xia zhi jiao	lower quarters; shacks
新天地	Xin Tian Di	Xin Tian Di redevelopment project
压锭	ya ding	smashing the spindles

CHAPTER 5 (LEE)

Chinese Characters	Pinyin Transliteration	Meaning
百忧解	baiyoujie	undoer of all worries
不开心 (不愉快)	bukaixin (buyukuai)	unhappiness
打假	dajia	to conquer counterfeiting
感情	ganqing	emotions of human concern
回扣	huikou	kickback
教授越教越瘦	jiaoshou yuejiao yueshou	the longer a professor teaches, the poorer he becomes
老黄牛	laohuangniu	old yellow cows
卖药	maiyao	selling drugs
难过	nanguo	feeling bad
气	qi	vital energy
七情	qiqing	seven emotions
全民经商	quanmin jingshang	everybody goes into business
人情	renqing	favor
神经衰弱	shenjing shuairuo	neurasthenia
瞎用药	xiayongyao	prescribe blindly
心理	xinli	psychological
虚	xu	weakness
血	xue	blood
压力	yali	stress
忧	you	worry
优	you	excellence
忧郁症/抑郁症	youyuzheng/ yiyuzheng	depression
灾后心理 （创伤后心理）	zaihouxinli (chuang-shanghou xinli)	post-traumatic psychology

CHAPTER 6 (WU)

Chinese Characters	Pinyin Transliteration	Meaning
道德资本	daode ziben	moral capital
非人	feiren	nonperson
夫妻冲突	fuqi chongtu	conjugal conflict
个人主义	geren zhuyi	individualism
公婆	gongpo	in-laws
家庭政治	jiating zhengzhi	family politics
农药	nongyao	pesticide

权力平衡	quanli pingheng	power balance
权力游戏	quanli youxi	games of power
委屈	weiqu	domestic injustice
现代性	xiandaixing	modernity
孝	xiao	filial piety
心理紊乱	xinli wenluan	mental disorder
抑郁	yiyu	depression
自杀预防	zishayufang	suicide prevention

CHAPTER 7 (GUO AND KLEINMAN)

Chinese Characters	Pinyin Transliteration	Meaning
艾滋病	aizibing	AIDS
安全	anquan	security
耻辱	chiru	shame
单位	danwei	work unit
道德常识	daode changshi	moral common sense
丢人	diuren	losing face
非人	feiren	nonperson
疯子	fengzi	crazy person
关系	guanxi	social relationships
家庭	jiating	family
检讨	jiantao	self-criticism
精神病	jingshenbing	mental illness
旧社会	jiu shehui	old society
礼钱	liqian	gift money
脸面	lianmian	moral face
面子	mianzi	social face
难堪	nankan	embarrassing
排斥	paichi	exclusion
批斗会	pidouhui	struggle sessions
歧视	qishi	discrimination
讨薪	taoxin	begging for salary
危险	weixian	danger
武疯子	wu fengzi	violent mentally ill person
新社会	xin shehui	new society
羞辱	xiuru	humiliate
威胁	weixie	threat
污名	wuming	stigma

CHAPTER 8 (KLEINMAN)

Chinese Characters	Pinyin Transliteration	Meaning
地位	diwei	status
好/善	hao/shan	good
快乐	kuaile	happiness
体验/经历	tiyan/jingli	experience
稳定	wending	stability
幸运	xingyun	fortunate
意义	yiyi	meaning
正义	zhengyi	justice
秩序	zhixu	order
尊重	zunzhong	respect

NOTES ON CONTRIBUTORS

GUO JINHUA is an assistant professor in the Department of Sociology, Peking University. A medical anthropologist, his research focuses on stigma related to mental illness and HIV/AIDS, healthcare reform, religion, natural disasters, and mental health in China.

JING JUN is a professor in the Department of Sociology, Tsinghua University, where he also directs the Center for Research on Public Health. He is the author of *The Temple of Memories: History, Power, and Morality in a Chinese Village* (1996) and the editor of *Feeding China's Little Emperors: Food, Children, and Social Change* (2000). He is the co-editor of *HIV in China: Understanding the Social Aspects of the Epidemic* (2010).

ARTHUR KLEINMAN is the Esther and Sidney Rabb Professor of Anthropology, Faculty of Arts and Sciences, and professor of medical anthropology and psychiatry, Faculty of Medicine, Harvard University. He is also the Victor and William Fung Director of Harvard's Asia Center. He is the author of *Patients and Healers in the Context of Culture* (1980) and *Social Origins of Distress and Disease: Depression, Neurasthenia, and Pain in Modern China* (1986). He is the coeditor of *Medicine in Chinese Cultures* (1974), *SARS in China* (2006), and *Japan's Wartime Medical Atrocities: Comparative Inquiries in Science, History, and Ethics* (2010).

SING LEE is a professor in the Department of Psychiatry and the director of the Hong Kong Mood Disorders Center, Faculty of Medicine, The Chinese University of Hong Kong. He is also a lecturer in the Department of Global Health and Social Medicine, Harvard Medical School. He was a Freeman Foundation Fellow in 1996–97. His principal research interests are mental health and social change in Chinese society. He is the author of "Higher Earnings, Bursting Trains, and Exhausted Bodies: The Creation of Traveling Psychosis in Post-Reform China" (*Social Science and Medicine*, 1998) and "Stigmatizing Experience and Structural Discrimination Associated with Treatment of Schizophrenia in Hong Kong" (*Social Science and Medicine*, 2006).

PAN TIANSHU is associate professor of cultural anthropology at the Fudan School of Social Development and Public Policy. He has conducted field research on global/local dynamics, local responses to threat of avian flu, homeowners' associations in Shanghai's gated communities, the impact of rural-urban migration on migrant-sending communities, and "Shanghai nostalgia."

WU FEI is an associate professor in the Department of Religious Studies, Peking University. He is the author of *Sacred Word over the Wheatland* (2001, in Chinese), *Suicide as a Chinese Problem* (2007, in Chinese), and *Suicide and Justice: A Chinese Perspective* (2009).

YUNXIANG YAN is professor of anthropology, University of California, Los Angeles. He is the author of *The Flow of Gifts: Reciprocity and Social Networks in a Chinese Village* (1996), *Private Life under Socialism: Love, Intimacy, and Family Change in a Chinese Village* (2003), and *The Individualization of Chinese Society* (2009).

EVERETT YUEHONG ZHANG is assistant professor of anthropology in the Department of East Asian Studies, Princeton University. He is the coeditor of *Governance of Life in Chinese Moral Experience: The Quest for an Adequate Life* (2011). He is the author of *Impotence in China: An Illness of Chinese Modernity* (forthcoming).

INDEX

lessness as virtue, 49–50; Sino-Japanese War and, 83. *See also* socialism

Communist Party, Chinese (CCP), 7, 17, 72n3, 99, 126; collectivist ethics of, 42; compulsory allegiance to, 182; divided self and, 287; homosexuality viewed by, 251; *People's Daily,* 108; politicization of mental illness and, 239; pornographic viewing by members of, 114; private sector encouraged by, 19; psychiatry and, 193; public trust in, 49; response to political traumas, 203; sex industry and, 130; Shanghai as birthplace of, 154, 162, 163; social control mechanisms of, 187; sociopolitical turbulence suppressed by, 178; terms of opprobrium for opposition to, 27; transition to modernity and, 30 *See also* party-state

Communist Youth League, 40, 41, 83, 97, 145

concubinage, 140

Confucianism, 6, 10, 182; collectivist ethics of, 42; Cultural Revolution and, 16; modernity and, 234–35; neo-Confucian tradition, 282; old-age security and, 207; patriarchal ethics of, 52; women's status and, 279

Confucius, 49, 51, 221

Cong Fei, 63–64, 66, 68, 73n5

construction, unsafe, 61, 73n4, 204–05, 283

consumerism, 18, 47, 54, 70; privileges of political elite and, 18; sex industry and, 124, 127, 129

contraceptives, 136–38

Corner Left Behind by Romantic Love, The (Zhang Xian), 134

corruption, 24, 39, 72n3, 207, 267, 287; in blood trade, 84; idealization of Maoist era and, 49; institutionalized, 62; Sichuan earthquake and, 204–5; suicide and, 200

counterfeiting, 186

courtesy stigma, 13

courts, 4, 28, 55, 93

crime, 109, 120, 122, 173, 207, 251

Cui Jian, 43

Cultural Revolution, 7, 23, 40, 50, 178, 183, 186, 276; blood donations during, 83; Confucianism shaken by, 16; consequences of, 270, 271; depression and, 183; as destructive period, 266–67; divided self and, 285; end of, 275; mental illness politicized during, 239; neurasthenic symptoms and, 181; peasant resistance during, 8; political trauma and, 203; psychiatrists/ psychologists and, 194, 208; public criticism sessions, 254; self-interest during, 42; sexuality during, 110–11, 115, 132–34, 137, 145; survivors of, 6, 263; violence of, 5. *See also* Maoism

Culture, Medicine, and Psychiatry (journal), 191

culture war, 49–51

cynicism, 24, 51, 70, 99, 185, 206, 273

Daoism (Taoism), 142, 239

dating, online, 20

Davis, D., 54

deaf people, 28–29

"debris," of socialist system, 157, 166, 167, 169, 172, 173

decollectivization, 14, 28

Deleuze, Gilles, 117, 144

democracy, 70, 115, 143

Deng Xiaoping, 44, 98, 152, 153, 191, 206

depression (mental illness), 12, 47, 177–212; Chinese politics of, 190–92; commercialization of, 192–97; drug (pharmaceutical) companies and, 197; increase in diagnosis of, 199, 206, 207; in Maoist era, 182; neurasthenia and, 179, 192, 277; social context of, 188–90; stigma of, 208; suicide and, 200–203; treatment of, 208; U.S.-China paradox of, 177–78

Falun Gong, 168, 209, 273

family, 3, 20, 22, 42; conflicts over food, 222, 223, 224; conjugal relationship in, 216; HIV/AIDS stigma and, 257; homosexuality and, 251; in-law conflicts, 224–28, 279; mental illness and, 244–48; prosperity and harmony of, 54; self connected to, 8; standard of living for, 10; suicide and, 13, 214–16, 232–33; support groups and, 283; trust and, 59

famine, 6, 64, 178, 266

favor, exchange of *(renqing)*, 197–200

Fei Xiaotong, 28, 50, 59, 214, 220

femininity, 39

feminism, 139, 281

Feng, J. C., 186

fengshui (geomancy), 161, 164

feudalism, 21, 30, 64, 239

filial piety, 36–37, 46, 48, 55, 220–23, 224, 251, 279

financial crisis, global, 152, 154, 207

floods, 203

food, family conflicts over, 222, 223, 224

food safety scandals, 57–59, 60, 207, 284

Foucault, Michel, 106–7, 136, 137, 144, 286

France, 80, 102n1

friends, networks of, 20

Gao Yaojie, 79

gated communities, 165, 166, 172–73

gays. *See* homosexuality

GDP (gross domestic product), 3, 138

Gemai, 123

gender, 19, 22, 279–80

gender equality, 141

gentleness *(wenrou)*, 38–39

gentrification, 156, 165, 166, 170–73

getihu ("individual household"), 17

gift giving, 62, 97–98

Gift Relationship, The (Titmuss), 79, 97

globalization, 25, 26, 70, 72, 74

Good Samaritans, extortion of, 56, 71

goudui business transactions, 111, 128

"granny cadres," 169–70, 173

Great Leap Forward, 6, 50, 178; birth rate and, 133; famine during, 266; forced labor during, 184–85; peasant resistance during, 8; political trauma and, 203

guanxi (personal connections), 37, 71, 245

Guattari, Félix, 117

Guo Jinhua, 13, 243, 259n4

Haizi, 213

Hamilton Depression Rating Scale, 199

Han chauvinism, 2

Han Han, 66, 73n6

Hanser, Amy, 280

happiness, pursuit of, 37, 48, 72, 206, 266–69; family tensions and, 233; sexual revolution and, 143–46; women's quest for valued status and, 279. *See also* meaning, quests for

Harrell, Stevan, 8

Harvey, William, 82

He Aifang, 79

health care system, 15, 153, 208, 248, 263

Heart of a Young Girl, The (anonymous novel), 109–10, 112, 113, 115

hepatitis, 81–82, 85, 98

History of Sexuality (Foucault), 106

HIV/AIDS, 13, 26, 79, 121, 207, 237–38, 263; "clustered infections," 89, 90; drive for profit and, 78; drug use and, 253–56; epidemic in central China, 80–82; first reported cases in United States, 80; "Four Free and One Care" policy, 249; government responsibility and, 95–99; homosexuality and, 251–53; sex workers and, 129; stigma associated with, 13, 93–94, 102n3, 123, 237, 240–42, 248–56; suffering of blood recipients and sellers, 87–95; trade and, 86–87

home ownership, 17, 45
homosexuality, 11, 120–24, 139, 140, 145,
	240, 251–53
Hong Kong, 7, 164, 194, 205; charities in,
	65; Pacific Plaza, 166; pop singers
	from, 16
Hoogewerf, Rupert, 64
"hooliganism," 120, 122
Hooper, Beverley, 57
Hope Project, 64
Horwitz, Allan, 189, 190, 191
household registration (*hukou*) system,
	19, 155, 162, 256
housing, 15, 19, 123; illegal, 159; Shang-
	hai housing market, 157; subsidized,
	153; "workers' new villages," 172;
	work units and, 253
Huang Xiaoju, 40–41
Huang Yongyu, 23, 285
Hu Jintao, 72
human nature, 11, 41, 46, 47
human rights, 2, 26, 129, 258–59
Hurun Philanthropy List, 64, 66
Hu Shi, 50

identity, 17, 157; identity cards, 37; iden-
	tity politics, 11; locality-based, 11;
	sexual, 107, 115, 121, 145, 251
ideology, 6, 16, 41, 43, 70, 169, 181–82,
	240–41, 259n3, 273
"I have nothing" (Cui Jian song), 43
Illness Narratives, The (Kleinman), 88
imipramine, 195
imperialism, 30, 180, 191
impotence, "epidemic" of, 115–18
individualism, 10, 11, 285; courtesy
	stigma and, 13; family politics and,
	232, 233; filial piety and, 220; insti-
	tutionalized, 61; Maoist criticism of,
	182; middle-class, 30; moral landscape
	and, 37; perception of moral crisis
	and, 51; property rights and, 46; quest
	for happiness and, 269; romantic love

and, 219–20; sexual desire and, 139;
	women's status and, 278
infrastructure projects, 152
in-groups, 21, 52
inheritance disputes, 54–55
in-laws, family conflicts involving,
	224–28
intellectuals, 6, 7, 267, 277, 285; divided
	self and, 8–9; Maoist suspicion of,
	200, 276; modernization and, 143;
	protest tradition and, 25; public
	morality and, 50
Internet, 4, 16, 19, 215, 282; chat rooms,
	29; as democratized social space,
	187; sexual materials and information
	on, 108, 112, 113, 120, 126; Sichuan
	earthquake and, 268; surveillance
	via, 24
"iron rice bowl," 153, 167, 168, 280
Islam, 273

Jacka, Tamara, 280, 281
Jacques, Martin, 278
Jankowiak, William, 62, 69
Japan, 1, 50; blood donation in, 79, 80,
	102n1; Sino-Japanese War, 178, 266
Jiang Zemin, 163
jiantao (self-criticism report), 254,
	260n12
Jing Jun, 11, 27–28, 71, 282
job security, 153
journalism, investigative, 58, 272
Judd, Ellen, 226
justice, quest for, 269–72

karaoke clubs, 188
kinship networks, 3, 20, 42; charity and,
	65; stigma of HIV and, 250; trust and,
	59
Kleinman, Arthur, 5–6, 13–14, 79, 192,
	196; on disease-related stigma, 243;
	neurasthenia study by, 180–81; study
	of depression, 185, 191

Kleinman, Joan, v, 72n1, 263
Korean War, 83, 267
Ku, Hok Bun, 69

labor laws, 28
Lady Chatterley's Lover (Lawrence), 113
landslides, 203
Landsteiner, Karl, 82
laoshi (honesty, obedience), 51–52
law, rule of, 61
Lawrence, D. H., 113
lawyers, 17, 62, 135
Lebaishi Group, 41
Lee, C. K., 45
Left Behind Love Letters, The [Yiqing Shu] (Muzi Mei), 111–12
Le Grand, Julian, 79
Lei Feng, 63, 68
leisure, 182, 267
leprosy, 237, 243
lesbians. *See* homosexuality
Lévi-Strauss, Claude, 97
Li, L., 44
Li, Z. S., 180
Liang Qichao, 8–9, 50
Liang Shumin, 50
life, meaning of. *See* meaning, quests for
life aspirations, 15–18
lifestyles, 3, 15, 18, 25, 54
Ling Mingyou, 276, 277
Lin Tsungyi, 276
Liu Junxiang, 102n2
Liu Quanxi, 84–85
Liu Wei, 79
Liu, Xin, 8, 69, 188
Liu Xinwu, 134
Liu Yanwu, 21, 279
Li Yinhe, 123
Lo, Victor, 163
Loss of Sadness, The (Horwitz and Wakefield), 189

love, romantic, 47, 132–35, 142, 217–20
Love Must Not be Forgotten (Zhang Jie), 134
Lu, H., 54

Macao, 164
Maoism, 4, 7, 16, 169, 284; blood donations under, 83–84; collapse of morality of, 71; collectivist vision and, 30; denial of individual under, 12; desexualization and, 145; divided self and, 9; emotions repressed under, 178; homosexuality repressed under, 120; ideology of serving the people, 282; individual identity denied under, 50; intellectuals and academics derided under, 276; labor market and, 14; political culture of, 47; pop culture and, 30; sexuality under, 124, 127; suicide in Maoist era, 200; transition to market economy, 267; urban planning scheme, 158, 167. *See also* Communist Party, Chinese (CCP); Cultural Revolution
Mao Zedong, 9, 11, 23, 42, 51; anti-imperialism of, 191; authority of, 61; dedication to, 132; idealization of life under, 49; "iron rice bowl" and, 280; neurasthenia and, 180; rule by stigmatization and, 258; sexuality and, 134
Marcuse, Herbert, 144
marriage, 10, 21, 22, 123, 220, 279; bride-wealth, 45–46; sex within boundary of, 133; women's attitudes toward, 48; work units and, 253
Marriage Law (1950), 45
martial arts, 29
Marxism, 4
materialism, 24, 44, 71, 273
Mauss, Marcel, 97
Ma Xiaonian, 118, 139
May Fourth movement (1919), 143

privatization, 15, 54
Problems of Social Policy (Titmuss), 79
professionals, white-collar, 5, 17, 111
property, private, 17, 44, 46, 54–55, 186
prostitution, 109, 124–28, 140; Communist Party view of, 239, 240; sexually transmitted diseases and, 130; *xiaojie* ("little elder sister"), 141
protest, popular, 25, 27–28, 44, 45, 272
Prozac, 193, 195, 196–97, 198
psychiatry/psychiatrists, 9–10, 26, 31, 177, 178, 180, 189; drug (pharmaceutical) companies and, 193–94, 195, 196; homosexuality classified as mental disorder, 120, 122; medical model of suicide and, 201–2; political abuse of, 210; quest for professional respect, 275–78; ratio of doctors to population, 209; support groups and, 283; terminology used by, 12
psychoanalysis, 29
psychotherapy and counseling services, 29, 187, 204, 208–9, 210, 264

qi (vital energy), 179, 209
qigong, 141, 142, 209, 273
QQ messaging tool, 109, 187
Qu Yuan, 200, 270, 288n2

racial stereotyping, 258
Redbud Pavilion, 172
Red Cross, Chinese, 64, 96
Reich, Wilhelm, 144
religion, 61, 71, 188, 265, 273–75
respect, quest for, 275–78
responsibilities, collective, 42, 46, 54, 61, 65
rights, 10–11, 40, 61; assertion of, 17, 44, 54, 62; consciousness of, 28; consumer, 57; emerging morality of, 43; individualism and, 68; property, 46
rock and roll, 141
Rofel, Lisa, 4, 47

Rolandsen, U.M.H., 67
Rose, Nikolas, 3
Rural Women (NGO), 214, 234
Rural Women in Urban China (Jacka), 280

sadness, normal, 189, 191
Sanlu Group, 57–58
Sanmao, 213
saohuang ("sweeping yellow") campaign, 127
SARS epidemic, 99, 243, 248, 263
scar literature, 6
schizophrenia, 193, 238, 259n1; political dissidents diagnosed with, 209–10; mentally ill people killed by relatives, 246–48; stigma associated with, 244–46; support groups and, 282; WHO International Pilot Study of, 276
science, 143, 190, 277
Scott, James C., 7, 153, 286
Selective Serotonin Reuptake Inhibitors (SSRIs), 195, 198–99, 205
self: alienation of, 51; Communist ethics and, 42; divided, 5–14, 23, 70, 285–88; enterprising, 4; moral education of individual, 29; social changes and, 152; socialist hierarchy and, 3
self-censorship, 6–7, 286
self-development, 4, 18, 29, 40, 47, 70
selfishness, 41, 46
self-sacrifice, 10, 16, 40, 44, 46
sex and sexual revolution, 4, 21, 46, 47, 53, 106–8; Chinese words relating to sex, 106–7, 139–40, 142–43; distinctive features in China, 139–43; happiness and, 143–46; "impotence epidemic," 115–18; one-child policy and, 10–11, 135–39; premarital and extramarital, 53, 126, 133, 139; public recognition of sexual desire, 108–9; reemergence of romantic love, 132–35; sex industry and sex workers, 88, 109, 111, 124–29, 188; sex tourism,

241; sexually transmitted diseases (STDs) and, 124, 129–31, 138, 207; suicide and, 216, 231, 232; women's desire, 48, 118–20, 146. *See also* homosexuality; pornography and erotica

Shanghai, city of: Bay Bridge neighborhood, 157, 161–70, 170–73; bridewealth in, 45; divorce rate, 22; French Concession, former, 11, 156, 158, 160–63, 166, 167; gay life in, 120; International Settlement, former, 11, 156, 158, 161, 162; lower quarters, 160, 165, 166, 170, 172, 174; Nanshi District, Old, 158, 159; psychological counseling by telephone in, 187; "Shanghai nostalgia," 11–12, 156–57, 166, 167; spatial reconfiguration in, 152–57; upper quarters, 158, 166, 170, 174

Shanghai World Expo, 1, 29, 153, 174, 266

Shao Jing, 79

Shen, D., 48

Shen Qijie, 199, 276

Shenzhen, city of, 11, 63, 100, 199, 201, 207

Shi, M., 130

shopping malls, 152, 166

Shui On Group, 163

Sichuan/Gansu earthquake (2008), 20, 36, 73n4, 101, 204–5; blood donations after, 101; philanthropic practices and, 65; public discussions unleashed by, 268

Sing Lee, 9, 238

Sino-Japanese War, 83

slave labor, 39

socialism, 2, 16, 132, 240; "debris" of, 166, 167, 172, 173; developmental logic and, 153; egalitarianism of, 18; gender equality and, 278, 280; ideals and values of, 40; mental illness and, 275; moral landscape and, 40; self-identity and, 3. *See also* Communism

social justice, 25, 27, 28, 30, 39, 114

Social Transformation of American Medicine, The (Starr), 189

sociology/sociologists, 10, 21, 56, 60, 107, 180, 274

"soft power," 1

soldiers. *See* military

Solomon, A., 190

somatoform disorders, 192

songbang ("to untie"), 14

Song Pingshun, 200

Soviet Union, former, 209

Special Economic Zones, 11

speech, freedom of, 30, 61

Starr, Paul, 189, 190

state-owned enterprises (SOEs), 15, 154; bankruptcy of, 166, 206; health care budget and, 195; restructuring of, 153; termination of, 165

stigma, 237–38, 256–59; of drug abuse, 253–56; of HIV/AIDS, 240–42, 248–56, 257–58; of mental illness, 238–39, 244–48, 258

strangers, society of, 59, 60, 61; blood donations and, 96; ethics and, 63; philanthropy and, 65, 66–67; public trust and, 71; social trust and, 20–21

students, 18, 96–97

style, 18

Subei people, 159

subjectivity, 29, 30, 174, 205, 225; expansion of, 288; incomplete modernity and, 215; sexuality and, 107

substance abuse, 26

suicide, 205, 207, 213–36; conjugal conflicts and, 216–20, 224; Cultural Revolution and, 5; as depression, 200–203; disease and, 233; family politics and, 214–16, 234; of famous people, 125, 213, 288n2; filial piety and, 220–23; increase in, 47; in-law family conflicts and, 224–28; mental disorder and, 229–31, 246; poverty

Text:	10/14 Fournier
Display:	Fournier
Compositor:	Integrated Composition Systems
Indexer:	Alexander Trotter
Printer and binder:	IBT Global